Lateral Preferences
and Human Behavior

Clare Porac
Stanley Coren

Lateral Preferences
and Human Behavior

With 21 Figures

Springer-Verlag
New York   Heidelberg   Berlin

Clare Porac
Department of Psychology
University of Victoria
Victoria, British Columbia
Canada V8W 2Y2

Stanley Coren
Department of Psychology
University of British Columbia
Vancouver, British Columbia
Canada V6T 1W5

The quotation on page 93 is from *The Thornbirds* by Colleen McCullough,
Copyright © 1977 by Colleen McCullough. Reprinted by permission of
Harper & Row, Publishers, Inc.

Library of Congress Cataloging in Publication Data
Porac, Clare.
 Lateral preferences and human behavior.

 Bibliography: p.
 Includes index.
 1. Left and right (Psychology) 2. Human behavior.
3. Laterality. I. Coren, Stanley. II. Title.
[DNLM: 1. Behavior. 2. Laterality. WL 335 P832L]
BF637.L36P67   152.3′35   81-8978
                  AACR2

The use of general descriptive names, trade names, trademarks, etc. in this publication,
even if the former are not especially identified, is not to be taken as a sign that such
names, as understood by the Trade Marks and Merchandise Marks Act, may accordingly
be used freely by anyone.

© 1981 by Springer-Verlag New York Inc.
Printed in the United States of America

9 8 7 6 5 4 3 2 1

ISBN 0-387-90596-0 Springer-Verlag New York Heidelberg Berlin
ISBN 3-540-90596-0 Springer-Verlag Berlin Heidelberg New York

To our parents,
Ben, Chesna,
Joseph, and Katherine

Preface

Lateral preferences are strange, puzzling, and on the surface, not particularly adaptive aspects of behavior. Why one chooses habitually to write or to brush the teeth with the right hand, while a friend or family member habitually uses the left hand, might be interesting enough to elicit some conversation over dinner or a drink, but certainly does not seem to warrant serious scientific study. Yet when one looks at human behaviors more carefully, one becomes aware that asymmetrical behaviors favoring one side or the other are actually a fairly universal characteristic of human beings. In the same way that we are right or left handed, we are also right or left footed, eyed, and eared. As a species, we are quite lopsided in our behavioral coordinations; furthermore, the vast majority of us are right sided. Considering that we are looking at a sizable number of behaviors, and at a set of biases that seem to be systematic and show a predictable skew in the population, the problem takes on greater significance.

The most obvious form of lateral preference is, of course, handedness. When studying behavioral asymmetries, this is the issue with which most investigators start. Actually, we entered this research area through a much different route. Around 1971 we became interested in the problem of eye dominance or eye preference. This is a behavior where the input to one eye seems to be preferred over that to the other in certain binocular viewing situations. Such asymmetries were, at the time, little understood in reference to vision. As our work continued over the next three years it began to take a new turn. The impetus for this change came from our increasing knowledge of the literature and from interactions with numerous colleagues. It seemed that there was a notion existing in the field that accepted the concept of sidedness, but assumed that all forms of sidedness were simply correlates of the same process that causes handedness. Thus, many of our conversations with colleagues were punctuated with responses such as "Oh, yes, the dominant eye is the eye on the same side of the body as the dominant hand, isn't it?" The problem was that we simply did not know enough about the issue to either agree or disagree. The question had never been directly addressed in our work. The literature was not particularly helpful either, so if we were to satisfy our curiosity about the issue of the relationship between eye and hand preference, it seemed that we had to gather our own data.

By 1975 we were committed to a much broader research effort. By then we had been inundated by large amounts of data that began to shed light on the relationship between the preferred eye and the preferred hand, and also on how these were related to the preferred foot and ear. Furthermore, we had started to recognize that these simple lateral preference behaviors might be related to many other aspects of human behavior, ranging from sensorimotor coordinations to cognitive skills and even to some aspects of the behavior of certain clinical populations. We also were reasonably sure that the issue was fascinating not only to us, but to many luminaries in the history of thought, including Plato, Benjamin Franklin, Charles Darwin, William James, John B. Watson, James Mark Baldwin, Paul Broca, J. Hughlings Jackson, Sigmund Freud, and many others drawn from the diverse areas of physiology, psychology, philosophy, anthropology, and even physics. Everyone, it seemed, at one time or another had a question to ask, a speculation to put forth, or some data that seemed to bear upon the issue of behavioral asymmetries in the form of lateral preferences.

This book represents the results of nearly a decade of interest in and research into the problems of lateral preference. We have concentrated on the preferences manifested in hand, foot, eye, and ear use. This study subsumes a mass of data and theory, but like all multifaceted research efforts, it ultimately raises more questions that it answers. However, it does contain a wealth of data and analyses from approximately 20,000 individuals. We believe that it gives an accurate picture of how lateral preferences are distributed in humans, how they manifest themselves, and how they are related to other aspects of behavior.

We have arranged the chapters of the book in a sequence that starts with the measurement and presentation of lateral preference norms for a large human sample, followed by chapters that deal with the major theoretical viewpoints concerning the formation of lateral preferences. The latter portion of the book focuses on the various behaviors that have been connected to lateral preferences and that have been thought to covary with them. We present our data in each chapter and discuss both patterns within each index of preference and patterns of sidedness relationships across the various preference types. Although most empirical and theoretical literature is dominated by papers dealing only with handedness, we have tried to give a balanced view by presenting in each chapter both data relating to and discussions of all four forms of lateral preference. In the service of literary as well as scientific ideals, we have streamlined the descriptions of methodological detail and statistical analysis, except in Chapter 2, where we set the methodological context. All of the figures, graphs, and tables are original and unique to this book. However, some of the data presented here have been published elsewhere, usually in an altered format. These sources have been cited where appropriate.

Because human lateral preferences, especially handedness, have been linked closely to processes of neural and cerebral lateralization of function, we know that many individuals who read this book will do so because of their interest in these topics. However, this is not a book about cerebral lateralization; it is a book about human sidedness behaviors. We deal with the topics of cerebral and neural lateralization because many of the theories concerning lateral preferences have emanated from a consideration of these processes. However, our emphasis throughout the book is on the *behavioral* rather than the *cerebral* asymmetry of function. Thus, our often brief discussions of many topics related to cerebral lateralization do not reflect a lack of awareness and knowledge of these areas; rather they reflect a purposive attempt to keep the discussion relevant to the topic of human behavioral asymmetries. In many instances, detailed discussions and descriptions of matters related to cerebral lateralization would have taken us far afield from lateral preference.

It should be obvious that an effort of this scope and duration could not have been completed by two people working alone. We acknowledge and express our gratitude to a number of sources of assistance, cooperation, and support. First, and most important, we thank the large numbers of subjects who participated in our various studies and who, in most instances, gave voluntarily of their time for no financial recompense. Many universities, colleges, community colleges, high schools, day care centers, senior citizens' organizations, hospitals, sporting federations, and athletic teams provided the points of contact that enabled us to collect the necessary data that form the basis of this monograph. These organizations and institutions are located not only in British Columbia, but throughout the United States and Canada, and unfortunately they are too numerous to mention individually. However, we thank the staff members and officers of the various organizations who assisted us in collecting the data and all of the individuals who chose to participate in our studies.

Second, our research could not have been accomplished without the cooperative efforts of the departments of psychology at both the University of Victoria and the University of British Columbia. Since the cities of Victoria and Vancouver, where our respective institutions are located, are separated by approximately 50 miles of water, travel between them is not as easily accomplished as it might be in another locale. For this reason, our collaborative efforts often required long absences from our respective universities. Not only were these tolerated willingly, but attempts were made in both departments to schedule departmental and teaching duties in a manner that enabled each of us to travel between institutions as often as needed. We are grateful for this consideration. We also acknowledge colleagues in both of these universities who either helped us in our data gathering efforts or who provided assistance during the preparation of the manuscript. They are Drs. Louis Costa, Pam Duncan, Otfried Spreen, and Frank Spellacy from the University of Victoria and Drs. Ralph Hakstian, Robert Hare, Geraldine Schwartz, James Steiger, and Jerry Wiggins from the University of British Columbia. We also thank other colleagues from as far away as Montreal, such as Dr. Yves Michaud, who assisted in testing and data collection. Our research efforts were a joint project of our two laboratories, and a number of conscientious research assistants spent long hours collecting, collating, coding, and analyzing these data on human lateral preferences. The research assistants who worked in the laboratory at the University of Victoria were Lorna McCrae, Janet Nicholby, Maxine Stoeval, Carole Behman Summerfeldt, and Wayne Whitbread, while those who worked in the laboratory at the University of British Columbia were Murray Armstrong, Miriam Blum, Kathy Cooper, Colin Ensworth, Jeannie Garber, Jean Porac, and Candice Taylor.

Third, our research has been supported by financial assistance from a number of granting agencies. They include the National Research Council of Canada, the Medical Research Council of Canada, the Natural Sciences and Engineering Research Council of Canada, the University of British Columbia, Natural, Applied and Health Sciences Research Committee, and the University of Victoria Committee on Faculty Research and Travel. In addition, one of us (S.C.) was assisted by a grant from the Killam Foundation during the writing of the manuscript.

Finally, a number of individuals at our respective universities provided the specific support needed to prepare the manuscript. We were assisted by several able typists, Doris Chin, Susan Dixon, Elizabeth McCririck, Susan Louie, and Linda Watson. Both the University of Victoria and the University of British Columbia granted us sabbatical leave for one year so that we could concentrate on the completion of the manuscript. In addition, we thank the department of psychology at the University of British Columbia for providing the facilities while the two of us worked in one locale. This allowed the manuscript to be completed more quickly and efficiently than would have been possible in other circumstances. After six years of traveling between Victoria and Vancouver, we appreciated and benefited from the opportunity to work together in the same institution. We give special thanks to Dr. Peter Suedfeld, head of the department of psychology at the University of British Columbia, for his special efforts in making this joint residence possible during the completion of the manuscript.

We both feel that this monograph represents a new phase of our continually evolving collaborative research effort. It emerged from an often argumentative and volatile relationship that nonetheless was always productive and enjoyable. We have often noted in our other publications, and will say here again for the record, that this work truly represents the equal and shared contribution of both of the authors.

Clare Porac
Stanley Coren

Contents

1

Human Sidedness

We are two-sided organisms, bilaterally symmetrical around the vertical axis of our bodies. There is no doubt that the two sides of the human body offer a balanced and harmonious appearance, yet upon closer scrutiny, we find that the apparent symmetry of the human form is a global illusion that arises from our habitual inattention to the many observerable structural inequalities in the body.

From an aesthetic viewpoint, symmetry has its opponents and proponents. Thus Weyl (1952) defined the concept of symmetry as a harmony of proportions, whereas Victor Hugo has been quoted as saying, "Nothing oppresses the heart so much as symmetry." The existence of asymmetries, however, is a characteristic quality of both the inorganic and the organic world, even at the atomic and subatomic levels. For example, the Nobel Prize winning physicist, Chienshung Wu, demonstrated that the flow of electrons in a magnetic field is predictably asymmetrical, giving a physical basis for the notion of right- and left-sidedness that has been incorporated into contemporary physical cosmology (Gross & Bornstein, 1977). There are numerous examples of the structural inequalities of the right and the left sides in living creatues, ranging from differences in right and left claw size in lobsters and fiddler crabs to the one-sided placement of the eyes in some species of fish. There are even systematic differences in the thickness of the hide obtained from the right and the left side of a cow (Fincher, 1977; Jackson, 1905).

Similar asymmetries in the human body are also common. Portrait artists note that each human face has a number of asymmetries. For example, the mouth may have a slight downward turn on one side, or there may be an indentation in one cheek only. When one closely examines the appearance of the eyes and the ears, it is not surprising to find that one eye is somewhat larger or is positioned slightly lower than the other. Also, the right ear is placed lower on the head than the left for the majority of individuals, and there are small but detectable differences in the size and shape of the ears. For these reasons, portrait artists argue that a truly symmetrical face is both unnatural and unlikely. In addition to facial asymmetries, other parts of the external body also show right-left differences. McManus (1976) reports that the right testicle is generally larger and higher than the left. There are also often differences in limb length or hand or foot size in many structurally normal children and adults (Harris, 1980; Jones, 1915; Levy & Levy, 1978).

Although there may be slight structural asymmetries between the members of the paired sense organs and limbs, each right and left limb or sense organ is morphologically similar. Each member seems to be constructed to serve the same purpose. Simple observation of the two hands reveals no structural differences that allow one to predict the complex of behaviors called handedness. Considerations of structural properties alone would never lead to the conclusion that one hand could competently draw and write, or skillfully manipulate small objects, whereas the other would be clumsy and awkward at these tasks. These behavioral differences that cause one limb or sense organ to be preferred for certain activities, despite the apparently insignificant differences in their morphology, constitute a problem that, in one sense or another, has fascinated scientists and laymen for centuries.

Fritsch (1968) describes human functional asymmetries in a way that clearly pinpoints the problematic nature of their existence. Humans have a right and a left hand. Small differences in size may exist between them, but in the absence of any deformity, the two hands are of a similar form. Both have four fingers and a thumb, and the left hand is a mirror image of the right. For a moment, imagine a species of humans, perhaps inhabitants of another planet, who possess two hands that differ in design. One is pincer shaped and the other is shaped like a hammer. In the presence of such structural dissimilarity, one would not be surprised to observe that these organisms habitually grab objects with the pincer-shaped limb but always use the hammer-shaped hand in situations that require the pounding or breaking of an object. The structural differences between two hands of this type clearly promote their functional differentiation, and each limb is used when its design qualities are demanded by a task. However, such is not the case in the species of humans that inhabits the planet Earth. We possess functional asymmetries, but for us they emerge from bilateral limbs and sense organs that apparently are structural mirror image twins with similar capabilities. This book is concerned with the functional and behavioral differences that manifest themselves in the differentiated use of the right or left hand, foot, eye, or ear. These differences emerge in the form of lateral preferences or, to be more general, behavior biases toward one side of the body or the other.

Lateral asymmetries in behavior are easily observed in many common activities. *Handedness* has been the most widely studied of the human lateral preferences. Usually it is defined as the differential or preferred use of one hand in situations where only one can be used. When an individual writes, throws a ball, or uses a toothbrush, the demands of the activity are met more efficiently if one hand, not two, is used. There are a number of such one-handed tasks, involving both fine and gross motor coordination, where handedness can be observed. These include drawing, sewing, grasping small objects, and unscrewing lids from jars. Habitually, the same hand is chosen to perform all or most of these activities. Thus, it is a rare occurrence to find an individual who can write with equal facility with the right and the left hand.

Given the nature of handedness, one easily can predict the characteristic conditions for the appearance of the three remaining human lateral preferences, footedness, eyedness, and earedness. They are also displayed in situations where only one limb or sense organ is required to perform an action or complete a task. Kicking a ball, grasping a small object with the toes, or stamping on a lit match are circumstances in which one can observe *footedness* or foot preference. *Eyedness* emerges in typically one-eyed tasks such as sighting through a telescope, a microscope, or a riflesight or, in any alignment of a near with a far object. *Earedness* manifests itself when an individual is asked to press an ear against a wall in order to hear a conversation taking place in an adjoining room or to place a single earphone from a portable radio into one of the ears. In all of these situations, an individual can choose either the right or the left member, but (as is the case with handedness) these lateral preferences also show habitual sidedness tendencies. A typical individual consistently chooses one side in all or in most of the situations that demand the use of only one foot, eye, or ear. When each type of lateral preference is considered separately, one can divide individuals into those who are right sided and those who are left sided. Although the population distributions of right- and left-sidedness differ for the varying preference indexes, humans are, as a population, predominantly right sided.

There is a long history of fascination with human lateral preferences. Early references to handedness can be found in the Bible and even in Egyptian tomb writings. The problem of hand preference has caught the attention of many illustrious historical personages, including Benjamin Franklin, Charles Darwin, and Thomas Carlyle. Also, many eminent psychologists, such as G. Stanley Hall, James Mark Baldwin, William James, and John Watson, have written on the subject. Although eyedness was discussed as early as 1593 by Giam Baptista del Porta, most of the theorizing and empirical investigation surrounding human functional asymmetries has concentrated on hand preference. One recent bibliography listed over 2500 publications concerned with handedness. This figure clearly outdistances its closest competitor, eye preference, by a ratio of approximately ten published papers to one. Foot preference has engendered even less scientific interest, and ear preference has been virtually ignored. A few reports present data on combinations of human lateral preferences, with the most commonly studied combination being the relationship between hand and eye preference. Overall, however, the published literature on eye, ear, and foot preference and on lateral preference combinations is dwarfed by the vast theoretical and empirical output concerned solely with handedness.

This concentration of interest on handedness has shaped the history of investigation into human sidedness, and several theoretical themes have emerged that have determined the nature of empirical investigations into all forms of human lateral preference. First is the question of the adaptive significance of sidedness behaviors. Why should humans be one sided? To many theorists, one-sidedness amounts to the loss of the use of one limb through neglect, and they have argued that the most natural and effective mode of coordination is ambilaterality or dual hand use. For example, in 1905 Jackson wrote an eloquent appeal for the promotion of dual hand use in Western societies. He abhorred the use of only one hand and condemned the promotion of this practice by educators, parents, and society at large. He argued that the symmetry of form in humans indicates a natural intention for equality of hand use. He contended that the polarity of right-handedness *or* left-handedness is forced and artificial. In his zeal, Jackson even formed the *Ambidextral Culture Society* in Great Britain to promote the use and training of both hands.

Another problem is the genesis of sidedness. Two schools of thought exist on this issue. One maintains that custom and the pressure of society force the use of only one hand, while the other maintains that genetic or physiologically based processes promote the establishment of one-handedness. This controversy is a prominent feature of the literature. There is an empirical fact, however, that has tended to argue strongly for more physiological and genetic approaches. Right- and left-handedness do not exist in equal proportions in human populations. Regardless of the country of origin of the measured sample, contemporary estimates of the incidence of right-handedness range from 80 to 95%. In addition, there is some evidence that this right-left disproportion has existed within human populations for many centuries, perhaps dating back to prehistoric periods (Wilson, 1885a,b).

The contention that man has been right-handed throughout history has important theoretical implications and thus needs verification. We attempted to provide this in a study that addressed itself to the study of the historical record of human activity provided by artists since the paleolithic era (Coren & Porac, 1977b). The reasoning behind our methodology was simple. To the extent that artists accurately represent the world that they observe, they should also represent hand use as they see it. If they normally observe the majority of individuals manipulating tools with their right hand, they will predominantly portray right-handed use. If either hand is used indiscriminately, artists will portray a random pattern of hand use. Thus, we reasoned that depictions of active right- and left-handed use, observed in the artwork of various eras, generally reflect the incidence of right- and left-handedness existing in the population at that point of historical time. Therefore, we examined pieces of art from European, Asian, African, and American sources for the occurrence of handedness in active tool or weapon use. We took care not to include art with stylized mirror image symmetry. Figures within each work of art were selected randomly, and we did not count more than one instance of handedness in each piece of art that we examined. We found 1,180 scorable instances of unimanual tool or weapon use in more than 10,000 examples that we examined.

Figure 1-1 illustrates how easily one can conduct such a handedness survey of art. It shows examples of pieces of art from three historical periods. Figure 1-1A is a relief from ancient Egypt (approximately 3500 B.C.), 1-1B is from 14th-century Germany, and 1-1C is a 19th-century French engraving. Right-hand use is seen clearly in each instance of writing and drawing.

Table 1-1 presents the results of our art survey. The percentage of right-handedness depicted is listed, along with the date when the artworks were

Table 1-1: Percentage of Right-Handedness Depicted in 1,180 Works of Art Spanning a 5,000-Year Period (based on Coren & Porac, 1977b)

Era	Sample size	Right-handedness (%)
Pre-3000 B.C.	39	90.0
2000	51	86.0
1000	99	90.0
500	142	94.0
0	134	97.0
500 A.D.	42	93.0
1000	64	89.0
1200	41	98.0
1400	50	88.0
1500	68	93.0
1600	72	94.0
1700	71	93.0
1800	101	94.0
1850	39	97.0
1900	77	92.0
1950	90	89.0
Mean		92.6

created. The incidence of right-handedness, as shown in art, ranges from 86 to 98%, with no apparent significant changes or trends over time. All of these incidence rates are similar to those reported for right-handedness in contemporary populations (see Chapter 3) and suggest that the population distribution of dextral versus sinistral hand use has not altered over a 5,000-year period. Dennis (1958) examined depictions of handedness in reproductions of murals from Egyptian tombs, dated at approximately 2500 B.C., and also reported that the depiction of handedness during skilled activities was primarily right handed.

The riddle of right-handedness in humans is even more puzzling given its apparent uniqueness. Many other species show consistent paw preferences in activities involving the use of only one paw. Lateral preferences in paw use have been reported for rats, cats, mice, squirrels, monkeys, chimpanzees, baboons, and gorillas (Brookshire & Warren, 1962; Cole 1955, 1957; Collins, 1977; Corballis, 1980; Downey, 1927; Finch, 1941; Fincher, 1977; Jackson, 1905). These results, however, differ from that found in humans. Each animal is either right or left pawed, but the overall incidence of right and left pawedness, respectively, approaches 50% for the population. Thus there is no rightward population bias in these species. The disproportionate population dominance of the right hand is apparently an exclusive property of the human species (see Jackson, 1905).

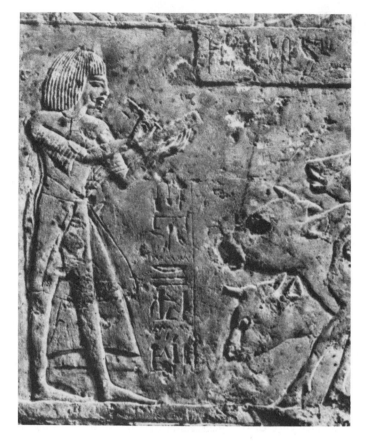

Fig. 1-1A

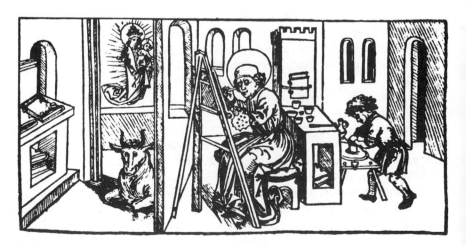

Fig. 1-1B

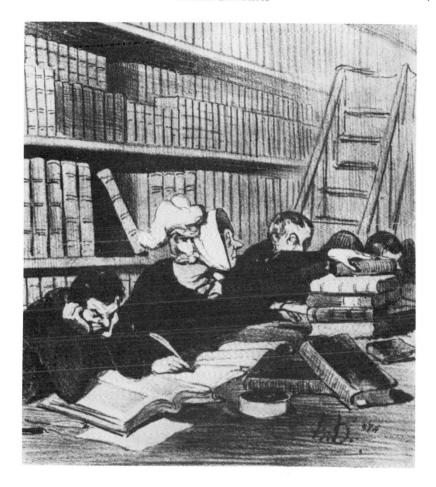

Fig. 1-1C

Figure 1-1. Some examples of right-handed implement use as depicted in art-works from three different historical eras: (A) Egyptian tomb relief (ca. 3500 B.C.); (B) German engraving of St. Luke (14th century); (C) French engraving by Daumier (19th century).

This right-sided bias in human populations, although it may arise from physiological or genetic sources, is thought to alter the environment in a manner that might further increase the population skew toward the right. Implements for everyday use are devised for the manipulative ease of the dextral majority. In effect, humans create a right-handed environment that causes an even greater degree of manifest right-handedness as left-handers are forced to switch because of covert or overt pressure. The correlation of right-handed biology with a right-handed environment has established the rationale for scores of investigative efforts into the specific mechanisms that cause human handedness.

Coincident with the study of the predominance of right-handedness have been attempts to explain the existence of the small but persistently recurring group of left-handers. One common assumption has been that left-handedness arises from some pathological condition that caused a deviation from the normal right-handed pattern. Advocates of this viewpoint have justified their position by pointing to scores of examples from numerous disparate cultures that associate left sidedness with evil, weakness, disease, or treachery, as opposed to the admirable qualities often associated with the right (see Fincher, 1977). They argue that these traditions reflect the underlying normality of right-handedness as opposed to the abnormality or pathology of left-handedness (Fritsch, 1968). Such ideas are even encoded into the very words used to describe left-sidedness. For instance, the word left comes from the Celtic *Lyft* meaning weak or broken. In French, left is *gauche*, which has been adopted in English with the meaning of awkward or gawky. The examples can be multiplied many times. *Sinister* is left in Latin, and in English the connotation is evil or unfortunate, as opposed to *dexter* for right, from which one gets the word dextrous. This line of reasoning has led to a number of damage hypotheses for the occurrence of left-handedness, which in turn, have fostered empirical attempts to verify that left-handedness arises from physical pathology or is associated with it in some way.

We have been outlining some of the themes that continually emerge in the study of lateral preference, yet we have not specified why so much attention has been given to this issue in the first place. Historically, probably the initial impetus came from simple concerns dealing with the relative motoric efficiency of the two hands. Soon, however, handedness, and by extension, footedness, eyedness, and earedness, were linked empirically and theoretically to a vast array of psychological processes. Most of the studies have been correlational and have produced a deluge of associations between lateral preference and other processes. It has been suggested that particular manifestations of lateral preference (or combinations of lateral preference behaviors) can predict, to name just a few,

1. musical ability	13. psychopathy
2. spatial cognitive ability	14. specific learning disabilities
3. verbal cognitive ability	15. dyslexia
4. problem solving ability	16. creativity
5. intelligence	17. balance and coordination
6. reading ability	18. skill at baseball
7. mathematical ability	19. skill at riflery
8. brain organization (cerebral specialization)	20. skill at basketball
9. level of neural development	21. alcoholism
10. presence of specific brain lesions	22. homosexuality
11. criminality	23. bedwetting
12. emotionality	24. strictness of childrearing

In addition, patterns of lateral preference have been linked to a variety of individual difference variables, including

1. age
2. sex
3. race
4. educational level
5. cultural milieu
6. historical era
7. nutrition

8. neurological integrity
9. birth order
10. birth stress
11. parental handedness
12. parental age
13. seasonal variation of time of birth
14. vegetarianism

and we could easily go on from here.

One's credulity is somewhat taxed by these lists. Can all of these relationships be true? If they are, what are the intercorrelations and where does lateral preference enter the picture?

Approximately 10 years ago, we became interested in the issue of lateral preference, specifically, in how it might predict variations in sensorimotor coordinations. As we studied the literature, we encountered numerous reports linking lateral preference to interesting behavioral phenomena and individual difference variables, such as those listed above, and our interest was captured by these reports. Since many investigations were based on clinical and/or causal observations, we also wondered about the validity and reliability of such reports for general populations. Thus, our research into the etiology of lateral preference behaviors and their relationships to other aspects of behavior began. Over this past decade we have developed, adapted, and validated a series of measurement techniques for the determination of limb and sense organ lateral preference. We have tested, questioned, observed, and measured over 20,000 individuals, who have ranged in age from 44 weeks to 100 years. They have included individuals from all socioeconomic levels, residing in both Canada and the United States. We have measured not only individuals, but also family groupings, and separate subsamples have been tested for cognitive abilities, sensorimotor coordinations, and other behaviors in order to ascertain their relationship to the lateral preference indexes. This book is a compilation of that research effort.

We have written the book so that the organization both within and among chapters has a coherent sequence. Chapter 2 is concerned with measurement problems. It describes the variety of methodologies that have been used to measure limb and sense organ preference and the empirical relationships among these various measurement techniques. The issues discussed in this chapter are important ones, since differences in assessment criteria have often resulted in discrepant results and heated theoretical controversies. Chapter 3 gives the general picture of the distribution of lateral preference behaviors in a contemporary North American population. Here, we present the method and the measurement instrument used to collect much of the data discussed throughout the book. Our normative population data for the four preference indexes are also presented. The empirical findings reported in this chapter are the basis of many of the discussions and arguments undertaken in later chapters. Chapters 4-6 detail the major hypotheses offered to explain the genesis of lateral preference behaviors. These include notions of physiological, biological, and cerebral asymmetries, as well as genetic, social, and environmental factors. In each chapter, we have outlined the various theoretical positions and, using data from the literature as well as those we have collected, we have attempted to assess the adequacy of these theories. We have not confined ourselves to handedness but have looked at the entire spectrum of lateral preferences and have tried to determine whether hypotheses concerning the formation of handedness can predict patterns in all four types of preference. Chapters 7 and 8 detail the major damage hypotheses that have arisen to explain left-handedness, and by extension, left-sidedness. Here we examine variations in lateral preference in groups that have suffered some form of physiological trauma, including studies of clinically affected groups. Chapters 9-11 discuss the relationship between patterns of lateral preference and cognitive and sensorimotor abilities in typical populations and in groups chosen for study because of specific skills, such as competitive athletes. Chapter 12 is devoted to the much-neglected topic of sense organ preference. Here, we present a rationale for the existence of eye and ear preference with supportive data. Finally, Chapter 13 is a critical overview of the book with some new conclusions and reformulations of old problems based on the pattern of empirical findings presented in each chapter.

Chapters 2-12 also share a common internal structure. Each chapter contains the results of studies that we have conducted. Some of this research has been published in various journals, and if so, we have given the appropriate reference. Occasionally, we have presented expanded or modified versions of data contained in work published in other sources. In other instances, our data are presented for the first time and the presentation and discussion of our findings are exclusive to this monograph. Besides the focus on our data, each chapter has another organizational theme. We attempt to examine similarities and differences in the empirical patterns displayed in each of the four indexes of lateral preference separately. These *within-index comparisons* are one point of emphasis. The second is provided by the treatment of the sidedness relationships among the various indexes considered together, or *across-index comparisons*. This thematic division will be found in most of the discussions of our data in the chapters that follow.

Over the years, the topic of lateral preference, especially handedness, has become associated with notions concerning cerebral lateralization of function. In fact, they have become so intimately linked that one of our colleagues, who is a clinical neuropsychologist, told us that human lateral preferences are of interest *only* if they can tell us something about neural or cerebral lateralization. However, this is *not* a book about cerebral lateralization; it is a book about human sidedness behaviors. Why does one choose consistently to use one limb or sense organ in many activities? What guides and maintains these choices, and what behaviors do patterns of lateral preference predict? Occasionally, we discuss theories derived from the literature on hemispheric specialization, but only in the context of how these theories have been used to study lateral preferences and the adequacy of their applications in this context.

We wrote this book in the hope that the data and the discussion contained in it would broaden our understanding of the mechanisms that promote and maintain human lateral preferences. Also we hope that it will demonstrate that human sidedness is an interesting behavioral phenomenon in its own right, irrespective of its connection to lateralization in the nervous system. We feel that our data offer perspectives that have not been possible when investigators have confined themselves to the study of handedness alone. In some instances, we discovered that the study of four indexes of lateral preference provided new insights into the adequacy of certain hypotheses concerning the etiology of functional asymmetries in humans. Occasionally, we found that our data challenged traditional assumptions and approaches but, in return, offered the opportunity to approach the problem of human sidedness in new and exciting ways. By studying hand, foot, eye, and ear preference, both in isolation and in their various combinations, we have begun an investigation into the meaning of "rightness" and "leftness," their similarity, their polarity, and their functional and behavioral significance.

2

Measurement

At an informal level, the assessment of lateral preference (at least of handedness) has a long history. A written account of a procedure for measuring handedness appears in the Bible (Judges 20: 15-16), where note was taken of the number of men of the tribe of Benjamin who used their left hand when throwing stones with a sling. In this first record of a measurement operation, it is clearly a combination of preference (and skill) at a unimanual task that determines the dominant or preferred hand. The first formal measurement of hand preference by a behavioral scientist may have been the work of Sir Francis Galton. He tested approximately 7,000 males who attended a health exhibition in 1884. The measure of handedness was a test of strength, in which each individual pressed a dynamometer with each hand in turn.

The notion that the preferred hand is better or stronger is implicit when one calls it a dominant hand. There has been a tendency to view skill, strength, and preference as relatively interchangeable indicators of the dominant hand; however, evidence suggests that they are separable aspects of behavior perhaps mediated by different mechanisms. Furthermore, measures of these separate dimensions often show low levels of concordance. In this book we are concerned predominantly with preference measures for determining the dominant or preferred limb or sense organ, and it is important to emphasize that data based on sensory or motor efficiency cannot be directly substituted for measures of preference. One can demonstrate this empirically by reference to the existing literature. Since the largest body of available data pertains to handedness, we will use it as the focus for reviewing some of the evidence that suggests that *skill, strength* (or general *proficiency*), and *preference* might be orthogonal dimensions.

Proficiency and Preference

The concept of lateral preference suggests an element of choice. The preferred hand is the hand *chosen* when only one hand can be used for a given activity; similarly, the preferred eye is the eye chosen for such uniocular tasks as sighting through a telescope. While one might suppose, on logical grounds, that the chosen member of paired limbs or sense organs would be the better or more proficient of the two, there is no necessity for this to be the case. Strength and dexterity, for example, can be affected by environmental factors and may be independent of preference.

There is much evidence that shows that preference and proficiency, while correlated, are not interchangeable concepts. For example, Satz, Achenbach, and Fennel (1967) reported that only 45% of their self-classified left-handers had a stronger grip in their left hand. Right-handers also showed some differences between strength and preference, with 13% demonstrating a stronger grip with their nonpreferred left hand. Provins and Cunliffe (1972) used two different grip strength measures and found that, on average, 35% of the individuals who classified themselves, via questionnaire, as preferring their right hand for most common activities showed stronger grip strength with their left hand. An amazing 75% of the left-preferent individuals actually showed greater grip strength and endurance with their right hand. This poor concordance between strength and preference measures for handedness has been replicated several times. For instance, Johnstone, Galin, and Herron (1979) report that the correlation between a dynamometer test for strength and questionnaire preference inventories is only 0.31, which although significant, accounts only for about 9% of the predictive variance.

If one shifts focus from pure strength and endurance measures to dextrality or skill, one still does not find a strong concordance with preference. Benton, Meyers, and Polder (1962), using a standardized manual dexterity test requiring manipulation of small items with a pair of tweezers, reported that 10% of declared right-handers were better at the task with their left hand, while 27% of the left-handers were better at the task with their right hand. Satz, Achenbach, and Fennel (1967) used a similar task and found that 26% of the left-handers scored better with their right hand and 17% showed no hand superiority. For the right-handers, 20% showed better manual dexterity with the left hand and 19% showed no difference. Provins and Cunliffe (1972) have reported similar findings.

One could argue that these manipulation tests are too complex and involve learned components. In a world dominated by right-handers, machines, tools, and implements often are designed for right-hand use. Perhaps the poor concordance between dexterity and preference measures results from left-handers having learned to use their right hand skillfully out of necessity. Similarly, bimanual use of many tools and machines could attenuate the measured skill and strength differences between the hands for both left- and right-handers. Greater concordance between preference and proficiency tests might be found if a very simple response, not clearly subject to learning, is used. One of the most popular tasks of this type involves a simple tapping response, where an individual is required to tap a telegraph key as rapidly as possible, or even more simply, to wiggle a finger up and down as rapidly as possible during a given time interval. However, there is little correlation between preference and proficiency measures even with such simple tasks. Satz et al. (1967) found that 35% of left-handers did better on tapping with the right hand, while 6% showed no difference between the hands. The difference was somewhat smaller for right-handers; however, 12% showed better tapping with their nonpreferred left hand and 1% showed no difference. Provins and Cunliffe (1972) reported that 10% of the right-handers performed better at this task with their left hand, while 40% of the left-handers did better with their nonpreferred right hand.

The concordance between proficiency and preference measures of handedness also seems to vary as a function of the specific index or measure used, even in such apparently simple tasks as finger tapping (Todor & Kyprie, 1980). For example, Peters and Durding (1979) found that when scoring the speed of tapping, all of their left-handers showed faster tapping with their nonpreferred right hand. However, with tapping regularity, rather than speed, as the dependent variable, 30% of the left-handers showed greater regularity with the right hand and 14% of the right-handers tapped more regularly with the left hand. Johnstone et al. (1979) reported that the overall correlation between tapping performance and preference is 0.6. While this value represents a respectable correlational level of association, it still indicates a misclassification rate of 26% if a dichotomous scoring procedure is adopted (Wiggins 1973).

Table 2-1 summarizes the results of several studies that compared skill, strength, or dexterity to preference measures of handedness. In order to provide

Table 2-1: Percentage Agreement between Preference and Proficiency Measures of Handedness[a]

Proficiency test	Agreement with preference classification (%)
Dynamometer (grip strength)	59[1-3]
Steadiness	85[1]
Small parts manipulation	74[2-4]
Tapping speed	80[1-3,5]
Throwing accuracy	60[1]
Cutting accuracy	78[4]
Tracing accuracy	71[6]
Twisting speed	80[1]
Aiming	79[6,7]
Mean concordance (%)	74

[a] Superscripts indicate sources: 1, Provins & Cunliffe (1972); 2, Satz et al. (1967); 3, Johnstone et al. (1979); 4, Benton et al. (1962); 5, Peters & Durding (1979b); 6, Stellingwerf (1975); 7, Lake & Bryden (1976).

a common measure, all of the values in the table are expressed as the percentage of individuals assigned the same sidedness (both right or both left) on the two tests, and this has been averaged across the indicated studies. When correlation coefficients were the only available statistic, the percentage agreement with the preference measures was estimated from the computational procedures provided by Wiggins (1973). As can be seen, the concordance rate is not high. The mean agreement between preference and skill or strength tests is only 74%. Thus, one of every four individuals is performing more proficiently with the nonpreferred hand than with the preferred hand. Also, the concordance between proficiency and preference is task specific. While a steadiness test gives a high degree of concordance with preference (85%), a grip strength test gives a very poor rate of agreement, misclassifying 41% of the individuals.

The lack of concordance between proficiency and preference is not surprising. Proficiency measures each require a specific set of responses. Variations on the basic responses required may affect the relative manual dominance measured by proficiency tests. For example, Steingrueber (1975) studied tapping and dotting. He systematically varied each in levels of difficulty and reported that manual asymmetries are greater when the task is easy. Todor and Doane (1977) found that preference and proficiency show the smallest correlations for difficult tasks. This agrees with Sheridan (1973) who reported that increasing movement precision requirements increases right-hand superiority, regardless of preference. Other data have suggested also that relative manual superiority may be affected by factors such as fatigue (Hellebrandt & Houtz, 1950), practice (Provins, 1967a,b), stimulus and response compatibility (Annett & Sheridan, 1973), and directional or timing properties of the specific movement involved (Brown, Knauft, & Rosenbaum, 1948; Downey, 1932; Flowers, 1975; Nakamura, Taniguchi, & Oshima, 1975; Reed & Smith, 1961; Shimrat, 1973; Vanderwolf, 1970).

These considerations suggest that there should be a low concordance between the various proficiency measures themselves. Table 2-2 shows the percentage agreement between various proficiency measures of handedness. As can be seen,

Table 2-2: Percentage Agreement between Various Proficiency Measures of Handedness[a]

	Dyn	St	SmP	Tap	Throw	PR	Twist
Dynamometer	—	54[1]	62[2]	62[1,2]	63[1,3]	—	—
Steadiness		—	—	58[1]	62[1]	—	—
Small parts manipulation			—	64[2]	—	—	—
Tapping speed				—	—	57[4]	57[4]
Throwing accuracy					—	—	—
Pursuit rotor						—	54[4]
Twisting speed							—
Mean agreement (%)	59						

[a] Superscripts indicate sources: 1, Heinlein (1929); 2, Johnstone et al. (1979); 3, Provins & Cunliffe (1972); 4, Buxton (1937).

the percentage of the samples congruently classified by the various proficiency measures of handedness is not high. For example, grip strength (measured with a dynamometer) has only a 54% agreement with a steadiness test for handedness. The mean percentage agreement across the eight tasks is only 59%. Thus, a given skill or strength measure for hand dominance may not measure the same thing as another proficiency test.

The lack of concordance among the various skill and strength measures for handedness may stem from the fact that hand proficiency measures are themselves multidimensional in nature. This is confirmed by Fleischman and Hempel (1954), who used 15 tests of manual dexterity and found only a median intercorrelation of 0.29. Fleischman and Ellison (1962) found that the median intercorrelation among 22 different measures of manual dexterity was 0.23. Factor analytic techniques used in these studies suggested that there were five independent dimensions of unimanual proficiency. More recently, Fleischman (1972) has modified his position to suggest that there may be as many as 10 separable dimensions. The implications of such suggestions for a strength- or skill-defined criterion of handedness are sadly obvious.

This survey suggests that, depending on the specific task employed, proficiency measures of handedness produce greatly varying results. Also, proficiency appears to be a dimension that is separable from preference. If such is the case for handedness, which is the most studied form of lateral preference, one can presume that the situation is similar for the preferred foot, eye, or ear.

One final consideration tends to distinguish proficiency from preference indexes. Populations of scores based on proficiency measures of handedness typically form normal distributions with a mean shift toward the right side (Annett, 1972; Benton et al., 1962; Ojemann, 1930; Satz et al., 1967). Thus, the distribution of the difference in scores between the left and the right hand might look like that pictured in Figure 2-1 as the solid line. The shape of the distribution of preference scores is different. When individuals are tested for their handedness, with an index based on the difference in the number of simple unimanual activities where each hand is preferred, the distribution of responses is J-shaped, as in the dotted line in Figure 2-1. This represents a bimodal distribution, with a principal peak indicating strong dextral preference and a smaller secondary peak representing consistent sinistral preference. Notice that ambilaterality is relatively rare in preference distributions. Such J-shaped distributions have been found in many studies using preference measures (Annett, 1970; Crovitz & Zener, 1962; Hull, 1936; Humphrey, 1951; Oldfield, 1971; Satz et al., 1967). Both the lack of correlation between proficiency and preference measures, and the distinct distributions that each produces, support the notion that these different measures represent separable dimensions of handedness and, by extrapolation, of sidedness.

Preference measures reflect the limb or sense organ chosen when only one can be utilized in performing a specific task. Typical manifestations of lateral preference include the hand selected to throw an object or the eye used to peek through a telescope. The most important aspect of such measures is that they involve an

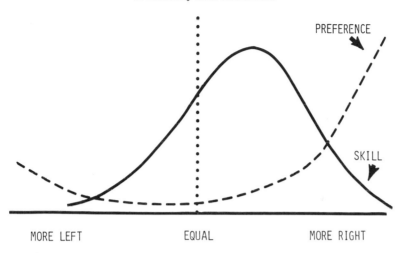

Figure 2-1. The typical J-shaped distribution found in preference measures of handedness (dotted line) compared to the typical right-biased normal distribution found for skill or proficiency measures of handedness (solid line).

aspect of choice. The preferred hand, for instance, is the hand that the subject *chooses* when faced with a task that can be accomplished by either hand. This does not necessarily imply that it is the better hand, nor the hand that could accomplish the task more efficiently or more expediently (as the previous discussion has demonstrated).

One can administer preference measures either through behavioral tasks, where an individual actually performs simple actions involving the choice of a limb or sense organ, or through self-report inventories. In general, preference measures show higher concordance with each other than do proficiency tests. For example, Buxton (1937) used four simple unimanual tasks—throwing an object, reaching for an object, picking up a small object, and brushing with one hand—and reported an average intercorrelation of 0.63, which is 94% classification concordance (Wiggins, 1973). Koch (1933) reported an average percentage agreement among 118 different hand preference tasks of 88% with a test-retest reliability of 0.81. Similar results are found for self-report inventories. For example, Porac, Coren, Steiger, and Duncan (1980) reported on average intercorrelation of 0.60 among a set of self-report items for handedness. This value is almost identical to that found by Buxton (1937) for behavioral measures of preference, and it represents a classification concordance of 93% (Wiggins, 1973). Bryden (1977) tested hand preference using self-report items from the batteries designed by other investigators. From a reconstruction of his correlation matrix, one can estimate the mean percentage concordance between any two indexes of hand preference to be approximately 87%. Coren and Porac (1978) and Coren, Porac, and Duncan (1979) broadened the scope of these preference measures to include indexes for the preferred foot, eye, and ear. They report an average within-index concordance of 92% among behavioral measures of preference and 90% among self-report measures. This overall pattern of results suggests that lateral *preferences* are less sensitive to specific task components than are lateral *proficiency* measures.

Each form of lateral preference manifests itself in a different manner. The same test cannot be used to ascertain the preferred hand and the preferred eye. We will consider separately some of the behavioral and self-report measures that have been used to assess lateral preference of the limbs and the sense organs. We also shall consider the reliability and validity of the various measures in turn.

Hand Preference

At first glance, the measurement of hand preference seems simple. One might argue that individuals know enough about their own behavior to categorize themselves into groups of left- or right-handers. Based on such presumptions, many investigators have utilized the simple technique of asking individuals "Do you consider yourself to be right or left handed?" At a psychometric level, one might guess that such global, ill-defined questions are unreliable and have little validity because such questions do not specify whether the response should pertain to hand preference, relative manual strength, or relative dexterity, or to some other proficiency measure. However, evidence suggests that subjects do not respond to a general handedness question by choosing the hand with the greatest dexterity. For example, Benton et al. (1962) and Satz et al. (1967) tested self-avowed right- and left-handers (determined by this global form of assessment) on a small parts dexterity test and found that 8% of the reported right-handers and 21% of the reported left-handers performed better with their nonpreferred hand. Benton et al. (1962) reported that 43% of the self-declared left-handers performed better on a cutting accuracy task with their right hand. Other data suggest that global self-report also does not represent relative manual strength. Satz et al. (1967) found that 24% of their subjects did better with their reported nonpreferred hand in a test of grip strength. Similar findings have been reported by Whipple (1914). It is unlikely, then, that simple dichotomous self-classification reflects proficiency measures of handedness.

Since preference and proficiency are relatively uncorrelated, one can suggest that individuals respond to the global question about their handedness in terms of hand preference. Although this is generally true, we still find a number of discrepancies. Satz et al. (1967) obtained self-reports about the hand used in a number of common activities, such as throwing a ball or holding a toothbrush, and compared them to global self-classification. An average of 7% of the sample performed more of these tasks with their reported nonpreferred hand. Similar results have been reported by Crovitz and Zener (1962), who also offered the observation that whenever individuals classify themselves as right or left handed, they also report that the corresponding hand is the hand with which they write. This suggests that individuals respond to the general question in light of this

single activity. Interestingly, the writing hand is the most frequently used criterion activity for determining an individual's handedness (see Annett, 1973;
Selzer, 1933). Unfortunately, the hand used to write is the handedness behavior
most apt to be subject to social pressure. Teachers and other socializing agents
have often forced individuals into right-handed writing, despite natural sinistral
tendencies (see, e.g., the opening section of Chapter 6). There are a number of
reports of individuals whose sole dextral activity is writing, while all other unimanual activities are conducted with the left hand, and conversely, of some
individuals whose sole sinistral activity is writing. To the extent that Crovitz and
Zener (1962) are correct, these individuals will misclassify themselves on a global
self-classification handedness question. Perhaps for this reason, most investigators have resorted to preference measurement techniques where hand use is
determined by a number of unimanual tasks.

Typically, hand preference assessment batteries have required individuals to
perform simple actions in a laboratory or clinical setting. Throwing a ball, picking up a small item, pointing to an object, drawing a circle with a crayon are
some examples of these activities. Any simple unimanual task seems to be usable,
and many have been tried. Since the tasks are so simple and familiar, many investigators have employed self-report questionnaire inventories rather than actual
behavioral measures. In other words, one is asked which hand is used to hold a
bottle opener, to throw a ball, or to hold a toothbrush rather than being asked
to emit the action.

Historically, there has been a good deal of repetition in the items used to
determine handedness by various investigators. Table 2-3 shows a composite battery based on the inventories of Annett (1970), Coren and Porac (1978), Coren,
Porac, and Duncan (1979), Crovitz and Zener (1962), Harris (1957), Oldfield
(1971), and Raczkowski, Kalat, and Nebes (1974). The actual wordings varied
slightly from inventory to inventory and the permitted responses often differed.
In general, however, observers responded to each question with "left" or "right,"
and in some instances with a form of an ambilateral response, such as "either" or
"both." Crovitz and Zener (1962) allowed a somewhat more graded response
where subjects responded "right hand always," "right hand most of the time,"
"both hands equally often," "left hand most of the time," and "left hand always." Overall, the questions in Table 2-3 are typical of most self-report inventories. By providing individuals with the actual apparatus referred to in each
query, one can readily turn these items into behavioral rather than self-report
measures of handedness.

If one uses similar items for both behavioral and self-report assessments of
hand preference, one can compare the results of the two types of measurement
techniques. To date, four studies have attempted to determine the validity of
handedness questionnaire items in this manner. These are Koch (1933),
Raczkowski, Kalat, and Nebes (1974), Coren and Porac (1978), and Coren,
Porac, and Duncan (1979). Although Koch's (1933) study is very extensive, she
did not report statistics for the individual handedness questions, so her data have
not been included in Table 2-3. As can be seen from Table 2-3, however, the

Table 2-3: Selected Self-Report Items for Measurement of Hand Preference, Their Mean Agreement with Behavioral Tests, and Their Reliabilities When Available[a]

Hand preference items	Agreement between self-report and behavioral tests (%)	Agreement between self-reports at 1-month retest[6] (%)	Agreement between self-reports at 1-year retest[2] (%)
With which hand do you:			
1. draw[2-6]	98[3,6]	96	100
2. throw a ball to hit a target[1-6]	98[3,6]	93	100
3. use an eraser on paper[2,3,6]	98[3,6]	92	96
4. remove the top card for dealing[1-3,6]	94[3,6]	100	96
5. write[1,2,4-6]	100[6]	96	96
6. hold a toothbrush[1,2,4-6]	97[6]	96	100
7. hammer[1,2,4,6]	97[6]	96	96
8. use a bottle opener[2,6]	100[6]	94	96
9. use a screw driver[6]	97[6]	95	—
10. use a tennis racket[1,4-6]	95[6]	96	—
11. use scissors[1,4-6]	94[6]	95	—
12. hold a match while striking[1,5,6]	94[6]	89	—
13. hold a spoon to stir liquids[5,6]	94[6]	100	—
14. pick up a salt shaker[6]	85[6]	100	—
15. guide a thread through a needle[1]	84[6]	78	—
16. use a knife[4,5]	—	—	—
17. hold a potato while peeling[b,4]	—	—	—
18. hold a bottle while removing its top[b,4]	—	—	—
19. hold a dish while wiping[b,4]	—	—	—
20. hold at the top of a broom while sweeping[1,5,6]	78[6]	—	—

[a] Superscripts indicate sources: 1, Annett (1970a); 2, Coren, Porac, & Duncan (1979); 3, Coren & Porac (1978); 4, Crovitz & Zener (1962); 5, Oldfield (1971); 6, Raczkowski, Kalat, & Nebes (1974). [b] Items are reverse scored.

overall concordance between behavioral and self-report assessment procedures based on the data from the three remaining studies is above 90% for the first 13 items. This suggests that individual behavioral tests are not necessary, since self-report batteries provide the same information. This is particularly convenient, since self-report inventories can be given rapidly to large numbers without individual testing.

Self-report measures of handedness are not only valid, but also seem to be reliable over repeated testing. Raczkowski et al. (1974) retested individuals on a self-report inventory after one month, and these results are listed in Table 2-3. The reliabilities are quite high, and most test-retest concordances are above 90%. McMeekan and Lishman (1975) performed a test-retest reliability study using two self-report inventories for handedness where subjects were classified according to a six-group system ranging from "consistently right" to "consistently left." After 14 weeks subjects were retested and although there were numerous changes in response to individual items, 84% of the subjects maintained the same handedness classification upon retest. Coren and Porac (1978) extended this reliability measure to a one-year interval. As can be seen from Table 2-3, even after this protracted period, the test-retest concordances are above 95%. Thus, one can conclude that self-report measures of hand preference behaviors are both reliable and valid indicators of the behaviors themselves.

Additionally, hand preference does not seem to be a multifactorial behavior, as is manual proficiency. Four studies have looked at the factorial structure of hand preference items and have shown that hand preference is described by a single factor. Richardson (1978) tested 160 subjects on an eight-item battery, and Porac, Coren, Steiger, and Duncan (1980) tested 962 subjects on a four-item battery; both studies found that all of their hand preference responses loaded upon a single factor. White and Ashton (1976) tested 406 subjects on Oldfield's 18-item battery, and Bryden (1977) tested 1,107 subjects on 14 items from Crovitz and Zener, as well as on 10 items from Oldfield. Once again, both studies reported a single major factor including all of the handedness items, with some additional variance accounted for by specific wordings of items.

Thus it appears that hand preference is a behavior that is easily measured, either with simple behavioral tests or with self-report inventories. Both types of procedures produce similar results and have high classification concordance. Proficiency measures of handedness show a complex, interactive structure. In contrast, hand preference displays a singular, unitary structure, and the various specific items and the techniques of assessment are highly correlated and uniform in nature.

Foot Preference

Measures of footedness are encountered much less frequently than are measures of handedness. Proficiency techniques have been used only rarely to determine the dominant or preferred foot. Peters and Durding (1979) used a tapping procedure, analogous to the finger-tapping task for the determination of handedness, to measure relative pedal efficiency, while Downey (1927) observed which foot was used to provide power when digging with a spade or a shovel. These are rare examples in which footedness has been assessed with only a test of strength or skill.

However, foot preference measures exist in both behavioral and self-report forms as part of several lateral preference test batteries. The footedness items in the Harris Inventory (1958) are typical of these. Here, the experimentor observes the foot that is used to kick a ball or the foot that stamps out an imaginary fire. Kovac and Horkovic (1970) suggest that in addition to ball kicking, one might assess footedness by observing the foot and leg that bear the weight during relaxed standing, the foot placed first on a chair when one is stepping onto it, or the foot used in one-legged hopping. The most frequently encountered foot preference self-report item (found in a number of inventories) is the question, "With which foot do you kick a ball?" (Clark, 1957; Friedlander, 1971; Koch, 1933; Oldfield, 1971). In both the behavioral and the self-report procedures, the elicited activities are relatively common and require the selection of one limb to perform the selected coordination.

Three studies have looked at the agreement between self-report and behavioral assessments of foot preference (Coren & Porac, 1978; Coren, Porac, & Duncan, 1979; Raczkowski, Kalat, & Nebes, 1974). The results of these assessments, shown in Table 2-4, indicate that the concordance between self-report and behavioral tests is above 80% for all of the items, with an average concordance of

Table 2-4: Self-Report Items for Foot Preference, Their Agreement with Behavioral Tests, and Their Reliabilities[a]

Foot preference items	Agreement between self-report and behavioral tests (%)	Agreement between self-reports at retest (%)
1. With which foot do you kick a ball?	95[1,2]	96[b]
2. If you had to step up onto a chair, which foot would you place on the chair first?	85[1,2]	—
3. If you wanted to pick up a pebble with your toes, which foot would you use?	85[2]	—
4. Which foot do you put a shoe on first?	83[3]	93[c]

[a] Superscripts indicate sources: 1, Coren & Porac (1978); 2, Coren, Porac, & Duncan (1979); 3, Raczkowski, Kalat, & Nebes (1974).
[b] One-year retest.[1]
[c] One-month retest.[3]

87%. The agreement between self-report and behavior is comparable to that obtained between various behavioral measures themselves. Coren, Porac, and Duncan (1979) computed the concordance between the behavioral versions of the kicking and the stepping items, and they found an 89% concordance between them. This is similar to the 87% overall concordance shown in Table 2-4. Few test-retest reliabilities are available for footedness measures. However, as can be seen in Table 2-4, the existing retest reliabilities on the self-report items are above 90%.

Evidence suggests also that foot preference, like hand preference, is a unitary dimension. In a factor analytic study, Porac, Coren, Steiger, and Duncan (1980) showed that the first three foot preference items listed in Table 2-4 all loaded on the same factor. This finding suggests a common factor measured by most foot preference items. Less is known about foot preference than is known about hand preference, but the empirical patterns appear to be similar. Foot preference measures are highly correlated with one another, and as in handedness, both self-report and behavioral measures are valid indicators of the preferred foot and tend to produce similar results.

Eye Preference

Hand and foot preference are manifestations of sidedness that have been recognized for centuries. People are often surprised to learn that the bilateral sense organs, the eyes and the ears, show lateral asymmetries and are subject also to differential preference behaviors.

The first formal description of a dominant or preferred eye was by Giam Baptista del Porta, in 1593, who described a test for determining the preferred eye. He recommended that a staff be held directly in front of the body. With both eyes open, the viewer aligns the tip of the staff with a mark or crack on a distant wall. When the eyes are winked alternately, the tip of the staff remains in good alignment when viewing with one eye; however, the viewer perceives the tip of the staff to be shifted to one side, apparently in misalignment when viewing with the other eye. Thus, the tip of the staff and the distant target have been aligned using the information from one eye's view, while the misaligned view of the other eye has been ignored or suppressed. The eye for which target and staff are in alignment is the preferred eye. This is just one of the many tests for eyedness that have been developed. Walls (1951) catalogued 25 different measures, Gronwall and Sampson (1971) employed 18 tests, and Coren and Kaplan (1973) utilized 13 tests; many others have appeared separately in the literature. One can divide these measures into the same two global classes that are used for tests of handedness and footedness, namely, proficiency versus preference measures.

The rationale offered for proficiency measures of eyedness is similar to the justification for strength measures of handedness. For example, Duke-Elder (1952) argues that "when the vision in the two eyes is unequal from some pathological or refractive reason or when strabismus exists, the better eye attains a position of marked supremacy, but when the two are approximately equal in visual acuity there may be little evidence of dominance." A series of tests for eye preference based on relative muscular efficiency, refraction, or physiological status has arisen from this viewpoint. Table 2-5 lists a number of these.

In contrast to ocular efficiency or proficiency tests, there are also a series of eye preference tests. Usually these are presented in the form of monocular sighting tasks, such as looking through a telescope, a microscope, or the sights of a rifle. Since only one eye can be used at any time, the individual must make a selection. The eye that is chosen is called the *sighting dominant eye*. Notice that determining the sighting eye is analogous to designating the hand preferred in unimanual tasks. A number of sighting or eye preference tests are listed in Table 2-6.

In dealing with eyedness, we can pose a question similar to that asked concerning hand (and foot) preference, namely, what is the relationship between the proficiency and the preference measures, and do they measure a similar

Table 2-5: Proficiency Measures of Eyedness

Eye proficiency test	Testing procedure
Relative acuity	Eye with better monocular acuity as measured with Snellen letters or Landolt C's (Duke-Elder, 1938; Woo & Pearson, 1927)
Phoria test	Eye with less or no deviation or phoria during binocular fixation (Crider, 1935; Dolman, 1920; Ogle, 1964)
Convergence test	Eye that maintains convergence better as a target is brought close to the face along median plane (Coren, 1974; Mills, 1925, 1928)
Vascularization	Eye with greatest blood flow (Kovac & Horkovic, 1970)
Wink test	Eye more difficult to wink (Danielson, 1930; Kovac & Horkovic, 1970)
Chromatic test	Eye in which colors appear more saturated (Pascal, 1926)
Dichoptic test	Eye whose view predominates when discrepant images are flashed briefly to the two eyes (Andercin, Perry, & Childers, 1973; Kephart & Revesman, 1953; Perry & Childers, 1972; Porac, 1974; Porac & Coren, 1975b)
Color rivalry	Eye whose view predominates when discrepant colors are presented stereoscopically (Cohen, 1952; Coren & Kaplan, 1973; Washburn, Faison, & Scott, 1934)
Form rivalry	Eye whose view predominates when discrepant forms or contours are presented stereoscopically (Cohen, 1952; Porac & Coren, 1978b; Toch, 1960)

trait? Fortunately, two studies have looked at the intercorrelation among a number of different eyedness measures, and both have produced a similar pattern of results (Coren & Kaplan, 1973; Gronwall & Sampson, 1971). Coren and Kaplan (1973) administered 12 eyedness tests to a single sample of subjects. The tests included seven proficiency tests and five sighting tests from among those described in Tables 2-5 and 2-6. They also included a test of handedness. The correlation among these 12 tests is shown in Table 2-7. The five sighting preference tests (items 1-5) are all highly intercorrelated, whereas the proficiency tests (items 6-12) show little intercorrelation. The two binocular rivalry tests are correlated with one another, and somewhat with visual acuity, while visual acuity and recognition of discrepant dichoptic stimuli also show some association.

Table 2-6: Sighting and Preference Measures of Eyedness

Eye preference test	Testing procedure
Telescope	Eye used to sight down a telescope (Harris, 1957; Walls, 1951)
Rifle	Eye used to sight down a rifle or along pistol (Cuff, 1930; Harris, 1957)
Hole[a]	Eye used to sight through a hole in a card (Porac & Coren, 1975a; Suchman, 1968)
Miles ABC[a]	Eye aligned with small hole when subject holds wide end of a truncated cone over face and views distant target (Miles, 1929, 1930; Updegraff, 1932)
Asher[a]	Subject holds a card in each hand and gradually brings them together until all that is seen in the slit is the experimenter's nose. The eye aligned with the slit is sighting eye (Asher, 1961; Coren & Kaplan, 1973)
Point[a]	Eye aligned with finger when subject points to experimenter's nose (Crovitz & Zener, 1962; Coren & Kaplan, 1973; Palmer, 1947)
Alignment[a]	Eye used to align wires set on opposite ends of an open tube (Coren & Kaplan, 1973; Crider, 1944; Cuff, 1930a)
Porta[a]	Pencil aligned with distant target; eye that maintains alignment when each eye is closed in turn (Crovitz & Zener, 1962; Gronwall & Sampson, 1971; Porta, 1593)
Hold card[a]	Eye on same side of body midline where a card is held when subject reads fine print (Gronwall & Sampson, 1971)

[a] Both eyes are open during testing.

Table 2-7: Correlations between Preference and Proficiency Tests for Eyedness (based on Coren & Kaplan, 1973)

	Preference tests							Proficiency tests				
	1	2	3	4	5	6	7	8	9	10	11	12
1. Point	—	0.64^b	0.65^b	0.64^b	0.69^b	0.06	-0.11	0.53^b	0.18	0.52^b	0.21	0.16
2. Alignment		—	0.64^b	0.74^b	0.51^b	0.07	-0.21	0.30^a	0.16	0.42^b	0.28^a	0.22
3. Hole			—	0.84^b	0.73^b	0.12	-0.01	0.35^b	-0.05	0.47^b	0.13	0.08
4. Miles ABC				—	0.68^b	0.06	-0.14	0.28^a	0.03	0.51^b	0.09	0.06
5. Asher					—	0.18	0.08	0.45^b	0.08	0.42^b	0.08	0.16
6. Form rivalry						—	0.41^b	0.16	0.17	0.17	0.00	0.41^b
7. Color rivalry							—	0.08	-0.04	0.01	-0.06	0.16
8. Chromatic								—	0.17	0.24	0.06	0.15
9. Dichoptic									—	0.08	-0.08	-.39^b
10. Convergence										—	0.20	-0.03
11. Wink											—	0.14
12. Relative acuity												—

^{a} $p < .05$.
^{b} $p < .01$.

Note. The various tests are described in Tables 2-5 and 2-6.

Other than these, there are no significant intercorrelations among the various proficiency tests, and only two proficiency tests (8 and 10) are associated strongly with the preference measures. The study by Gronwall and Sampson (1971) showed a similar pattern; they also found the highest intercorrelations to be among the sighting tests. Coren and Kaplan (1973) explored the structure of eyedness tests further by factor analyzing the data. They found three distinct factors, with a major factor that accounted for 67% of the common variance. This factor contained all of the sighting preference tests. The binocular rivalry tests loaded on a separate factor, and acuity and dichoptic recognition on a third. Thus, the largest coherent cluster of eyedness tests is composed of the sighting preference measures.

These results are reminiscent of those observed for handedness measures. When considering a population of individuals, there is a suggestion that preference and proficiency are related; however, the intercorrelations are low. Preference measures are associated strongly with another but not with proficiency measures. Proficiency meaures, on the other hand, do not predict each other very well. Once again preference measures emerge as a unitary phenomenon separable from proficiency measures.

Questionnaire items also exist for the assessment of eye preference, and these self-report devices have been validated against behavioral assessments of eyedness. Coren and Porac (1978) and Coren, Porac, and Duncan (1979) compared sighting preference behaviors to the results obtained from a series of self-report items. The items used and the concordance between self-report and behavioral tests are indicated in Table 2-8. Items 1-3 show high concordance between self-report and behavior. The other items show weaker classification agreement, although (except for the winking question) all remain statistically significant. Coren and Porac (1978) retested individuals on these questions after a one-year interval. The percentage test-retest agreements, as shown in Table 2 8, are not as high as those observed for the retest of hand and foot preference items, but they are all statistically significant. Overall these results suggest that eyedness, defined as the preferred eye used in sighting coordinations, can be measured validly and reliably with self-report techniques.

Ear Preference

Of all of the indexes of lateral preference, the least is known about earedness. However, one can define preference and proficiency measures for this index as have been done for handedness, footedness, and eyedness. As in the case of the other preference types, ear preference measures demand the selection of one of the two ears in situations where both cannot be used simultaneously. Examples of such tasks involve pressing an ear against a clock to hear its ticking, or pressing an ear to a door to hear sound in the adjoining room. Self-report items seem to be as efficient as behavioral tests for determining ear preference in a manner analogous to the other lateral preference types. Coren and Porac (1978) and

Table 2-8: Self-Report Items for the Measurement of Eye Preference, Their
Mean Agreement with Behavioral Tests, and Their Reliabilities[a]

Eye preference items	Agreement between self-report and behavioral tests (%)	Agreement between self-reports at year retest (%)
1. Which eye would you use to peep through a keyhole?	86[1,2]	83[1]
2. If you had to look into a dark bottle to see how full it was, which eye would you use?	87[1,2]	76[1]
3. Which eye would you use to sight down a rifle?	84[1,2]	76[1]
4. Which eye do you use when looking through a telescope?	78[1,2]	73[1]
5. Suppose you are bending to look under a bed, which eye would be closest to the floor?	64[1]	—
6. Most people carry their head with a slight tilt. Do you carry your head tilted to the left or right?	60[1]	—
7. If someone asks you to wink your eye, which one do you wink?	52[1]	—

[a] Superscripts indicate sources: 1, Coren & Porac (1978); 2, Coren, Porac, & Duncan (1979).

Coren, Porac, and Duncan (1979) measured the relationship between behavioral demonstrations of ear preference and answers to questions concerning ear preference behaviors. The questions and resulting classification concordance are shown in Table 2-9. The magnitudes of these values suggest that ear preference can be measured using self-report procedures.

One can define two types of proficiency tests for earedness that are analogous to those described for eyedness, the other form of sense organ lateral preference. The first is relative ear performance during dichotic listening. In a dichotic listening paradigm, discrepant auditory stimuli (usually words, nonsense syllables, or numbers) are presented to the two ears simultaneously and an assessment is made of the relative efficiency with which each ear processes its input. For example, if greater amounts of the right ear input are recalled, right ear preference is displayed under these conditions. Dichotic listening, then, is the auditory version of the visual binocular rivalry or dichoptic flash tests described in Table 2-5. An alternative proficiency measure, analogous to visual acuity, is to assess the relative threshold sensitivity of each ear. The ear with the lowest threshold is the preferred ear.

Table 2-9: Self-Report Items for the Measurement of Ear Preference and Their Agreement with Behavioral Tests[a]

Ear preference items	Agreement between self-report and behavioral tests (%)
1. If you wanted to listen to a conversation behind a closed door, which ear would you place against the door?	87[1,2]
2. If you wanted to hear someone's heartbeat, which ear would you place against the person's chest?	81[1]
3. Into which ear would you place the earphone of a transistor radio?	84[1,2]

[a] Superscripts indicate sources: 1, Coren & Porac (1978); 2, Coren, Porac, & Duncan (1979).

Unfortunately, only one study has looked at the relationship between ear preference, seen in one-eared situations, and ear proficiency as defined by auditory processing asymmetries (Bilto & Peterson, 1944). Therefore, we conducted a study with the assistance of Dr. Frank Spellacy of the University of Victoria. We measured ear preference in 227 subjects with the self-report items described in Table 2-9, and we also assessed sensory efficiency in two ways. First, we determined the threshold acuity for each ear separately. Then we used a dichotic listening task where discrepant English words were presented to each of the ears simultaneously. The words were presented in groups of six items (three to each ear) and subjects reported as many as possible on each trial for a total of 22 trials. This experiment explored three measures of earedness for each subject; preference in a one-eared situation, auditory acuity, and dichotic listening.

We found only a 54% concordance between the preferred ear as determined by the questions and the more acute ear as measured by threshold sensitivity, a value that is not significantly different from chance. However, the preferred ear does appear to extract slightly more information than does the nonpreferred ear during dichotic listening. The percentage concordance between the side of one-ear preference and the side of dichotic listening preference was 57%. While statistically greater than the 50% chance expectation, this value does not represent a high degree of association. Most likely the two measures do not share much of a common mechanism. In addition, there seems to be little association between the two measures of aural efficiency. The obtained classification concordance between threshold sensitivity and dichotic listening was only 47%. Our conclusions about earedness are in accord with those reached for handedness, footedness, and eyedness. Ear preference is relatively independent of aural efficiency and can be measured using behavioral or self-report procedures.

Quantification of Lateral Preference Behaviors

Once one decides on an assessment technique, a number of issues still remain concerning the scoring and the classification of lateral preference responses. Since we will present a great deal of data in the chapters to come, it is important to discuss these problems with the aim of clarifying the scoring and classification procedures that we have chosen for the presentation of our own data.

In assessing the various forms of lateral preference, psychometric theory suggests that multiple measures be used because they provide a higher degree of measurement reliability (Guilford 1954). Multiple administrations of a given test, or data from the administration of several different measures of lateral preference, require some methodological decisions. With multiple assessment procedures, lateral preference indexes can be treated as continuous variables, where consideration is given to the strength as well as to the side of the behavior. One can devise scoring techniques based on the premise that manifestations of lateral preference have both a sidedness and a strength dimension, which reveal themselves through the consistency or inconsistency of response patterns over repeated trials or questions. One procedure that has been used in a number of studies (Coren & Porac, 1978, 1980a,b; Coren, Porac, & Duncan, 1979; Porac & Coren, 1979) assigns a *+1* to each right-sided response, a *-1* to each left-sided one, and a *0* to each response that shows no preference (ambi-sided). Algebraic summation of the values creates a scale where larger positive numbers indicate more right-sidedness and larger negative numbers indicate more left-sidedness. One can normalize this index by dividing the algebraically summed scores by N or the number of items in the preference inventory. This normalization procedure allows one to compare results across research efforts that have used different numbers of items. This procedure reduces to the formula $(R-L)/N$, where R represents the number of right responses, L the number of left responses, and N the total number of items in the assessment battery. Ambi-sided responses do not need to be entered into the numerator, although all items appear in the N. This scoring method has an upper bound of +1 and a lower bound of -1 regardless of the number of items employed. Multiplication by 100 converts the results to a scale with a range of ±100. Preference scales similar to this have been utilized in a number of studies (Durost, 1934; Falek, 1959; Oldfield, 1971).

Historically, lateral preferences have often been viewed as dichotomous factors. Such a viewpoint maintains that only the side, not the degree, of lateral preference is relevant. Thus it maintains that individuals are either left or right sided on any index, and this description sufficiently characterizes their lateral preference. The simplest procedure for establishing a dichotomy classifies any individual with a predominance of right-sided over left-sided responses as dextral, whereas an individual with more left-sided responses is classified as sinistral. The problematic issue of ambi-sided individuals can be avoided by using an odd number of items and restricting the response alternatives to left and right. Alternatively, one can assign ambilaterals arbitrarily to either the left or the right category. Since the usual classification of such individuals is with the left-preferent group, the dichotomy is actually one of right-siders and non-right-siders.

Another technique halves the number of ambi-siders and assigns one half to the sinistral group and one-half to the dextral group (Humphrey, 1951; Witty & Kopel, 1936).

The placement of ambi-sided individuals within any scoring scheme raises another problem. The definition of ambi-sidedness or no preference is, in itself, ambiguous. Many investigators have chosen to call individuals who are not consistently sided (all right or all left responses) "mixed dominant," "ambi-lateral," or "ambi-sided." Rife (1940) maintained that any deviation from consistent dextrality indicated left preference. Thus individuals were classified as left if they gave only one left response out of 10 items. Similar procedures for determining left-sidedness have been used by Komai and Fukuoka (1934) and Pelecanos (1969). This procedure implies a classification of cases into a dichotomy of consistently dextral versus not consistently dextral, as opposed to that of right versus left. In this scheme, a nominally left-sided individual might actually perform more tasks with the right hand than with the left. Thus, when dealing with dichotomized preference data, it is important to understand the assignment criteria for the right- and left-sided groups.

Some investigators have tried to avoid these problems by using a trichotomous classification scheme that divides individuals into left, right, and mixed groups. This procedure is a gradual movement toward a continuum of side and strength, once again. To see how this might operate, consider the next logical step, a polychotomous division, such as "strong right," "weak right," "mixed," "weak left," "strong left." This five-point graded system encodes both side and strength. Many investigators prefer such gradations to simple dichotomies. This suggests an implicit assumption by many researchers that lateral preference varies along both these dimensions.

This discussion has clarified the fact that each investigator can choose a scoring technique and a quantification scheme from a number that exist within the literature. This choice rests ultimately on the theoretical considerations and the empirical questions that guide the investigator's efforts. However, one can assess the significance of preference data patterns only if one is certain about the scoring techniques that have been used. This also serves as a warning to the reader, who must ascertain the particular scoring procedure used by a given investigator. Many of the discrepancies observed in the literature, such as those pertaining to the number of left-handers in the population, may be artifacts of the particular categorization procedure rather than indicative of actual differences in the performance of the subjects tested (see McManus, 1980). Before deciding that two studies disagree in the direction of the results, it is important to determine whether they used the same scoring procedures. For the consumer of laterality data, as in the marketplace, there is a *caveat emptor,* where reading the fine print in the methodology section may be as important as reading the main text.

3

Population Characteristics

Before one can begin to understand the function and etiology of lateral preference, the prevalence of such behaviors in the general population must be determined. What is the distribution of dextrality and sinistrality for hand, foot, eye, and ear, and what are the relationships among the various manifestations of lateral preference within individuals? Do individual difference variables alter the distribution of these preference behaviors? This chapter will provide a normative description of lateral preferences in an attempt to answer these questions.

There is an extensive literature pertaining to the distribution of handedness and eyedness, with empirical efforts dating back to the early 19th century. Unfortunately, the existing estimates often do not agree, and wide discrepancies exist in the reported percentages of right- and left-sidedness obtained by various investigators. Data on hand preference distributions illustrate this point very well. The earliest attempt to assess the distribution of right- and left-handedness is found in the Bible (Judges 20:15-16), where it is stated that there were 700 left-handed or ambidextrous men against 26,000 right-handed men in the tribe of Benjamin. This means that 97% of this population showed dextral handedness. More recent reports yield percentage incidences of right-handedness varying from maximum rates of 98-99% (Baldwin, 1911) to minimum levels of 70-71% (Parsons, 1924; Woo & Pearson, 1927). This variability is probably due largely to the different methods used to define the preferred hand, as was explained in Chapter 2. For instance, in our biblical example handedness was based on the arm used to hold a slingshot, while contemporary estimates have been based on dozens of different measures. Many researchers have relied upon self-reports of hand use during various unimanual skilled activities or upon the direct observation of hand use during these activities. Others have used sensory tests that involve the subjective judgment of weight differences when weights are suspended from the index fingers of each hand (van Biervliet, 1897), the determination of differences in the lengths of the radius and ulna of each arm (Jones, 1915), the assessment of differences in the grip strengths of each hand (Woo & Pearson, 1927), or the determination of the habitually placed top thumb or arm during hand clasping or arm folding (Kobyliansky, Micle & Arensburg, 1978). Even covert measures, such as noting the hand used to carry common objects like umbrellas and handbags (Wile, 1934), have been employed as ways of determining the distribution of handedness in the general population. As the previous chapter noted, there is often little correlation among these measures, since they include the full gamut of proficiency and preference assessment techniques, as well as many other nonbehaviorally validated indicators. As also indicated in Chapter 2, various researchers have used different criteria for classifying an individual as right or left handed. In one study, a left-hander might be any individual who shows at least one non-right-sided response; in another study, all responses might be required to be left sided for such a designation. For these reasons, one should actually expect, rather than be surprised by, such a diverse range of estimated percentages of right-handedness.

These methodological considerations pose problems to an investigator who wants to obtain normative estimates of lateral preference distributions. One solution might be to limit literature-based estimates to studies that have utilized uniform measures. In our case, since we are interested in preference aspects of sidedness, we could base our estimates on studies that have used self-report inventories or simple performance batteries when determining sidedness patterns. For handedness, population percentages could be obtained easily from the numerous questionnaire studies that exist in the literature. Unfortunately, narrowing our criterion to this smaller set of measurement techniques does not solve the methodological problems. Many self-report studies of handedness have been based on the single index of the writing hand. This index, as noted in Chapter 2, may be subject to social and cultural pressure. Data from self-report inventories that have employed larger batteries of questions may still be questionable methodologically, since there have been only a few attempts to establish the validity and reliability of questionnaire items for handedness (Coren & Porac, 1978; Coren, Porac, & Duncan, 1979; Koch, 1933; Razckowski, Kalat, & Nebes, 1974). In addition, there have been only three attempts to correlate behavioral and self-report items for the other indexes of lateral preference, and two of these have been conducted only recently (Coren & Porac, 1978; Koch, 1933; Coren, Porac, & Duncan, 1979). These studies show that although valid and reliable questionnaire items (as determined through comparisons to behavioral tests) can be selected, many questions are too poorly correlated with actual behavioral tests to be classified as valid indicators of preference. Several such items have been quite popular and they often appear in lateral preference batteries. Since item-by-item analyses are seldom given in published reports, one cannot remove suspect items from the composite data; thus, the reported population percentages must be viewed as uncertain. A final problem rests with the fact that the available data seldom assess more than one type of lateral preference, namely, handedness. Although over the years several investigators have measured three or four indexes of preference in the same sample (Clark, 1957; Downey, 1927; Koch, 1933; Thompson, 1975), they have confined themselves to the study of relatively small samples of circumscribed age groups. There are no existing reports that have looked at the population characteristics of the four types of lateral preference on a large scale, so that norms can be established on the sidedness relationships within and among the various preference types. For this reason our ability to describe certain patterns of behavior, such as the congruency of sidedness across indexes of lateral preference, is severely limited. The only remedy is a new data-gathering effort that elimates the methodological problems and empirical limitations that we have described. Therefore, we conducted a study oriented toward achieving this aim.

Several considerations dictated the choice of our methodology. Because we wanted data from a sample large enough to form stable population estimates, we selected a self-report inventory technique to collect our data. We required each item used in the questionnaire to have a demonstrated high rate of concordance with results of behavioral testing on similar actions. In addition, each item was required to have a reasonably high retest reliability. Also, we wanted to measure all four indexes of lateral preference (hand, foot, eye, and ear) simultaneously. The questionnaire battery that we chose to use is shown in Table 3-1. The items were selected from Raczkowski, Kalat, and Nebes (1974), Coren and Porac (1978), and Coren, Porac, and Duncan (1979); the average concordance between

Table 3-1: Behaviorally Validated Self-Report Inventory Used to Assess Lateral Preference Distributions

Hand preference
  1. With which hand would you throw a ball to hit a target?
  2. With which hand do you draw?
  3. With which hand do you use an eraser on paper?
  4. With which hand do you give out the top card when dealing?

Foot preference
  1. With which foot do you kick a ball?
  2. If you wanted to pick up a pebble with your toes, which foot would you use?
  3. If you had to step up onto a chair, which foot would you place on the chair first?

Eye preference
  1. Which eye would you use to peep through a keyhole?
  2. If you had to look into a dark bottle to see how full it was, which eye would you use?
  3. Which eye would you use to sight down a rifle?

Ear preference
  1. If you wanted to listen in on a conversation going on behind a closed door, which ear would you place against the door?
  2. If you wanted to hear someone's heart beat, which ear would you place against their chest?
  3. Into which ear would you place the earphone of a transistor radio?

Note. Items were presented in mixed order, and not identified as to purpose. Responses were "left," "right," or "both."

these items and behavioral tests is approximately 90% with an average retest reliability of 91%.

We measured a large heterogeneous population of individuals who were contacted through various educational and community organizations, sports and recreation groups, senior citizens' associations, high schools, universities, and colleges. We attempted to obtain respondents from a broad range of socioeconomic categories, all living in the United States and Canada. Potential respondents were contacted by mail and asked to complete the inventory shown in Table 3-1. In addition, they were asked to supply some medical history and socioeconomic data. Approximately 20,000 individuals were contacted in this manner, and complete data (defined as answers to all aspects of the questionnaire) were obtained from 5,147 individuals. The final sample ranges in age from 8 to 100 years and in composed of 2,391 females and 2,756 males. The age and gender composition of the sample is shown in Table 3-2.

Distributional Characteristics within Indexes of Lateral Preference

To arrive at an overall estimate of the distribution of the lateral preferences in a general population, we used a simple dichotomization procedure. Subjects responded to each question in the battery with an answer of "left," "right," or "both." Data were transformed by means of the formula $(R-L)/N$ where R is the number of "right" responses, L the number of "left" responses, and N the total number of items used to measure any given type of lateral preference. This preference index varies from ± 1, where negative values represent a predominance of left responses and positive values represent a preponderance of right responses. For the purpose of this initial analysis, all ambilateral responders (with a preference score of 0) were classified as left sided. This group is a very small percentage of the sample; however, the implication of this method of dichotomization is to classify the sample into right-sided versus non-right-sided groups. Table 3-3

Table 3-2: Age and Gender Composition of Lateral Preference Normative Sample

Age group (years)	Total sample	Females	Males
8-15	292	179	113
16-25	3,409	1,527	1,882
26-35	468	200	268
36-45	278	124	154
46-55	361	176	185
56-65	213	124	89
66-75	89	43	46
75-100	37	18	19
Total	5,147	2,391	2,756

Table 3-3: Percentage of Population Classified as Right-Sided for the Four Indexes of Lateral Preference[a]

Preference type	Total sample (N = 5,147)	Females (N = 2,391)	Males (N = 2,756)
Hand	88.2	90.1[b]	86.5[b]
Foot	81.0	86.0[b]	76.7[b]
Eye	71.1	69.1[b]	72.9[b]
Ear	59.4	64.6[b]	54.8[b]

[a] All percentages are significantly greater than the chance expectation of 50%, $p < .001$.

[b] Significant sex difference, $p < .01$.

presents the resulting percentages of right-sidedness for our normative sample. All four indexes show a predominance of right-sided preferences; however, there are differences among the various indexes in the prevalence of dextrality. Handedness shows the largest degree of right-sidedness, followed by footedness, eyedness, and earedness, respectively.

That humans are predominantly right sided in all manifestations of lateral preference could lead to the belief that there is a single process that biases the population toward dextrality. This fact might also lead to the expectation that the degree of right-sidedness would be the same for all four indexes. However, we find that comparisons across the indexes shows that the degree of right-sidedness varies significantly among these manifestations of lateral preference. This could be evidence that all of these preferences do not share the same causal mechanism, an issue that we will discuss more fully in Chapter 4.

Many investigators have looked for possible sex or gender differences in the incidence of lateral preference (at least in handedness). Gender is an obvious individual difference variable, and if it affects the process under study, it may have a bearing upon both physiological and environmental theories of lateral preference. In general, the existing literature suggests that when sex differences for handedness are found, a higher percentage of males are shown to be left handed than are females (Bryden, 1977; Clark, 1957; Dawson, 1972; Enstrom, 1962; Hardyck, Goldman, & Petrinovich, 1975; Harshman & Remington, 1975; Levy, 1976; Le Roux, 1979; Pringle, Butler, & Davie, 1966; Oldfield, 1971; Wold, 1969). Unfortunately, the differences between the sexes are often quite small, a 1-5% difference favoring increased left-handedness in males. If the gender difference is of this magnitude, it is not surprising to find reports of no sex differences in handedness (Annett, 1970; Porac & Coren, 1978a, 1979a; Searleman, Tweedy, & Springer, 1979). Few researchers have looked for sex differences in the other indexes of lateral preference, although Porac, Coren, and Duncan (1980a) have provided some evidence suggesting the existence of sex differences in the relative dextrality of foot, eye, and ear. In this sample we also analyzed our data as a function of the sex of the respondent, as can be seen in Table 3-3. There are significant sex differences for all four indexes. Consistent with earlier research, we find that females, as a group, show more right-handed-ness than do males; however, it is an incidence difference of only 3.6%. That the difference is so small may well explain why there are discrepant reports in the literature as to whether or not such a sex difference exists for hand preference. Overall, females manifest 9.3% more right-sidedness than do males. A small sex difference is found in eye preference. This difference is interesting because it shows the reverse of the pattern for hand, foot, and ear, with females being somewhat more left-eyed (3.8% difference) than are males. The relative prepon-derance of left-eyed females replicates a previous report by Porac, Coren, and Duncan (1980a).

When we use dichotomous division of subjects into right versus left, we have information only about the direction or side of preference. No indication of the consistency or strength of the preference remains. In order to see how lateral preferences vary in strength in the population, we can return to the scoring index of $(R-L)/N$, and consider the occurrence of each possible preference scale value in our sample. As mentioned earlier, these values vary between ± 1, with a +1 indicating consistently right preference on all response items and a -1 con-sistently left responses. Scores between these endpoints represent intermediate strengths of lateral preference, with 0 indicating complete ambilaterality. We can derive a picture of the distribution of preference behaviors in terms of both strength and direction by plotting the percentage of the sample receiving each possible scale value. This is done for the four types of preference in Figure 3-1.

Figure 3-1 shows that consistent or strong lateral preference behavior pat-terns are more likely than the mixed or ambi-sided patterns. This manifest itself by the J- or U-shaped functions of Figure 3-1. For example, 72% of our sample gave consistent right-handed responses. There is a rapid drop-off as one moves toward ambilaterality, and for preference scale values between -0.75 (moderate left-handedness) and 0.25 (weak right-handedness), the incidence hovers around 2% or less. There is a slight upswing at -1, indicating consistent left-sidedness with a rise to a secondary maximum of 5.3%. The distributional pattern is more U-shaped for eye and ear. For eye preference, approximately 54% of the popu-lation is consistently right sided, 14.5% is consistently left sided with intermedi-ate values of about 5%. Ear preference shows a peak incidence of consistent right-sidedness of 35% and of consistent left-sidedness of approximately 15%. Intermediate values are more common for ear preference than they are for the other indexes, averaging about 10%. Foot preference deviates slightly from the other patterns. It shows the usual mode at consistent right-sidedness, accounting for 46% of the sample. However, rather than showing the usual secondary peak at consistent left-sidedness, the incidence rate diminishes steadily as one moves toward more negative scale values and consistent sinistrality. The number of consistent left-footed individuals is only 3.9%.

The bimodality of three of these distributions suggests that left- and right-sided individuals may represent distinct groups. It also suggests that dichotomous classification of the side of lateral preference behaviors presents a reasonable picture of the underlying distribution of scores for some types of preference but not for others. Actually, dichotomous classification seems to produce groups

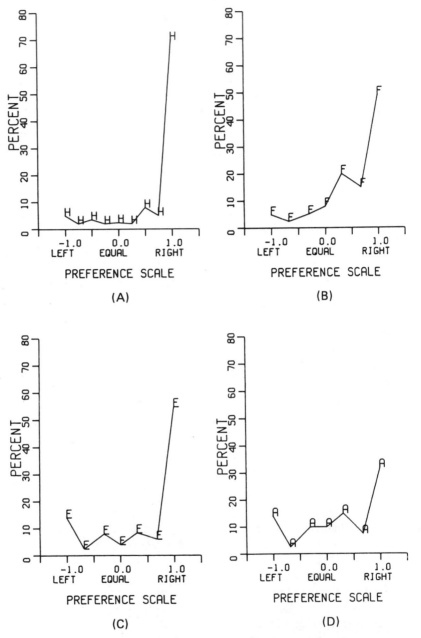

Figure 3-1. Distribution of lateral preference scores for the four indexes of preference (H is hand; F, foot; E, eye; A, ear). Scores are based on $(R-L)/N$ where R is right responses, L, left responses, and N the total number of items.

that differ in terms of consistency as well as side. In the group dichotomously called "left handed" only 45% are −1. The results are similar for the other indexes, with the sample of right-sided subjects always containing a higher percentage of consistent individuals than the sample of left-sided subjects.

We can analyze mixed responders as a separate group. This, at least, segregates the consistent right- and left-sided individuals from those showing a weaker sidedness. This is done by separating those individuals who show consistent sidedness (a scale value of +1 or −1) from those individuals showing some mixed or ambilateral tendencies. An interesting finding emerges when we segregate the consistent responders and analyze for gender differences. Females show significantly more consistency in their lateral preferences than males on all preference indexes, as seen in Table 3-4. Males and females differ not only in side, but in strength or consistency of preference.

The results of the dichotomous scoring technique have revealed that our sample is predominantly dextral in both limb and sense organ preference. Because of our sample size, we feel that we can generalize and state that the contemporary North American population is predominantly right sided. The dextral bias varies across the four indexes and is stronger for females than for males for three of the four preference types. In addition, the incidence rates of consistent and mixed response patterns differ for the various indexes as well as for right- and left-sided individuals. This supports the notion that right- and left-siders form distinct groups and that lateral preference response patterns for the various indexes may not stem from a common mechanism. When we considered the strength of the preference, in isolation from its displayed sidedness, we found that females are significantly more consistent in their sidedness patterns than are males. This difference holds for all of the preference types.

Lateral preference behaviors also seem to vary as a function of age. As usual, most of the available data pertain to handedness. Over the last 100 years, numerous investigators have been interested in the problem of changes in handedness patterns as a function of age. The results of all of these studies indicate that there is a developmental trend in the establishment of handedness patterns.

Table 3-4: Percentage of Sample Showing Consistent Preference as a Function of Sex

Lateral preference type	Percentage consistent (lateral preference index ±1)	
	Females (N = 2,391)	Males (N = 2,756)
Hand	80.6	74.0
Foot	57.7	42.2
Eye	72.4	65.4
Ear	53.7	46.4

Note. All sex differences significant with $p < .001$.

Although infants appear to exhibit inherent hand preferences at an early age, these asymmetries increase in consistency with a gradual shift toward habitual right-handedness with increasing age (Baldwin, 1890; Bethe, 1925; Cernacek & Podivinsky, 1971; Coryell & Michel, 1978; Darwin, 1877; Gesell & Ames, 1947; Giesecke, 1936; Hall, 1891; Hildreth, 1949, 1950; Ingram, 1975; Jones, 1931; Ramsay, 1979; Ramsay, Campos, & Fenson, 1979; Roos, 1935; Seth, 1973; Watson, 1925; Woolley, 1910). In addition, a number of recent studies have shown that the age-related rightward trend in hand use continues into adulthood (Coren & Porac, 1979b; Fleminger, Dalton, & Standage, 1977; Porac, Coren, & Duncan, 1980a). Little work of this type has been reported for foot, eye, and ear preference. However, Porac, Coren, and Duncan (1980a) used an indirect procedure to extract possible age trends from the published literature. They tabulated the incidence of dextrality of hand, foot, and eye that had been reported in a number of studies published over the past 90 years. The criterion for inclusion in the survey was the use of a preference measure to assess handedness, footedness, or eyedness (unfortunately, there are too few studies of ear preference to make meaningful age comparisons). Table 3-5 is based on their survey. The data in this table suggest that there may be age trends for hand, foot, and eye preference. The pattern is similar in each instance, with adults apparently more dextral than children. The most systematic changes appear in handedness, where the adult samples seem to be about 12% more right handed than the infant samples. Eye preference shows a 9% rightward shift from infancy to adult-

Table 3-5: Age Trends in Hand, Foot, and Eye Preference Suggested by a Survey of Published Studies

Index	Age range of sample	Number of studies reviewed	Right-sidedness (mean %)
Hand	Infant	3	79.9
	Preschool	4	82.6
	Elementary school	24	92.7
	High school/college	15	90.0
	Adult	20	92.3
Foot	Infant	—	—
	Preschool	—	—
	Elementary school	6	84.6
	High school/college	4	64.7
	Adult	3	90.5
Eye	Infant	1	62.0
	Preschool	3	60.5
	Elementary school	18	65.6
	High school/college	9	69.6
	Adult	15	71.0

hood, while the dextral trend in footedness, although somewhat more erratic, is about 5%.

Our normative data allow us to assess directly whether there are life-span age trends in all four forms of lateral preference. Analyses were performed on the lateral preference scale values $(R-L)/N$. First, the data were collapsed across the sex variable, since there were no significant age by sex interactions. Multivariate statistical analyses revealed an overall effect of age on lateral preference and indicated that the various age trends are not parallel. There is a significant trend toward increased right-sidedness with increasing age for both handedness and footedness. Statistically, there is also a trend toward increasing right-eyedness as a function of age, although it is rather weak. Ear preference also changes with age; however, its age trend is opposite in direction, shifting toward increased left-sidedness with advancing age. These overall age trends are shown graphically in Figure 3-2, where each data point represents the mean percentage incidence of right-sidedness for every 10-year block.

A compact way of summarizing these trends is to correlate age with the dichotomized score for each type of preference (values less than or equal to zero are scored as 1, and those greater than zero are scored as 2 for each individual for each form of lateral preference). A positive correlation indicates a rightward shift as a function of increasing chronological age, while a negative correlation indicates a leftward trend. These correlations are presented in Table 3-6 for the entire sample, and for each sex separately. The correlations are small, but except for the age trend in eye preference for females, all significantly differ from zero. As expected from the earlier trend analyses, the correlations for

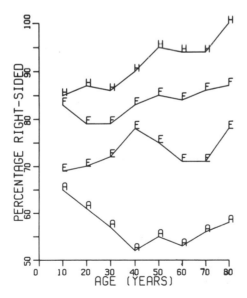

Figure 3-2. Percentage of the sample classified as right sided as a function of chronological age (H is hand; F, foot; E, eye; A, ear).

hand, foot, and eye are positive, while the leftward shift in ear preference mani-fests itself as a negative value. None of the correlations obtained for males and females differ from each other, indicating that there are no significant sex differ-ences in the rate of change in lateral preference as a function of age. This is the case despite the earlier observed baseline differences in the sidedness distribution of preferences for males and females (Table 3-3).

We can assess statistically the rate at which these age-related shifts are occur-ring in the population by computing the slopes of the regression lines for each of the age trends shown in Figure 3-2. This computation serves as an index of the rate of change per year for each form of preference. Such an analysis reveals that the rightward shift in handedness occurs at a rate of 0.22% per year; for foot preference the rate is 0.16% per year, and for eye preference it amounts to 0.09% per year. The sample becomes more left sided in ear preference at a rate of 0.30% per year. While apparently small, these changes accumulate into a substantial shift over the life span; for example, there are 15% more right-handers in the oldest as opposed to the youngest age group.

Age-related changes in lateral preference, such as we have observed, can arise from a number of different factors. For example, the apparent rightward shifts could result from a decrease in the total number of left-sided individuals, or from a slight rightward shift of individuals of mixed preference response pat-terns. The re-analysis of the data presented in Table 3-7 allows us to differenti-ate between these two possibilities. Here we dichotomized the age variable by forming two groups. The first is composed of the four younger age categories, seen in Figure 3-2, and the second is made up of the four senior age categories. In other words, we divided the sample into those less than or equal to 45 years and those older than 45 years. In addition, we trichotomized the lateral prefer-ence responses into three groups in order to classify individuals as right, left, or mixed on each index. Only those subjects with a preference scale of +1 (all responses right) were called right-sided in this form of analysis, while those with a scale value of −1 (all responses left) were denoted as left sided. All others were classified as mixed. As can be seen from Table 3-7, the age trend for hand and foot seems to be based on both an increase in the number of individuals classi-

Table 3-6: Correlation Coefficients for Age versus the Side of Lateral Preference

Lateral preference type	Total sample ($N = 5,147$)	Females ($N = 2,391$)	Males ($N = 2,756$)
Hand	.073[b]	.073[b]	.073[b]
Foot	.065[b]	.064[b]	.066[b]
Eye	.032[a]	.029	.035[a]
Ear	−.055[b]	−.064[b]	−.048[b]

Note. Positive values indicate a rightward shift with increasing age.
[a] Significantly different from 0.0, $p < .05$.
[b] Significantly different from 0.0, $p < .01$.

fied as consistently right sided and a halving of the number of individuals classified as consistently left sided. There is also a decrease in the number of individuals classified as mixed. This pattern is consistent with the interpretation of
a general rightward shift of the entire sample, perhaps as a result of the adoption
of additional right-sided activities. This would shift a number of mixed-preferent
individuals toward consistent dextrality and reduce the percentage of consistent
sinistrals. A similar pattern emerges for eye preference, except that here the shift
just misses statistical significance (p=.06). The pattern is somewhat different for
ear preference, which manifests a leftward age trend. This trend seems to occur
as a result of an approximate doubling of the number of individuals classified as
consistently left eared. However, there is no concomitant decrease in the number
of individuals classified as consistently right sided. Thus, for ear preference the
shift seems to be completely due to changes in those individuals who had previously been classified as mixed preferent, with these individuals becoming more
left with advancing age. There is also a shift in the relative consistency of side
preference. The proportion of the population classified as consistently preferent,
regardless of side, increases significantly with age for hand, foot, and ear, as can
be seen from the "total" columns in Table 3-7. This consistency increase holds
for all four indexes, although the slight percentage increase in eye preference is
not statistically significant.

An overview of the preceding data on the distributional qualities of each
index of lateral preference indicates that two major individual difference variables, gender and age, must be taken into account when examining human sidedness. Also, it appears that the four types of lateral preference do not exhibit the
same trends and distributions in either the preferred side or strength and consistency. Some of the hypotheses proposed to explain these sex and age effects will
be discussed more fully in Chapter 6.

Table 3-7: Consistency of Lateral Preference as a Function of Age (Percentage
Measures)

| Lateral preference type | Younger than 45 years | | | | Older than 45 years | | | |
| | Consistent | | | | Consistent | | | |
	Right	Left	Total	Mixed	Right	Left	Total	Mixed
Hand[b]	70.7	5.9	76.6[a]	23.4	78.2	2.0	80.2[a]	19.8
Foot[b]	43.2	4.1	47.3[b]	52.7	59.9	2.0	61.9[b]	38.1
Eye	53.6	14.8	68.4	31.6	58.3	12.3	70.6	29.4
Ear[b]	34.5	13.8	48.2[b]	51.7	36.0	22.5	58.5[b]	41.5

[a] Significantly different, $p < .05$.
[b] Significantly different, $p < .01$.
The overall age difference for hand, foot, and ear is statistically significant.

Distributional Characteristics across Indexes
of Lateral Preference

Delacato (1963) has said, "Right-handed humans are one sided, i.e., they are right-eyed, right-footed, and right-handed. . . ." This statement reflects a common belief, namely, that the various manifestations of lateral preference are aligned along the same side of the body, and that this is the normal arrangement. Surprisingly, there are very few empirical data to either support or refute this contention, since, as we have mentioned previously, only a few investigators have explored more than one index of lateral preference in the same sample. It is not the purpose of this section to detail the theoretical basis of the expectation that humans are congruently right-sided; this will be done in Chapter 4. Rather, here we will present a first attempt at an empirical assessment of this belief by using the data from our normative sample to explore the patterns among the various indexes of preference.

In the previous section, we dichotomized individuals into right- and left-sided groups in each of the four indexes of lateral preference. Now we can consider the indexes in a pairwise fashion (e.g., hand versus foot). If an individual is classified as either right preferent on both indexes or left preferent on both indexes under consideration, this person is called *congruent* for this pair. Individuals are *crossed* preferent if one index displays right-sidedness and the other left-sidedness. If individuals are completely right or left sided on all four indexes, they are called *totally congruent.* Such rescoring allows one to examine the pattern of sidedness relationships across indexes.

The left portion of Table 3-8 presents the percentages of obtained congruency for the six pairs of lateral preference types and for all four indexes combined. This is shown for the total sample and for males and females separately. Generally, the incidence rate of obtained congruency is greatest for the limb preference pair and smallest for the sense organ preference pair. In addition, there are significant gender differences in five of the six possible pairwise comparisons; females are more congruent for the pairings of hand-foot, hand-ear, foot-ear, and eye-ear, while males display greater congruency in the hand-eye pairing. The female group also shows a significantly higher incidence of total congruency in sidedness when all four indexes are considered together. Thus, females are not only more consistent in their within-index response patterns but they are also more totally congruent in their across-index patterns than are males.

Casual scrutiny of the congruency values for each pair of lateral preference behaviors and for all of the indexes combined could lead one to state that the rate of congruency is generally very high, especially for the various pairings, although the incidence rate of total congruency is less than 50%. To a certain extent, these data support the notion that humans tend to be ipsilateral (same sided) in their preference patterns, as Delacato (1963) has maintained. However, one would like to examine statistically the obtained rates of congruency in order to assess if individuals are more congruent than one might expect based on some

Table 3-8: Percentage of Sample Showing Congruent Lateral Preference for Paired Indexes[a]

Lateral preference pair	Obtained			Theoretical		
	Total sample (N=5,147)	Female (N=2,391)	Male (N=2,756)	Total sample	Female	Male
Hand-foot[b]	84.0	89.2	79.4	73.7	78.9	69.5
Hand-eye[b]	73.8	72.0	75.4	66.1	65.3	66.7
Hand-ear[b]	63.0	68.2	58.5	57.2	61.7	53.5
Foot-eye	70.0	70.3	69.7	63.1	63.8	62.2
Foot-ear[b]	65.6	68.6	63.1	55.8	60.5	52.6
Eye-ear[b]	61.8	64.1	59.9	54.0	55.6	52.2
Totally congruent[b]	44.0	46.7	40.8	30.0	35.0	27.4

[a] All obtained values are significantly greater than the theoretical values, $p < .01$.
[b] Significant sex difference in obtained percentages, $p < .01$.

chance or theoretical expectation. We know that most of the individuals in our sample are right sided on the four indexes; therefore, by chance alone, a sizable proportion of our sample should manifest congruency. We can assess whether the congruency rates are better than would be expected on the basis of random assortment in a right-sided population by borrowing procedures from probability theory and applying them to our data along with certain assumptions. For any lateral preference index, there are two possible sidedness outcomes, right and left. However, the probabilities of obtaining right- and left-sidedness are unequal. The right-sided outcome is more probable than the left-sided, given the properties of our sample. Using handedness as an example, the data in Table 3-3 show that the probability of a left-handed individual is only .12. If we use the proportions of right- and left-sided individuals in Table 3-3 as probability values, we can compute theoretically expected congruency proportions against which we can evaluate the obtained values in Table 3-8. To do this, we must make an additional assumption. We will assume that the various indexes of lateral preference operate independently and that the probability of being right- or left-sided on one preference type does not alter the probability of being right- or left-sided on another, and then test to see if such a hypothesis is tenable. The probability of being right sided on both of two indexes is equal to the probability of being right sided on one of them multiplied by the probability of being right sided on the other. In the case of the hand-foot pair, for instance, we can use the values in Table 3-3 to compute a theoretically expected probability value of observing congruent right-handedness and right-footedness. This is $.882 \times .810 = .71$. We must also add to this value of .71 the probability of observing congruent left-handedness and left-footedness in order to obtain the expected value for general congruency (regardless of side) for the hand-foot preference pair. Thus, our computations are $(.882 \times .810) + (.118 \times .19) = .737$. In a general form, our formula for all of these calculations is

$$\text{theoretical congruency value} = p(R_1) \times p(R_2) + p(L_1) \times p(L_2)$$

where $p(R_1)$ and $p(L_1)$ are the obtained proportions of right- and left-sidedness on index 1, while $p(R_2)$ and $p(L_2)$ represent the values for the second index.

This computation is the basis for all of the calculated values presented in the right portion of Table 3-8. We computed the theoretically expected percentage congruency figures for each pair of indexes and for total congruency (this is done by extending the general formula to the four-index case). We used the values in Table 3-3 to compute theoretical expectations for the total sample and for males and females separately. We then compared the actually obtained percentage of congruency for each subsample to its appropriate theoretical value. As can be seen from Table 3-8, all of the obtained congruency rates are significantly greater than those expected if the various preference indexes are independent of one another. Thus, individuals are more ipsilateral in their sidedness patterns than expected by chance alone.

The preceding analysis looked at only the direction of lateral preference, using the dichotomized scoring procedure. An alternative analysis involves the continuous scoring procedure based on the preference scale values (as shown in Figure 3-1). Since these measures are continuous, or at least ordinal, we can compute correlation coefficients between various pairs of indexes. This provides a statistical mechanism for directly assessing the degree of association between each pair of preferences in terms of the amount of predictive variance explained by each cross-index relationship. This alternate analysis is shown in Table 3-9.

First, consider the correlation matrix for the total sample. All of the correlation coefficients are statistically greater than zero and are positive, suggesting some common relationship among all of the indexes of sidedness. However, the amount of variance explained by these correlations is not large. Except for the relationship between hand and foot (accounting for 28% of the variance), each of the remaining correlations accounts for only 10% of the predictive variance. Second, although the overall pattern of correlations for males and for females is similar, there are some individual differences in correlational magnitude. These differences involve the relationship between hand preference and the other classes of side preference. Females have significantly higher correlations than do males for the hand-foot and the hand-ear pairs. Males show a somewhat higher degree of association between the hand-eye pair.

Since age affects the individual manifestations of sidedness, one can ask if it also affects the cross-index relationships. To answer this question we created a variable based on the congruency of preference for any pair of indexes. We scored congruency as a dichotomized variable. Congruent preference on a given pair of indexes was given a value of 2, while a crossed side preference was scored as 1. In the case of establishing a score for total congruency, we made same-sidedness on all four preferences equal to a score of 3, congruent-sidedness on

Table 3-9: Pearson Product Moment Correlation Coefficients Computed among the Indexes of Lateral Preference[a]

	Total sample (N=5,147)			
	Hand	Foot	Eye	Ear
Hand	—	.527	.310	.247
Foot		—	.264	.354
Eye			—	.216
Ear				—
	Females (N=2,391)			
Hand	—	.590[b]	.275[b]	.292[b]
Foot		—	.253	.353
Eye			—	.217
Ear				—
	Males (N=2,756)			
Hand	—	.478[b]	.349[b]	.204[b]
Foot		—	.290	.336
Eye			—	.224
Ear				—

[a] All correlations are significantly greater than 0, $p < .01$.
[b] Significant sex difference, $p < .01$.

three of the four indexes equal to a score of 2, and incongruent-sidedness, where two indexes are on the left side and two on the right, equal to a score of 1. Thus, for total congruency, we established a trichotomous classification scheme. Based on these procedures, we computed the correlations of chronological age with the congruency scores. Increasing congruency with age should manifest itself as a positive correlation, while decreasing congruency is demonstrated by a negative correlation. The results of this analysis are shown in Table 3-10.

Table 3-10 reveals that there are some significant age-related trends in cross-index congruency. The likelihood that the preferred hand is on the same side as the preferred foot increases with age, as does the likelihood that foot and eye preference will be congruent. Hand-eye congruency is relatively invariant with age, while the association between ear preference and any of the other indexes tends to drop with increasing chronological age. This is probably due to the gradual loss in dextral ear preference in the population with increasing chronological age. This loss in dextral ear preference, when contrasted with the increasing right-sided preference for handedness, footedness, and eyedness, results in the significant negative correlations between the congruency of ear preference with the other three indexes as a function of age. The divergence of the age trends among the various indexes also may account for the significant negative correlation between total congruency and age; thus, individuals are becoming more incongruent in their sidedness patterns with advancing age.

Table 3-10 also shows that the patterns of age shift are quite similar for males and for females; none of the correlation coefficients differ significantly as a function of sex. However, some of the individual age trends differ in statistical significance within the male and the female portions of the sample. Also, females show a significant loss in total congruency with increasing age, a trend that is not apparent in the male group.

In considering the within-index normative data, we presented analyses based upon a consideration of both the side and the strength of the displayed preference. This same task is difficult to accomplish for the cross-index comparisons, since the two possibilities of consistent and mixed response patterns must be considered across the six pairs of preference indexes. Since there are many possible combinations of mixed and consistent patterns within each pair, such analyses produce an extremely large number of tabular presentations that, for reasons of clarity and length, cannot be presented here. However, we can look at one possible strength outcome, namely, the observed percentage of individuals who have scored the most extreme value (± 1), on the same side, for the four preference types. This is the most strongly congruent right- and left-sided group combined. Sixteen percent of our sample produced responses of this type. Since Table 3-8 shows that 44% of our sample is classified as totally congruent under a dichotomous procedure that considers only sidedness, this finding indicates that the majority of individuals displaying congruent sidedness (28%) are doing so based on patterns of mixed and consistent responses across the four indexes. Thus, the norm for total congruency is not an extreme response pattern across the four indexes. In addition, we found an interesting and significant gender difference; 19% of the female sample as opposed to 12% of the male group is classified as strongly and totally congruent. As we have found in other analyses, females continue to show a more extreme overall preference pattern than that observed in males.

Table 3-10. Correlation Coefficients of Age versus Congruency

Lateral preference pair	Total sample ($N = 5,147$)	Females ($N = 2,391$)	Males ($N = 2,756$)
Hand-foot	$.055^b$	$.047^a$	$.060^b$
Hand-eye	$.012$	$.010$	$.015$
Hand-ear	$-.064^b$	$-.079^b$	$-.052^b$
Foot-eye	$.033^b$	$.022$	$.046^b$
Foot-ear	$-.069^b$	$-.092^b$	$-.048^b$
Eye-ear	$-.008$	$-.019$	$.003$
Total congruency	$-.053^b$	$-.062^b$	$-.025$

Note. Positive values indicate increasing congruency.

[a] Significantly greater than 0, $p < .05$.

[b] Significantly greater than 0, $p < .01$.

In this chapter, we have tried to present a picture of the relative distributions of lateral preference types in a large sample that represents a general North American population. The emerging pattern is one in which a clear bias toward dextral preference patterns for hand, foot, eye, and ear is apparent. The degree of manifest right-sidedness in our sample, however, varies as a function of the particular index under consideration. Handedness shows the most extreme right-left dichotomy, followed by footedness, eyedness, and earedness. In addition, although there is congruency of sidedness across the various indexes, it differs as a function of the pair under consideration; also, fewer than 50% of our respondents show total sidedness congruency.

There are also clear individual difference variables that affect the observed sample patterns. However, these age and sex effects are not uniform for all of the indexes. In general, females are more consistent in their response patterns within indexes and show stronger preference scale values. Females also show greater total sidedness congruency across indexes, although this does not hold for all of the paired-index comparisons. There are also marked age differences that are divergent for the four indexes of preference. Handedness and footedness tend toward greater dextrality, and there is some indication that eyedness also becomes more dextral with age. The opposite age trend appears for earedness, with the population becoming gradually more left sided with age. There is a general age trend suggesting that individuals lose total sidedness congruency with increasing age.

In many respects, this chapter forms the center of the book, since we will be referring to these data repeatedly as we attempt to explore the theoretical and functional implications of these preference patterns in later chapters. Given our normative findings, a number of questions remain to be resolved. Why do populations appear to be predominantly dextral in sidedness patterns? What is the basis of the observed sex differences in lateral preference? What is the basis of the association between indexes of preference? As we deal with these issues in the succeeding chapters, we hope to move toward answering the most intriguing question: What is the significance of lateral preference behaviors?

4

Physiological, Biological, and Cerebral Asymmetries

The apparent physical symmetry of the human body has led scientists, philosophers, and researchers to puzzle over and theorize about the mechanisms that give rise to the functional asymmetries seen in the common displays of handedness and the other lateral preferences. For centuries investigators have postulated various asymmetrical developmental processes and structures that could induce functional inequalities in a seemingly symmetrical organism.

Physiological Asymmetries

Perhaps the first theory of bodily asymmetry emanates from ancient Greece, where any deviation from symmetry was viewed as another example of man's ungodlike imperfection. Aristophanes declared that man had been created as a sphere, with his face toward heaven and his buttocks to the ground. Thus, there was no right or left side. However, man grew arrogant and angered Zeus, who, as a result, split man into halves. He tossed the halves to Apollo, who turned the newly made face and genitals of each raw hemisphere forward, creating a right and a left side. Furthermore, Zeus warned, "If mankind continues in its impertinence I shall split them once more and they will then hop along on one leg!" (Yakovlev, 1973).

Although not as imaginative, theorizing over the past 200 years has often focused on types of structural imbalances that could lead to a favoring of one side of the body. For example, there have been a number of theories that postulate asymmetrical size, strength, weight, blood flow, and so forth to account for laterally biased behaviors. We reviewed the asymmetrical strength and dexterity issue in Chapter 2, since these approaches are intricately bound to the problem of the measurement of lateral preferences. Having found that strength or dexterity is not always predictive of lateral preference, we now consider the relevance to lateral preference of other asymmetrical structure theories.

A number of investigators have proposed that limb preferences can be predicted from asymmetries in the relative size, weight, and blood supply to the two sides of the body (see Harris, 1980, for a review of early work). For example, Jones (1915) proposed that measurement of the length and the size of the limbs was a good way to distinguish and classify individuals into pure, or "natural," right- and left-handers. He argued that the longer and wider limb is the naturally preferred one. A number of investigators became interested in this approach, and some forensic scientists have even suggested that patterns of bone development might be used as indexes of hand preference when examining skeletal remains (Schulter-Ellis, 1980).

There have also been a number of more global hypotheses, involving general bodily asymmetries. These have a long history and have engendered vigorous debate. For example, one theory maintained that limb preference is fostered and maintained by differences in the blood flow to the two sides of the body. This theory was offered as early as 1516 by Rhodognus and was carefully considered by many of the early theorists, such as Browne (1646), Bell (1833), and Hyrdl (1860). All of these theorists addressed themselves to the issue of handedness, contending either that there was more vascularization to the right arm, or that the blood flow from the heart was more direct and forceful in the right arm, thus biasing the population toward right-handedness. The most convincing line of counterargument to this position focused on the other index of limb preference: Dwight (1870) pointed out that the abdominal aorta divides into ileacs to the left of the body midline, which would favor blood flow to the left leg, and should result in a population bias toward left-footedness. As we saw in Chapter 3, however, 80% of the population is right-footed as well as right-handed. Other theorists resorted to more general considerations, including the distribution of the mass of the body and its organs. Typical of this approach was Buchanan (1862), who contended that asymmetry in the number of lobes in the lungs, plus the position and weight of the liver, pulls the center of gravity of the human body toward the right side and the back. This shifts the balance to the left side, leaving the right leg and arm free for action and thus more likely to be preferred. Some empirical findings verified that the body was heavier on the right side (Moorhead 1902; Struthers, 1863), yet the linkage of this aspect of bodily asymmetry with limb preference remains tenuous. The most embarrassing data for this position were discussed as early as 1871 by Pyre-Smith, who noted that in individuals with *situs inversus* (i.e., the location of whose body organs is ler-right inverted), right-handedness still predominates.

Although the search for gross differences in bodily dimensions as an underlying explanation for lateral preference continues to the present (see Levy & Levy 1978), most researchers have lost interest in these approaches. Although they engendered much debate and speculation, convincing empirical support for the correlation between such bodily asymmetries and behavioral differences is lacking (see Harris, 1980). Contemporary researchers have shifted their attention to theoretical positions that deal with neural control systems and with early cellular development.

Cerebral Asymmetries

Perhaps the major reason most contemporary researchers have abandoned the search for gross bodily asymmetries is that the search for the physiological substrate of lateral preferences has shifted to the brain. In the decade between 1860 and 1870, it became apparent that there are lateral asymmetries in the brain. Each hemisphere of the brain exerts primary motoric and sensory control over the contralateral half of the body. Thus the left cerebral hemisphere controls the motor movements of the right hand and foot, and may also be the primary locus of right ear inputs. That some higher cognitive functions, such as speech control, also seem to be represented differentially in the two halves of the brain offered a potential link between lateral preference and other aspects of behavior (Subirana 1969). Unlike the former reasoning, this approach did not require the existence of overt and measurable structural differences between the limbs and sense organs as a mechanism to account for behavioral preferences, since differences in the organization and location of neural control would suffice.

When researchers became interested in the connection between cerebral factors and the formation of lateral preferences, this interest was accompanied by some shifts in research strategy. First, most of the attempts to find size, weight, and vascularization differences between the two sides of the body, and to relate these differences to behavioral preferences, shifted from the limbs or body core to the brain. The second shift was of a theoretical nature, and is somewhat more complex. That the left cerebral hemisphere controls the action of the right hand *and* contains the primary speech centers for the majority of individuals seemed to many researchers to be more than mere coincidence. Numerous attempts to link these two facts were made, and the presumption that lateral preference (especially handedness) is associated with language and other forms of cognitive function colors much contemporary research. The earliest notions of a connection between the linguistic functions of one hemisphere and handedness probably arose from reasoning by analogy. It was argued that the presence of speech functions in one hemisphere (the left) somehow made this hemisphere *dominant.* Is it not logical to assume that the limbs controlled by this half of the brain are also dominant or preferred? Thus, the left hemisphere is speech dominant for most individuals and the preferred hand is contralateral to the dominant cerebral hemisphere; hence the right hand is dominant. According to Subirana (1969), this doctrine was unquestioned for many years and its acceptance altered the course of investigation into the problem of lateral preference. If one accepts these basic premises, then left-handedness is associated with a reversed neural organization, so that the speech dominant hemisphere is the right half of the brain. If such were not the case, then one would have to assume that some neural disruption or physiological assault had disrupted the normal connection of the dominant (left) hemisphere to the dominant (right) hand.

The emphasis on the notion of dominance not only engendered specific types of research, but it also suppressed other types. For example, it was assumed further that the preferred hand link to the dominant contralateral hemisphere is such a strong relationship that it influenced the determination of sidedness in the other types of preference. Thus, humans should be naturally one sided (most likely, right sided), with the preferred foot, eye, and ear on the same side as the preferred hand. Handedness became, at least for purposes of empirical investigation, the primary form of lateral preference. Most investigators therefore addressed themselves to handedness, to the virtual exclusion of the other three types of lateral preference, and all other forms of preference became merely other indexes of the same process. This is clearly shown by the fact that it is not unusual to find questions ascertaining the "foot used to kick a ball" averaged into an index that supposedly indicates right- or left-handedness (Giannitrapani, 1979; Weybrew & Noddin, 1979). This is permissible only if one assumes that all forms of lateral preference are manifestations of handedness or are caused by the same process that causes handedness.

Structural differences that might account for lateral preferences were no longer sought at the periphery (at the level of the limb or sense organ itself), but rather in the structure of the two halves of the brain. Hemispheric organization was postulated to be directly responsible for the existence of lateral preferences. The initial research effort followed predictable lines. Since the majority of individuals are right handed, and the right hand is controlled by the (speech dominant) left hemisphere, one should expect structural evidence suggesting physiological dominance in this side of the brain, and the early work seemed to show that such asymmetries existed. Broca (1877), de Fleury (1865), Lombroso (1903), Lueddeckens (1900), and Ogle (1871) presented evidence consistent with the presumption that the blood supply is greater to the left hemisphere; that the left hemisphere is heavier or has greater size or density than the right (Bastian, 1869; Boyd, 1861); that the left hemisphere has more convolutions and a greater complexity of convolutions than the right (Bateman, 1869; Cunningham, 1902); and finally, that there are substantial differences in the fissure lengths, specifically the Sylvian fissure, on the left as opposed to the right side of the brain (Cunningham, 1892; Eberstaller, 1884).

Contemporary theorists have followed similar lines of reasoning and investigation. Perhaps the most influential observation was by Geschwind and Levitsky (1968), who noted that the posterior temporal lobe regions of the left hemisphere (known to be involved in language functions) are larger than the homologous regions of the right hemisphere in the majority of individuals. Other left- versus right-sided differences also were found. These included the observations that the anteroparietal region is larger on the left side, as is the posterooccipital region, while the prefrontal region is larger on the right side. There is evidence that the occipital horn is larger in the left ventricle, which in turn suggests that there is more occipital tissue on the right side. There are larger pyramidal motor tracts on the right side, and there is evidence that the patterns of vascularization differ between the halves of the brain (Galaburda, LeMay, Kemper, & Geschwind, 1978; Geschwind, 1974; Witelson, 1977a, 1980).

While the existence of left-right differences in the brain is interesting, it cannot readily be related to lateral preference behaviors. To say that one section of the brain is larger on the left side in the majority of the population, and that the right hand is also preferred in the majority of the population, does not provide evidence of a link between the two processes. If some aspect of the neural substrate is correlated with the development of lateral preference, then evidence must indicate that variations in lateral preference behaviors directly covary with the manifestation of these anatomical differences.

With this object in mind, a number of investigators have looked at selected aspects of brain anatomy and have compared the data obtained for right- versus left-handed subjects. Presumably, if the differences in the physiological structure of the two sides of the brain are responsible for manifest lateral preference, then lateral brain asymmetries will be observed and those seen in right-handers will be on the side opposite to those found in the left-handers. Table 4-1 contains the results of a series of physiological measures of various parts of the brain obtained separately for both right- and left-handed subjects. The entries in the table represent the percentage of each experimental sample showing differences in the left or the right hemisphere for each of the regions or aspects considered. The left hemisphere does not appear to show the expected anatomical superiority in all indexes, even in the right-handed group. Thus, although the left parietal operculum is larger, as is the left occipital lobe, the right frontal lobe is generally larger and blood pressure and volume are greater in the right hemisphere than in the left in dextral individuals. Thus, the left hemisphere does not manifest physiological superiority in either mass or blood supply. While some measured indexes are greater on the left, others are greater on the right.

If one supposes that handedness is caused by the anatomical asymmetries manifest in Table 4-1, a number of other questions arise. For example, the observed asymmetries should predict the preferred hand. Yet, as Table 4-1 shows, on average, 15% of the samples show no discernible difference between the hemispheres, and, on average, 23% of these samples show asymmetries directionally opposite to the majority difference. Additionally, a convincing theoretical outcome would have been one where left-handers show cerebral anatomical asymmetries that are the mirror image of those observed in right-handers. The data tabulated in Table 4-1 are not consistent with these expectations. In many instances, the observed cerebral asymmetries are in the same direction for both sinistral and dextral subjects. When these groups differ, there are many reversals and failures to find any asymmetry. The largest difference between the left- and the right-handed groups resides in the size of the observed anatomical asymmetries. The right-handers show marked differences between the two hemispheres. Thus if we simply take the mean of the absolute difference between the percentage of the sample showing a left versus a right bias in the data of Table 4-1, we find that this difference is 53% for the right-handers and only 18% for the left-handed group. Right-handers are three times more likely to manifest a cerebral structural asymmetry than are left-handers, a difference that is statistically significant. The table also reveals that an average of 10% of the tested right-handers fail to show brain asymmetries, while 20% of the left-handers show no significant cerebral asymmetries. Again, this difference is statistically significant.

These data indicate that lateral preference, at least for hand, is not predictable directly from, nor strongly correlated with, anatomically definable asym-

Table 4-1: Comparison of Anatomical Differences between Right and Left Sides of Brain

Aspect measured	Right-handers[a]			Left-handers[a]			Technique
	Left+	Right+	Equal	Left+	Right+	Equal	
Parietal operculum size[1]	67	8	25	22	7	71	Arteriogram
Parietal operculum size[2]	86	5	9	17	11	72	Arteriogram[b]
Frontal lobe size[3]	19	61	20	40	27	33	Tomography
Frontal lobe size[3]	14	66	20	36	37	27	Bone protrusion
Frontal lobe size[3]	25	39	36	42	26	32	X-ray
Occipital lobe size[3]	66	9	25	38	27	35	Tomography
Occipital lobe size[3]	77	13	10	36	47	17	Bone protrusion
Occipital lobe size[3]	68	10	22	35	33	32	X-ray
Occipital posterior horns[4]	60	10	30	38	31	31	Pneumoencephalogram[c]
Pyramidal fibers (number)[5]	16	73	10	14	86	–	Count of fibers after decussation
Venous drainage[6,7]	59	–	41	38	–	62	Vein of Labbe greater than vein of Trolard
Arterial blood pressure[8]	11	76	13	41	18	41	Systolic ophthalmic pressure[c]
Hemispheric blood volume[9]	25	62	13	64	28	8	Radioactive trace[c]

Note. Superscript numbers refer to sources: 1, Hochberg & Le May, 1975; 2, Le May & Culebras, 1972; 3, Le May, 1977; 4, McRae, Branch, & Milner, 1968; 5, Kertesz & Geschwind, 1971; 6, Di Chiaro, 1962; 7, calculations from Witelson, 1980; 8, Carmon & Gombos, 1970; 9, Carmon, Harishanu, Lowinger, & Lavy, 1972.

[a] Plus sign means greater; entries represent percentage of sample.

[b] Presumably right-handed group is an unselected population.

[c] Left-handed group includes ambidexters.

metries in the brain. There are, however, some detectable differences between the groups. Right-handers have more asymmetrical brain structures as a population. Left-handers are less likely to show the patterns of asymmetries found in dextrals, and they are more likely to show no differences between the left and right side of the brain. However, left-handers are not the mirror images of right-handers when one considers asymmetries in cerebral structure. If brain asymmetries and lateral preference behaviors are correlated, we cannot conclude from this survey that individuals are right handed *because of* physiological superiority of the left cerebral hemisphere. Perhaps right-handedness is more likely to be a consequence of (or a correlate with) an organized, asymmetrical brain structure, whereas left-handedness is more likely the result of a less differentiated, symmetrical brain structure.

Lateral Preference and Language Specialization

At the beginning of this chapter, we pointed out that the finding that the left hemisphere controls the motor function of the right hand, in addition to being the primary mediator of language function in the majority of individuals, resulted in speculations that language development and lateral preferences are associated processes. The nature of this association has never been very clear. Some speculations as to neurological, developmental, or even evolutionary factors have been offered to substantiate this linkage (see Herron, 1980). To justify such conclusions, the data must show direct covariation between the cerebral locus of language control and the specific pattern of lateral preference manifested by the subject.

The original belief was that the localization of language processes occurs in the hemisphere contralateral to the preferred hand; thus, it would be in the left hemisphere for right-handers and in the right for left-handers. As the data began to accumulate, however, it became clear that only the former assumption is true. A number of investigators looked at patients with various forms of brain damage and assessed the nature and distribution of language loss (Milner, Branch, & Rasmussen, 1964; Roberts, 1969; Zangwill, 1967). They concluded that virtually all right-handers are left lateralized for language. This result has been verified by using injections of sodium amytal, which can selectively inactivate one hemisphere while leaving the other one unaffected (Wada & Rasmussen, 1960). Such testing has indicated that left-handers are not as easily classified, and seem to be a much more mixed group. The results of both clinical and experimental techniques indicate that 50-67% of left-handers manifest right hemisphere language processing. However, an appreciable number apparently have bilateral language function (Ettlinger, Jackson, & Zangwill, 1956; Goodglass & Quadfasal, 1954; Hecaen & Piercy, 1956; Hecaen & Sauget, 1971; Humphrey & Zangwill, 1952; Milner et al., 1964; Zangwill, 1960). Additionally, there is evidence that the bilaterally represented groups can be subdivided on the basis of whether both hemispheres have the same or a different language function (Rasmussen & Milner, 1976).

Satz (1980) used a mathematical treatment to fit several models to the available clinical data on aphasia (a class of language disorders associated with damage to the cerebral speech and language centers) to see if left- and right-handers manifest different cerebral organizations for language. He concludes that "A unilateral model represents the best estimate of brain lateralization in right-handers and a more complex model of bilateral and variable unilateral speech represents the best estimate of brain lateralization in left-handers" (Satz, 1980, p. 196). It is interesting to compare this conclusion to our own, derived from looking at anatomical organization of the brains of right- and left-handers as summarized in Table 4-1. On the basis of these types of data, Kimura (1976) has stated that the early view that speech functions and handedness were always controlled from the same hemisphere is not correct, although she still maintains that, most probably, the two are related in some way. Although the level of certainty that pervaded earlier investigations is no longer apparent, new research and theories based on the assumption that language function and handedness emanate from the same neural control system continue to appear. In order to remain consistent with the disconfirming data, however, the recent models are more complex and often involve additional variables.

Levy (1973) and Levy and Reid (1976, 1978) proposed a theory that contends that alternative cerebral speech organizations can be directly predicted from individual *patterns* of handedness behaviors. Although this hypothesis assumes an intrinsic connection between the hemisphere specialized for speech functions and manifest handedness, it deviates from the previous doctrine, which maintained that the relationship between the controlling hemisphere and the preferred hand must always be contralateral in nature. This viewpoint proposes that the nature of the preferred hand and speech hemisphere connection can be determined by the posture an individual assumes while writing. The handwriting postures studied by Levy and Reid (1978) are shown in Figure 4-1. Basically, an individual can be either an inverted or a straight, noninverted writer. A noninverted or typical writer holds the writing implement so that its top is oriented toward the bottom of the paper, and the hand is held below the writing line. A writer using the inverted posture rotates the hand so that the top of the pen or pencil points toward the top of the piece of paper and the hand is held at the level of or above the line of writing. Within each of these types of postures, an individual can display either right- or left-handedness as shown in Figure 4-1.

Levy and Reid (1978) offer the usual hypothesis that the hand is controlled by the hemisphere that is dominant for speech and language functions. However, that hemisphere is not necessarily contralateral to the hand. They argue that contralateral hand control is found only in subjects with the more common straight handwriting postures. They contend that there is ipsilateral cerebral control for inverted writers. Therefore, in a straight right-hander, the hypothesized neural control path would be between the right hand and the left hemisphere. Since it is assumed that the preferred hand is controlled by the hemisphere specialized for speech functions, this means, by definition, that speech functions are localized in the contralateral left hemisphere. The population of left-handed inverted writers would also have a speech dominant left hemisphere

LEFT-HANDED RIGHT-HANDED

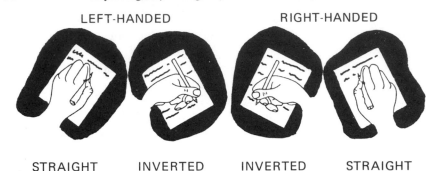

STRAIGHT INVERTED INVERTED STRAIGHT

Figure 4-1. The inverted and straight (or noninverted) handwriting postures for left- and right-handed writers.

(in the same fashion as right-handed noninverters), since in their case the control is assumed to be ipsilateral. Straight left-handed and right-handed inverted writers have right hemisphere speech function. The interesting aspect of this approach is that it not only assumes that the cerebral speech organization and displayed hand preference are intrinsically connected, but it also uses an overt lateral preference behavior to predict individual differences in cerebral speech organization. According to this line of reasoning, then, the population incidence of the various handedness and speech hemisphere relationships can be determined from the observation of handwriting posture.

Table 4-2 presents data from a study conducted by Coren and Porac (1979b) who queried approximately 2,000 individuals concerning their handwriting posture. Individuals were asked to match their writing posture to pictures of the left- and right-handed inverted and straight positions. The pictures were similar to those shown in Figure 4-1. As can be seen from the table, 81% of the respondents use the straight right-handed writing position, while 5% of the sample have inverted left-handed writing positions. It follows from the Levy and Reid (1978) theory, then, that approximately 85% of this sample should have primary speech functions that are localized in the left hemisphere.

If the Levy and Reid theory is correct, it could have important implications in that it directly links aspects of handedness with the lateralization of speech processes. However, some difficulties have emerged that raise doubts about its adequacy. Levy and Reid (1978) have used data from studies on dichotic listening (where a subject listens to discrepant inputs in the two ears) and from visual half-field presentations (where the visual stimuli are presented to the right or to the left of the retinal midline) to support their position. These techniques are thought to present information directly to only one hemisphere. Of course, the information is transmitted through the corpus callosum and the cerebral commissures to the contralateral hemisphere in normal observers, but it is argued that the relative speed and accuracy of performance can serve as an indicator of the hemisphere that is best organized for particular types of information processing. For example, visual and auditory linguistic stimuli should be more quickly

Table 4-2: Distribution of Handwriting Positions (based on Coren & Porac, 1979b)

Handwriting position	All cases (%)	Females (%)	Males (%)
Noninverted right	80.9	82.8	76.6
Inverted right	8.2	6.7	10.1
Noninverted left	6.0	6.3	5.6
Inverted left	4.9	4.2	5.7
Total right	89.1	89.5	88.7
Total left	10.1	10.5	11.3
Total noninverted	85.8	89.1	84.2
Total inverted	14.2	10.9	15.8
Number of cases	1758	956	802

and efficiently processed in the hemisphere specialized for verbal and linguistic functions. Unfortunately, these are very indirect measures, and if a specific function can be processed in an interactive manner by both hemispheres, which is suggested by analyses and data from Rasmussen and Milner (1976) and Satz (1980), the validity of the technique can be questioned. Even if these techniques are reliable indicators of the locus of speech lateralization, one must still be cognizant of a number of unsuccessful attempts to replicate the results of Levy and Reid (1978) that have failed to find visual half-field or dichotic listening asymmetries that support the direction of functional specialization predicted by the theory, at least for left-handers (Herron, 1980; Marlowe, 1977; McKeever, 1979; McKeever & Hoff, 1979; McKeever & Van Deventer, 1980).

There are aspects of the data on handwriting position itself that lead one to doubt its validity as an accurate predictor of speech lateralization. For instance, in line with the tenets of the Levy and Reid (1978) theory and the data in Table 4-2, one should expect that approximately 10% of right-handers have right-hemisphere speech function (which is a considerably greater percentage than that usually obtained), while fewer than 50% of the left-handers have left-hemisphere speech (which is much less than that reported in the literature). In addition, there are a number of individual difference variables that interact with handwriting position. For example, males are more apt to display inverted writing postures, as shown in Table 4-2 and in other reports (Allen & Wellman, 1980; Coren & Porac, 1979b; McKeever, 1979; McKeever & Van Deventer, 1980). Coren and Porac (1979b) and Allen and Wellman (1980) also have reported systematic age differences, with fewer inverted writers in the older age groups. Based on the Levy and Reid (1978) hypothesis, this finding would suggest that cerebral speech organization changes over the life span. Shanon (1978) has shown cross-cultural differences in handwriting posture, and Peters and Pedersen (1978) have found that hand posture is often taught directly. Both

Peters and Pedersen (1978) and Shanon (1978) have argued for the influence of training and experiential influences in the determination of handwriting posture and against a strictly physiological mechanism of control. Thus, although the Levy and Reid (1976, 1978) approach is an attempt to incorporate individual differences in manifest hand preference into a theory based on the localization of speech function, it has been unable to account for some systematic variations in the behavioral phenomenon. Thus, the connection between cerebral asymmetries, particularly for speech and language functions, and manifestations of lateral preference remains obscure.

Biological Asymmetries

In order to explain the functional asymmetries that we call lateral preferences, a number of investigators have attempted to find theoretical mechanisms that could account for the broad spectrum of physiological asymmetries observed in living organisms. Perhaps the most influential and best-conceived of these theories has been presented by Corballis and Beale (1976) and Morgan (1977). Their theoretical position is based on an analysis of developmental processes that might result in structural asymmetries in humans. The underlying notion is that structural asymmetry will result in functional asymmetry.

Evidence suggests that the universe is asymmetrical. Even at the molecular level, one finds that some molecules agree with others in chemical constituents and general shape, with the sole difference residing in the directional torque with which the components are arranged. In other words, one molecule may be a mirror image of another. Such molecules, differing only in the direction of their asymmetries, may not be treated equivalently by organic systems. Thus, Fritsch (1968) mentions a number of instances in which one such molecule may be completely innocuous, whereas the other may produce a fatal reaction in various species. Asymmetry is a characteristic of living organisms. For example, Pasteur (1874) speculated, "I am convinced that life, as it manifests itself to us, is a function of the dissymmetry of the universe or of the consequences of this dyssymmetry." Although this may be a philosophical overgeneralization, it is the case that asymmetries are visible in the human embryo only 14 days after conception (Moore, 1973). Boklage (1980) has even presented some evidence suggesting visible asymmetries in humans as early as the first cellular cleavage during development. This indicates that asymmetry is a preprogrammed property of our species and its development.

Asymmetries may be found in a variety of organisms. At least for vertebrates, these asymmetries are varied and suggest an underlying gradient that favors the left side. For example, almost all vertebrate species show a displacement of the heart toward the left. The single tusk of the narwhal (often said to be the prototype for the mythical unicorn) is actually an enlargement of a tooth on the left side (Gardner, 1964). Nottebohm (1971, 1972) presented evidence that the neural control of bird song in chaffinches is predominantly mediated through the left hypoglossal nerve. In the previous section we noted a number of asymmetries in the human brain that favor the left side, such as the size of the parietal operculum. Similar asymmetries are also often found in simian species. Thus, Groves and Humphrey (1973) reported that the left side of the skull is typically enlarged in the African mountain gorilla. Yeni-Komshian and Benson (1976) reported that the Sylvian fissure in the temporal lobe of the chimpanzee is longer on the left than on the right, and Le May and Geschwind (1975) have found similar asymmetries in the orangutan. Numerous other examples can be found in Corballis and Morgan (1978), Morgan (1977), and Morgan and Corballis (1978). Of course, as demonstrated by Table 4-1, this left side advantage is not universal. There are numerous assymetries that seem to favor the right side, at least for brain structure.

Corballis and Morgan (1978) and Morgan and Corballis (1978) have offered an interesting hypothesis to explain the appearance of such physiological asymmetrics, which they attempt to use to explain the functional asymmetries observed in humans. They point out that the coding of lateral asymmetries in the structure of organisms poses a particularly difficult example of the general problem of morphological differentiation. Contemporary theorists maintain that the various cells of the body, whether they develop into heart, liver, or any other organic tissue, contain exactly the same genetic material. There is no evidence that suggests that the cells on the left side of the body differ genetically from those on the right side. Thus, if these cells are to develop differentially (or to express some sort of lateral asymmetry), it must be that they find themselves in different environments. There seems to be a gradient in the cytoplasm of the unfertilized egg that could provide such a difference (Lepori, 1969; Morgan, 1977; Spemann & Falkenberg, 1919). The nature of this gradient is such that cells on the left and the right side develop at different rates, and Corballis and Morgan (1978) argue that this cytoplasmic difference results in a developmental gradient that favors the left side.

This asymmetrical developmental gradient is thought to be particularly important in the development of cerebral and neural control systems. They contend not only that the left side (particularly the left side of the brain) develops faster, but also that with its head start it actually exerts an inhibitory influence on right-hemisphere cerebral development. If this were the case, there would be positive feedback in the system, such that the asymmetry would become increasingly pronounced with age, and there are reports of such increasing physiological asymmetry as a function of age. For example, Wada, Clarke, and Hamm (1975) studied the asymmetry of the temporal planum in 100 infant brains and 100 adult brains. They found that an asymmetry in size, favoring the left, was present in the brain even in the youngest infants studied (19th week of gestation). However, they report that the asymmetries found in the brains of the adults were more extreme than those found in the brains of the infants. An interesting aspect of this theory is the contention that the dominant side actually inhibits the development of the nondominant side. The notion that the asymmetries may be associated with active inhibition of one side by the other has been supported in a number of organic systems. Thus Romer (1962), in a study of the development of the ovaries of avian species, found that removal of the larger left organ in the adults seems to release the vestigial right organ from inhibition, with the result that it rapidly increases in its rate of growth. Similar examples can be seen in the asymmetrical development of claw size in the crab (Wilson, 1903).

In terms of the development of lateral preference, this asymmetrical maturational gradient is important if one argues that lateral preferences arise from inequalities of neural control, whereby the stronger, better developed left side seizes control. This is particularly important when dealing with the left hemisphere, since it controls the motor behavior of the right hand and foot. Left-sided neural dominance causes the right hand and foot to become the dominant or preferred limbs, an argument that is really an extension of the same sort of reasoning discussed in the previous section. The hypothesis is that right-handedness results from dominance of the left side of the brain. Here, however, a specific mechanism for this left hemisphere dominance has been offered.

Unfortunately there are a number of difficulties with the Corballis and Morgan (1978) position, even if one could allow unquestioned their presumption that hemispheric dominance is a direct cause of lateral preference. One problem arises from the fact that there are a number of instances in which the right side not only seems to be favored but also appears to develop more quickly than the left. For instance, the right testicle in man is heavier and develops earlier (Chan, Hsu, Chan, & Chan, 1960; Morgan & Corballis, 1976). Mittwoch (1976) reports that even in human fetuses as young as 18 weeks of age, the right gonad is consistently heavier and contains more DNA. This lateral asymmetry in the distribution of DNA is present in both males and females and it implies that more cell divisions must have occurred on the right side. This would seem to indicate a growth gradient favoring the right rather than the left.

Another difficulty with this approach is that handedness and cerebral structural lateralization in man should be perfectly correlated if both are based on the same maturational gradient. As we saw in the previous sections, they are not. Thus, although differential maturational gradients may interact in the formation of physiological asymmetries, they may be independent of functional asymmetries. Differential development may produce statistically predictable differences in structure that may be relatively independent of the functional differences expressed in the form of lateral preferences.

One-Sidedness

An interesting by-product of the unicausal physiological approaches to lateral preference formation, whether they are based on presumed cerebral dominance or on developmental asymmetries, is the notion that individuals should display congruent sidedness. That is to say that all aspects of lateral preference should align themselves on the same side of the body (Delacato, 1963; Orton, 1937; Parsons, 1924). This line of reasoning implies that there is a primary sidedness factor and that the mechanisms that cause and support it subsequently influence the direction of handedness and the formation of all of the other expressions of lateral preference.

There are several reasons why human lateral preference is not described adequately as a unitary dimension with a single origin. Although the physiological considerations that we have discussed in earlier sections suggest that the hands and the feet share a similar locus of motor control, such a clearly lateralized control system does not exist for the eyes and the ears. Visual information from the two eyes is available to both hemispheres, since there is only partial decussation of the optic fibers at the chiasma. Similarly, auditory information from both ears is also bilaterally available at all stages of the auditory pathways beyond the superior olive (see Coren, Porac, & Ward, 1979). Thus, based on anatomical considerations, the inductive leap from hemispheric control processes to lateral preference expressed in the limbs cannot be extended directly to lateral preference in the sense organs. A strong physiological foundation for the assumption of a generalized dimension of lateral preference seems to be absent.

Still, even without a physiological justification for such an assertion, the belief that, at least behaviorally, there is cross-index congruency of lateral preferences persists. Empirically, there are some justifications for this. Several studies have reported significant, although low, correlations among the four indexes of lateral preference behaviors. For example, Table 4-3 shows the mean intercorrelations among the four indexes of lateral preference from several studies that we have conducted. As can be seen, all of the correlation coefficients are positive, which might indicate some underlying common factor. However, when one looks at the magnitude of the correlations, only that between hand and foot accounts for more than 10% of the predictive variance. Thus, if there is some general factor accounting for all manifestations of lateral preference, it must be rather weak.

Table 4-3: Mean Intercorrelations between Indexes of Lateral Preference[a]

	Hand	Foot	Eye	Ear
Hand	—	.55 $(.06)^{b}$	.21 (.12)	.24 (.02)
Foot		—	.29 (.05)	.32 (.04)
Eye			—	.23 (.03)
Ear				—

[a]Each table entry is based on a minimum of four and a maximum of seven published reports. Studied used in the compilation of this table: Coren & Kaplan (1973); Porac & Coren (1975a); Porac, Whitford, & Coren (1976); Porac & Coren (1978b); Porac & Coran (1979a); Porac, Coren, & Duncan (1980); Coren & Porac (1980a).
[b]Standard deviations.

Actually, looking only at the simple correlation matrix does not reveal whether or not the various types of lateral preferences represent a unidimensional, and hence perhaps a unicausal, system. To determine this, one must employ multiple measures representing each form of lateral preference behavior and use multivariate analytic techniques to explore the data. Such procedures attempt to explain the sources of covariation in an observed system of variables in terms of a smaller number of hypothetical dimensions or factors. Previously, such techniques have been used to explore the dimensional structure within a set of tests for a single form of lateral preference. For example, in Chapter 2 we reviewed studies showing that handedness, as measured through preference inventories, could be viewed as representing a unidimensional process (Barnsley & Rabinovitch, 1970; Bryden, 1977), whereas eyedness tests represented three separate dimensions (Coren & Kaplan, 1973). If all manifestations of lateral preferences are part of a generalized dimension, one ought to find, when conducting a multidimensional analysis of preference behaviors, a single global factor representing this dimension.

In order to test this hypothesis, Porac, Coren, Steiger, and Duncan (1980) administered the self-report inventory presented in Table 3-1 to 962 individuals, ranging in age from 10 to 75 years. The intercorrelations among the 13 items that they obtained are shown in Table 4-4. Again, all of the correlations are positive, suggesting some shared component; however, some interrelations are much larger than others, and the magnitudes of the correlations follow a definite pattern. Specifically, the handedness and footedness items (questions 1-7) are more closely related to each other than they are to any of the measures of sensory preference. Eyedness and earedness do not appear to be strongly related to limb preference or to each other. Given this pattern, Porac et al. (1980) reasoned that a better understanding of the interrelationships among these lateral preference variables could be obtained by applying factor analytic techniques to this correlation matrix. In such statistical procedures, one reduces the relationships represented in a correlation matrix to a smaller set of uncorrelated, nonoverlapping components. These components are then interpreted as the separable dimensions of lateral preference. When we conducted a principal component analysis of the data, the results revealed three distinct factors, as shown in Table 4-5.

Each of the entires in Table 4-5 represents the correlation between the row variable (actually a lateral preference self-report item) and the derived dimension. This value is called the factor loading. A simple criterion for ascertaining whether an entry is significant enough to warrant concern requires consideration of only those entries that account for 10% or more of the variance (the entry must be .33 or greater). These have been marked with an asterisk in Table 4-5. The significant factor loadings form simple interpretable patterns. On the first factor one finds high loadings for only the handedness and the footedness questions. The second factor shows significant loadings for only eyedness questions, while the third produces significant loadings only for earedness items. To the extent that each of these extracted factors represents a dimension of lateral preference, one can interpret these results as showing *three* dimensions of lateral preference,

Table 4-4: Correlations between Lateral Preference Questionnaire Items Based on a Sample of 962 Individuals

	1	2	3	4	5	6	7	8	9	10	11	12	13
1. Ball (hand)	—	.80	.74	.43	.63	.44	.34	.25	.27	.31	.19	.20	.25
2. Draw (hand)		—	.84	.39	.53	.41	.32	.25	.27	.31	.16	.17	.23
3. Eraser (hand)			—	.41	.58	.41	.31	.23	.26	.28	.16	.18	.25
4. Card (hand)				—	.40	.27	.24	.17	.19	.19	.17	.14	.17
5. Kick (foot)					—	.44	.37	.26	.28	.29	.23	.21	.26
6. Pebble (foot)						—	.30	.21	.24	.18	.20	.24	.27
7. Chair (foot)							—	.23	.20	.21	.24	.25	.25
8. Keyhole (eye)								—	.83	.60	.24	.20	.17
9. Bottle (eye)									—	.61	.22	.21	.21
10. Rifle (eye)										—	.19	.23	.14
11. Door (ear)											—	.72	.51
12. Heart (ear)												—	.45
13. Earphone (ear)													—

Note. See Chapter 3; based on Porac, Coren, Steiger, & Duncan (1980). All correlations are significant with $p < .001$.

Table 4-5: Results of Principal Component Analysis of Lateral Preference Questionnaire Items

	Factors		
	I	II	III
1. Ball (hand)	.87*	.13	.09
2. Draw (hand)	.87*	.14	.03
3. Eraser (hand)	.87*	.11	.05
4. Card (hand)	.57*	.08	.10
5. Kick (foot)	.73*	.18	.16
6. Pebble (foot)	.56*	.11	.22
7. Chair (foot)	.42*	.14	.31
8. Keyhole (eye)	.13	.90*	.12
9. Bottle (eye)	.16	.90*	.12
10. Rifle (eye)	.22	.78*	.09
11. Door (ear)	.09	.12	.88*
12. Heart (ear)	.10	.12	.86*
13. Earphone (ear)	.22	.06	.71*
Variance of component	3.80	2.38	2.24

Note. Based on Porac, Coren, Steiger, & Duncan (1980).
*Variable that predicts at least 10% of component's variance.

rather than the *one* that has been hypothesized previously. One dimension represents limb preference, which includes both handedness and footedness, while the remaining two dimensions are formed by eye and ear preference, respectively.

Sex and age are two individual difference variables that have been shown to interact with manifestations of lateral preference (Bryden, 1977; Clark, 1957; Fleminger, Dalton, & Standage, 1977; Hecaen & de Ajuriaguerra, 1964; Hildreth, 1949, 1950; Peters & Pedersen, 1978; Porac & Coren, 1975a; Porac, Coren, & Duncan, 1980a). These interactions were demonstrated in the data of Chapter 3. Therefore, we conducted similar principal component analyses for males and females independently. The separate solutions for the male and the female portions of the sample are shown in Table 4-6. The three-component solution for both genders is highly similar to that obtained for the entire sample. Statistical comparisons that look at the degree of similarity between the male and the female component solutions confirm that they show similar structures. When we subdivided the sample into three age categories, youth (ages 10-20 years), young and middle adulthood (age 21-55 years), and senior adulthood (ages 56 and above), we once again found a three-dimensional structure, similar to that shown in Table 4-5, for each age group. Statistical comparisons between the groups showed that the component solutions were highly similar regardless of the age of the subsample. Although gender and age might affect the degree to which one displays right or left preference, they do not seem to affect the underlying relationships among the preference behaviors.

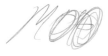

Table 4-6: Results of Principal Component Analysis of Lateral Preference Questionnaire Items for Males (*N*=453) and Females (*N*=509) Separately

	Males			Females		
	I	II	III	I	II	III
1. Ball (hand)	.83*	.18	.09	.87*	.08	.14
2. Draw (hand)	.90*	.13	.05	.91*	.11	.07
3. Eraser (hand)	.84*	.12	.05	.91*	.10	.09
4. Card (hand)	.44*	.13	.14	.45*	.09	.11
5. Kick (foot)	.58*	.22	.16	.69*	.14	.15
6. Pebble (foot)	.43*	.14	.22	.49*	.15	.16
7. Chair (foot)	.28	.16	.25	.41*	.15	.21
8. Keyhole (eye)	.18	.86*	.15	.11	.88*	.12
9. Bottle (eye)	.18	.91*	.18	.16	.89*	.07
10. Rifle (eye)	.30	.53*	.11	.20	.69*	.15
11. Door (ear)	.05	.14	.86*	.14	.09	.89*
12. Heart (ear)	.12	.11	.81*	.13	.10	.77*
13. Earphone (ear)	.18	.09	.54*	.25	.12	.53*

*Variable that predicts at least 10% of a component's variance.

If we had stopped our analyses at the stage of simple correlations, we might have concluded that there is a primary or general congruency between types of lateral preference, as is often assumed by theories based on a single mechanism, since all of the correlations between the questionnaire items are positive and statistically significant. However, the multivariate analyses indicate that more than one dimension is needed to adequately describe the relationships among the various types of lateral preference.

In this chapter we looked at various physiological asymmetries that theorists have attempted to associate with lateral preference behaviors. It is useful to stop and consider the conclusions that can be drawn from the data we have reviewed. First, simple physiological asymmetry does not seem to be predictive of lateral preference behaviors. Second, when one considers cerebral structure, some aspects of the brain show left-sided superiority while others show a bias toward the right in typical right-handed groups. The only predictable difference toward right- and left-handers on observable cerebral variables seems to be that populations of left-handers will tend to show less asymmetry, regardless of type, than dextrals. Third, the link between lateral preference and hemispheric specialization for speech also seems tenuous. Most right-handers and many left-handers show speech processing in the left hemisphere. Thus, the contralateral relationship between location of the speech centers and the side of the preferred hand is not always present. Since the developmental gradient hypothesis is designed to provide an explanation for a left hemisphere dominance, with the formation of lateral preference as a secondary consequence of this dominance, it also suffers from the same difficulties as the hemispheric specialization hypothesis.

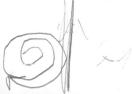

Each of the foregoing hypotheses presents a unicausal physiological mechanism to explain the existence of lateral preferences. None of them works particularly well. Perhaps they fail not so much because the hypothesized mechanisms have nothing to do with the formation of lateral preferences but because of their unicausal nature. In this chapter we have presented data that suggest that all forms of lateral preference do not seem to be based on a single process or mechanism. Lateral preferences are multidimensional, and although limb preferences may share a mechanism, eyedness and earedness seem to be separable. A single factor explanation for all manifestations of preference seems to be an oversimplification. Perhaps a single mechanism cannot explain even one form of lateral preference. Many different variables seem to play a role in the formation of these behaviors. As will be shown in the following chapters, we may be forced to abandon parsimonious explanations for more complex but accurate ones.

5

Genetic Approaches

In the search for a mechanism for laterally biased behaviors, theorists have been fascinated by the right-sided bias in human populations. This bias appears for hand, foot, eye, and ear use, as shown in Chapter 3, and appears to be a statistical constant for our species. Evidence available in the historical record suggests that humans have displayed a relatively constant proportion of right-handedness since the Paleolithic era, as noted in Chapter 1. Also, the proportion of right-handedness is relatively constant, regardless of geographical considerations (see Chapter 6). Such consistency, despite cultural and historical factors, leads to the suspicion that dextral lateral preference behaviors are part of our biological heritage and are therefore of genetic origin.

The knowledge that a trait is determined genetically is not always theoretically enlightening. For example, it is obvious that humans possess two hands, two eyes, and only one head because of genetic programming. To state this fact, however, sheds little light upon the functional properties of hands, eyes, or heads. The genetic determination of these traits is of little interest because *all* humans normally have two hands, two eyes, and one head. Genetic theories add to our knowledge only if we are dealing with traits that vary in their individual expression. When individual differences exist, knowledge of genetic mechanisms may allow one to predict how, and why, certain individuals express a given characteristic while others do not. When this argument is directed toward lateral preferences, we ask whether there are genetic reasons for one person's preferring the right hand or foot while another prefers the left. Simply stated, we want to know if there is a genetic component in the observed deviation from the norm that expresses itself as left-sidedness.

Genetic approaches to lateral preference have often been incorporated into the physiological and cerebral asymmetry theories discussed in Chapter 4. Since handedness has received the most attention, we can use it to acquaint ourselves with the general arguments in support of this approach and with the data that have resulted from it.

Genetic Explanations for Hand Preference

The informal observation that handedness apparently runs in families prompted early interest in developing possible genetic models of human handedness, and one can identify two traditions in the research literature. The first stems from geneticists, who have applied population genetic techniques in an attempt to estimate the frequencies within the population of what they presumed to be the right- and left-handedness gene. This *single-gene* approach presumes that a simple genetic model will account for hand preference. Most of these studies have treated handedness as a discrete, dichotomous variable and have focused on dominant-recessive models of genetic transmission. The second tradition is derived from the work of physiological and behavioral psychologists, who have treated handedness as a continuous variable. Generally speaking, these are not pure genetic theories because they assume that the actions of several genetic *and* nongenetic factors are at work. However, the genetic involvement is *polygenetic*; in other words, more than one gene is involved in determining handedness.

Single-Gene Approaches

Geneticists have often considered handedness to be a relatively simple trait. They have presumed that right-handedness is a different entity than left-handedness and that the two phenotypic manifestations are mutually exclusive and non-overlapping. In addition, the relatively low incidence of left-handedness (approximately 10-15% of the population) has led them to postulate that handedness is inherited and transmitted by genes in a dominant-recessive relationship where left-handedness is the recessive trait.

According to the basic principles of Mendelian genetics (Cavalli-Sforza & Bodmer, 1971), individuals possess two hereditary factors (genes), one originating from each of their parents, for each heritable trait. These two genes compose the *genotype* that in turn determines a particular observable trait or *phenotype.* Each gene may exist in two or more alternate forms, called *alleles.* In our case, geneticists would talk in terms of handedness being determined by a single genetic locus of control (actually one site on a chromosome) with two alleles. One (which we will designate as *L*) gives rise to left-handedness and the other (*R*) to right-handedness. Given one gene from the father and one from the mother, three types of individuals (*RR, LL,* and *RL*) can emerge; *RR* and *LL* genotypes emerge from pairings of identical alleles. The *RR* and *LL* genotypes are called *homozygous* because the union of gametes (sex cells) is identical for one pair of genes. A genotypic *RR* individual is presumably phenotypically right handed, whereas the genotype *LL* is phenotypically left handed. The third type of genotype is an *LR* individual, who is heterozygous because the genes are not identical and the two alleles at this genetic locus differ. Whether the individual is manifestly right or left handed depends on the type of genetic process that exists. In the case of a dominant-recessive mode of genetic transmission, where the gene for right-handedness (*R*) completely dominates the phenotypic expression of the trait, an *LR* individual displays right-handedness. Thus, *LR* and *RR* individuals, although genetically dissimilar, are phenotypically indistinguishable. The transmission process whereby certain offspring genotypes are formed from the combination of various parental genotypes, and the resulting distributions of phenotypes, are shown in Table 5-1.

Theoretically, it is possible to estimate the prevalence of a specific gene in a population by using the *Hardy-Weinberg theorem*. This theorem is named after its two originators, the English mathematician G. H. Hardy and the German physician W. Weinberg. It assumes that the frequencies of the phenotypes (the observed trait) are the same as those of the genotypes (the genetic combination). It further assumes that a population undergoing random mating (of the types shown in Table 5-1) reaches, in one generation, a distribution of genotype frequencies expressed mathematically as $(r+l)^2$. For the purposes of our discussion, *r* and *l* are the frequencies of the *R* and *L* genes. The expansion of this formula into the three terms r^2, $2rl$, and l^2 gives the relative frequencies of the three genotypes *RR, RL,* and *LL*, respectively, and allows us to estimate the genotype frequencies within the population as a result of the different parental mating combinations. By attempting these estimates, one can try to derive the proportion of a set of offspring who are expected to display each of the three genotypes. Given the simplifying assumption that genotype will be directly expressed in the phenotype, this procedure provides an estimate of the proportion of phenotypic right- and left-handers emerging from different parental mating combinations. The appendix to this chapter demonstrates the method for calculating

Table 5-1: Typical Mating Patterns and Resulting Genotypes and Phenotypes in a Single-Gene Transmission of Handedness

Mating type	Father's genotype	Mother's genotype	Possible offspring genotype	Resultant handedness phenotypes
Homozygous	RR	RR	RR RR RR RR	100% Right
Homozygous	LL	LL	LL LL LL LL	100% Left
Heterozygous	RL	RL	RR RL LR LL	75% Right, 25% Left
Homozygous-heterozygous	RR	RL	RR RL RR RL	100% Right
Homozygous-heterozygous	RL	RR	RL RR RL RR	100% Right
Homozygous-heterozygous	LL	RL	RL LL RL LL	50% Right, 50% Left
Homozygous-heterozygous	RL	LL	RL RL LL LL	50% Right, 50% Left
Homozygous cross	RR	LL	RL RL RL RL	100% Right
Homozygous cross	LL	RR	RL RL RL RL	100% Right

Note. *R* is a completely dominant trait and *L* a completely recessive trait.

the expected frequencies of different parental mating combinations and shows the expected proportion of offspring of these pairs who will display each of the three handedness genotypes. If one assumes that the total proportion of right-handedness is .87 (as given in the normative data in Table 3-3), one can derive the proportion of each genotype that is expected in the offspring generation with the Hardy-Weinberg procedure. This example is actually worked out in the appendix for those who want a more complete explanation.

Such computations are characteristic of the procedure used by theorists in the single-gene tradition. First, they postulate a specific type of genetic determination, and then they look for congruence between the values derived from the prescribed genetic model and the observed values found within a population (see Trankell, 1955). This type of model fitting can be more or less successful, depending on the various assumptions that are made. For example, when the homozygous RR and heterozygous RL individuals are assumed to be phenotypically identical, the predicted proportion of right-handed offspring, based on the data in Table 3-3, is .99. However, when the heterozygotes are assumed to be phenotypically mixed, with half of them displaying right-handedness and the other half left-handedness, then the predicted proportion of right-handedness in the offspring generation is .87. As can be seen, this second assumption leads to a better fit with the observed data.

The assumption concerning the relationship between genotype and phenotypic expression is a crucial part of the single-gene theorizing and model fitting procedure. For example, an alternate set of expected values may be derived from the same data if other assumptions are made. Suppose we based calculations on the premise that the RR genotype would most likely result in the phenotypic expression of consistent right-handedness. Our normative data provide this as the proportion of individuals who give right-handed responses for all of the questionnaire items, or .72 of our sample. Analogously, the frequency of the LL genotype is represented by the proportion of consistent left-handed responders, or .05. One can then assume that the remaining proportion of mixed responders, .23, is the frequency of the heterozygous RL genotype. If one assumes that the RL genotype results in an equal frequency of phenotypic right- and left-handedness, the derived expected proportion of right-handers is .84. Based on the premise that RR and RL individuals are phenotypically identical right-handers, the expected proportion is .97.

These estimates are quite discrepant, with one predicting 13% more right-handedness than the other. Each different set of assumptions results in a different set of estimates. The task that single-gene theorists have set for themselves is to try various models and assumptions. These are then statistically compared to the observed lateral preference proportions within the population. The model, with its underlying assumptions, that provides the best fit for the observed data is then proposed as the most likely to describe the nature of the genetic transmission of the trait.

In the preceding paragraphs we have outlined the research methodology that characterizes the single-gene approach, using the simplest possible dominant-recessive genetic model. Unfortunately, this simple approach does not work well.

The most obvious difficulty arises in situations where there is a mating of two left-handed parents. Since the left-sided gene is presumably recessive, the mating of two individuals with *LL* genotypes can result only in *LL* offspring, as we saw in Table 5-1. However, Table 5-2 presents the percentage of right-handed offspring observed as a function of parental mating patterns in a number of family studies. The expectation that all offspring of two left-handed parents will be left-handed is not confirmed, since on average 60% of the offspring of the left-handed matings are right-handed.

This difficulty with the single-gene approach was recognized quite early, and in 1911 Jordan commented,

> In what way or by what principle this inheritance acts remains obscure. . . . The writer does not delude himself—nor does he wish to leave the impression of attempting to mislead his readers in this matter—that left handedness even appears (on the basis of the limited data presented) to follow Mendelian principles of inheritance. (pp. 122, 123)

Despite such problems, a number of investigators have attempted to salvage the simple Mendelian approach and to provide models for the genetic transmission of handedness. These attempts generally involve additional assumptions to account for discrepancies in the observed data. Two typical examples are the efforts of Ramaley (1913) and Trankell (1955). These researchers attempted to explain the overrepresentation of right-handers in Left by Left matings by invoking the notion of social pressure, which might be expected to make a certain percentage of *LL* individuals appear as phenotypic right-handers. In addition, they introduced the notion of *partial penetrance*, suggesting that in *RL* individuals

Table 5-2: Percentage of Observed Right-Handedness in Offspring as a Function of Parental Handedness Mating Combinations

Study	$R_f \times R_m$	$R_f \times L_m$	$L_f \times R_m$	$L_f \times L_m$
Ramaley (1913)	87	—	—	14
Chamberlain (1928)	96	86	90	54
Rife (1940)	92	79	82	45
Merrell (1957)	81	69	50	80
Falek (1959)	90	63	87	84
Annett (1973)	90	71	86	65
Bryden (1979)	90	80	84	76
Porac & Coren (1979a)	94	—	—	—
Coren & Porac (1980b)	82	69	86	—
Carter-Saltzman (1980)	89	76	73	—
McGee & Cozad (1980)	81	66	71	58
Mean	88	73	79	60

Note. *R* means right, *L* left; subscripts f and m mean father and mother, respectively.

the *R* gene is not always dominant. With these new assumptions, the Hardy-Weinberg law can be used to generate estimates that reasonably approximate the actual observed frequencies of right- and left-handedness in an offspring population. However, these modifications result in a major shift at the theoretical level, since the investigator must abandon the presumed direct link between an individual's genotype and phenotype. Thus, an overt right-hander might actually be an *LL* genotype, while a manifest left-hander could be *RL*. Thus, to increase the adequacy of the single-gene model, one must forego the ability to predict individual differences in lateral preference behaviors from a knowledge of genotypic estimates, which goal provided the original impetus for exploring genetic models.

Despite these difficulties, the single-gene approach continues to appear in the contemporary literature. Most recently, however, in order to make the predictions agree with actual observations, the action of an *R* gene is assumed to be more indirect. The most usual hypothesis now is that the direct action of the gene is not in the determination of the preferred hand but rather in the determination of the hemisphere dominant for speech. The arguments for lateral preference then follow the line of reasoning encountered in Chapter 4, where cerebral specialization of one hemisphere for speech processing was linked to handedness. In addition, some investigators have suggested that this process might be modified by the action of at least one other gene. This allows a correction of the predictions so that one can account for the high frequencies of dextrality in pure sinistral matings. Models proposed by Levy and Nagylaki (1972) and Annett (1964, 1978a,b) typify this approach.

Levy and Nagylaki (1972) proposed that there are two genes, with two alleles each, that separately determine cerebral language localization and handedness. For example, they contend that one gene determines the hemisphere that is specialized for language processing, with left hemisphere organization dominant over localization in the right hemisphere. The other gene determines whether hand preference is contralateral or ipsilateral to the speech dominant hemisphere, where contralateral control dominates over ipsilateral. Thus, this model proposes that left-handers with language function in the right hemisphere are separate in genotype from left-handers with language function in the left hemisphere.

This model bases its estimates not only on the incidence rates of manifest right- and left-handedness, but also on data that deal with rates of recovery from aphasia. Brain injury in the speech processing regions of the left hemisphere may cause types of speech and language disruptions known as *aphasias*. If a left-handed individual is injured in this cerebral region and does not suffer from aphasia, or shows good recovery after an original temporary aphasia, it is concluded that speech function is shared to a large extent by, or even localized in, the right hemisphere. The same line of reasoning is applied to right-handers who have also suffered damage in the speech regions of the left hemisphere. Based on published accounts of aphasia recovery rates and other published reports of familial handedness patterns, Levy and Nagylaki (1972) attempted to estimate the proportion of each handedness type that had right and left hemisphere speech function. They then applied their model to family handedness data provided by Rife (1940) and found a reasonable fit, at least for the obtained percentages of right- and left-handers in his study.

The Levy and Nagylaki (1972) model has engendered a good deal of controversy. This controversy has illustrated some of the difficulties associated with single-gene approaches. First, there is a circularity inherent in these procedures. As we saw earlier, and is evident in the examples in the appendix, the original estimates of gene frequencies are based on some existing set of data. Expected values are derived from these observed values. This derivation is obtained by manipulating the data through a set of assumptions. This resultant "model" is then used again to predict the observed values. Thus it is not surprising to find that the model shows reasonably close fits to the observed data. However, this congruency is usually specific to one set of data. Hudson (1975) applied the Levy and Nagylaki (1972) model to the family handedness data obtained by Chamberlain (1928). He found, perhaps not surprisingly, that the fit was not as satisfactory as that obtained by Levy and Nagylaki (1972) for the data of Rife (1940). Similarly, when tested against a family study on handedness by Annett (1973), the model produced poor agreement. In reply, Levy (1977) suggested that problems may arise from different definitional criteria for left-handedness or from potential social pressures on left- versus right-hand use that may have biased the data in one or another of these studies. It seems likely, however, that the difficulty is also a methodological one, residing in the post hoc method of model building characteristic of the single-gene approach.

Annett (1972, 1978a,b) has supplied a modification of the strict single-gene analysis of handedness. This approach incorporates some of the features of the Levy and Nagylaki (1972) model in that it links the determination of handedness to cerebral speech localization. In some respects, however, this model is different from the others. It emanates from considerations of differences between the two hands in skills, rather than directly from lateral preference behaviors. Annett assumes that skill and preference covary (Annett 1976); hence, she uses these two types of data interchangeably. As we noted in Chapter 2, skill and preference measures cannot be directly equated, so we must be cautious in interpreting a theory that does this.

Annett's (1972, 1978a) model contains two components; one is genetic, and the other is environmental or at least accidental. She contends that a single gene accounts for a "right shift" in the developing organism. This factor is supposedly the one responsible for left-hemispheric speech representation, with right-handedness arising as a by-product of this aspect of neural organization. The right-shift gene does not have two directional alleles ($Right$ or $Left$); rather, it manifests itself as a bias toward the right, or the absence of a bias toward the right. When this right-shift factor is absent, accidental or random factors determine whether an individual is right or left handed. These chance factors also affect the strength of handedness and when considering differences in skill between the hands, produce a normal distribution in the population with a rightward bias (see Figure 2-1).

Annett's (1972, 1978a,b) model is a single-gene model that presumes the link between hemispheric factors and handedness (with all of the attendant difficulties discussed in Chapter 4 pertaining to this presumption). However, it also allows for nongenetic factors to influence sidedness. In addition, unlike the other single-gene models, it looks at handedness as a continuous, rather than a discrete dichotomous, variable, and in this respect it is similar to the polygenetic models that we will discuss shortly. However, whereas polygenetic models ascribe variability in the manifestation of sidedness to genetic factors, Annett (1972, 1978a, b) presumes that the continuous variation in handedness arises from nongenetic, random factors. Annett's (1972, 1978a,b) model does have one major advantage over other single-gene approaches. Since left-handedness supposedly arises from an absence of a right-shift factor (plus some chance pressures toward the left), the model can account for the high percentage of right-handed offspring in matings of two left-handed parents. The offspring of such matings have not been endowed with any bias toward the right; therefore, one expects to find approximately equal numbers of left- and right-handed offspring of such pairings. As Table 5-1 shows, 60% of the children of such matings are right handed, perhaps because in a predominantly right-handed world there are implicit pressures that push relatively unbiased individuals toward dextrality.

Hudson (1975) and Corballis (1980a) have described a major problem inherent in postulating single-gene determination of handedness. Twins, even monozygotic (MZ) twins, who supposedly share identical genotypes, are not perfectly

Table 5-3: Percentage of Reported Concordance in Handedness in Monozygotic (MZ) and Dizygotic (DZ) Twins

Study	Concordant MZ (%)	Concordant DZ (%)	Concordant nontwin siblings (%)
Siemens (1924)	73	–	–
Weitz (1924)	61	–	–
Lauterbach (1925)	83	78	–
Dahlberg (1926)	83	88	–
Verschuer (1927)	80	74	–
Newman (1928)	60	–	–
Wilson & Jones (1932)	81	81	–
Stocks (1933)	86	83	–
Rife (1940)	79	77	–
Rife (1950)	78	79	–
Carter-Saltzman et al. (1976)	75	69	–
Springer & Searleman (1980)[a]	77	78	–
Coren & Porac (1980b)	–	–	–
Sister-Sister	–	–	78
Brother-Brother	–	–	79
Sister-Brother	–	–	75
Mean concordance	76	79	77

[a] Based on summary data reported by authors.

concordant in their handedness patterns. For example, Table 5-3 shows concordance rates in both monozygotic and dizygotic (DZ) twin pairs as reported in a number of published studies. Monozygotic twins are offspring of the same fertilized egg, and they are assumed to be genetically identical. Therefore, if handedness is determined solely by genetic composition, MZ twins should always be perfectly concordant as to the sidedness of their preferred hand. Dizygotic twin pairs are used as a control group, since they share the womb at the same time and are of the same chronological age, mother, and familial upbringing. However, since they are the result of the fertilization of two ova, they are assumed to have only 50% genetic commonality, the same percentage of genetic overlap as any pair of siblings. As can be seen from Table 5-3, the concordance of handedness between MZ and DZ twins is approximately equal. In addition, average handedness concordance rates between siblings of approximately equal age, which we have observed in our work, does not differ from that for twins, as Table 5-3 also shows. Furthermore, the concordance between twins does not differ from the value expected if we compute the conditional probability of handedness concordance based on the random pairing of two unrelated individuals (.77) from the data in Table 3.3.

A number of investigators have made similar comparisons between MZ, DZ, and sibling pairs. Their conclusions are similar to those reported here. MZ twins show no greater correspondence in terms of handedness than do other groups (Collins, 1970; Corballis, 1980a; Rife, 1950; Springer & Searleman, 1980). A simple genetic model for the determination of handedness has difficulty explaining this lack of perfect concordance in genetically identical individuals. Some of the single-gene theorists have countered by arguing that MZ twins are not an appropriate group to use to test hypotheses about handedness. They contend that twins do not show the same population distributions of right- and left-handedness as do individuals who are single births. For instance, there are reports that the incidence of left-handedness may be twice as large in twin as opposed to singleton samples (Carter-Saltzman, Scarr-Salapatek, Barker, & Katz, 1976; Stocks, 1933). They argue that this high incidence of left-handedness results from the phenomenon of *mirror imaging*. If embryonic division into two individuals occurs at certain specific periods, the resulting twins manifest peripheral characteristics that are mirror images of each other. Thus, the shape of the right ear of one twin may match the shape of the left ear of the other. Such mirror-imaging differences may occur for facial features, hair whorls, or handprints (Dahlberg, 1926; Newman, 1937). This type of reversal during development could explain why one MZ twin is right handed while the other is left handed and could thus account for the lack of complete handedness identity (Nagylaki & Levy, 1973). This argument is weakened by the fact that all of the asymmetries that result from mirror imaging seem to be peripheral. The location of the organs is not reversed, and standard patterns of neurological specialization (e.g., left hemisphere speech) are found in the brains of mirror-imaged twins. Boklage (1980) has argued that mirror imaging of function does not seem to be a necessary consequence of this quirk of embryonic development. Thus the MZ twin data that show approximately 25% handedness discordance (Table 5-3) remain an embarrassment to a single-gene approach to the development of lateral preferences.

Although the simplest genetic models have many problems, this does not mean that one must abandon all hope of finding a genetic component to lateral preferences. For example, Table 5-2 showed that the percentage of right-handed offspring is reduced in mating pairs with one left-handed parent. The overall effects are greatest if the mother is left handed, although a sinistral father also lowers the overall incidence of dextrality. If both parents are left handed, the likelihood that the offspring will be left handed is increased even more. Data such as these, although not proving a genetic component to handedness, are at least consistent with such a hypothesis.

Simple Mendelian models may be inadequate for several reasons. Behaviors as complex as lateral preferences are not likely to be explained by the action of a single gene. It is more likely that we are looking at the interaction of a number of genetic contributions. Second, simple single-gene models require a discrete dichotomous trait, with one clear-cut manifestation for each allele. As demonstrated in Chapter 3, lateral preferences vary in strength, as well as side, and are dichotomized only as a methodological convenience. Polygenic approaches that deal with a graded manifestation of lateral preference, caused by several interacting genes, may provide a more successful description.

Polygenetic Approaches

A number of investigators suggest that genetic involvement in the formation of lateral preference behaviors follows a polygenetic mode of transmission. In other words, it is likely that a number of genes act together to determine variations in the side and in the strength of hand preference. Like the single-gene tradition, the polygenetic approach also has assumptions and analytic techniques that must be understood (see Plomin, DeFries, & McClearn, 1980).

Polygenetic models assume that phenotypic variation is due to both genetic and nongenetic influences. The goal is to estimate the proportion of phenotypic variance that can be attributed to genetic involvement. It is assumed that a number of alleles, or even genetic loci, contribute to the trait, and that their effect in forming the phenotype is additive and dependent on the number and type of genes that an individual has received. For this reason, polygenetic theorists talk about *additive genetic variance* within a population. Relatives are assumed to share varying proportions of additive genetic variance, depending on the type of their relationship and the proportion of common alleles that they are assumed to share. All first-degree relatives, such as parents and offspring and full siblings (the familial pairs most commonly studied in relation to handedness), are assumed to be 50% genetically similar. Half of the genetic material of an offspring comes from each parent, giving the offspring 50% of the genotype of each parent, as demonstrated in Table 5-1. Thus, 50% of the genetic variance is shared between one parent and an offspring, giving rise to within-family similarities. The remaining 50% does not covary and results in within-family differences.

The concept of shared genetic variation can be statistically translated into the degree to which there is shared covariance between distributions of related individuals measured on a particular trait. Generally, covariance is computed by summing the cross-products of deviations from the means of two distributions (i.e., the distribution of scores from mothers and the distribution of scores from daughters) and then dividing by the size of the sample. Numerical covariance estimates are derived, then, by computing a score (a deviation score) that places each individual in the distribution in relation to the mean of that distribution. Unlike single-gene approaches (which are more interested in the individual case or individual family), polygenetic approaches are concerned with the properties of phenotypic distributions found in samples of related individuals. They assume that if, for example, parents and offspring are sharing additive genetic variance in handedness, each parent-offspring pair will be similarly placed relative to the means of their respective distributions. Thus, a parent with a handedness score above the mean of the parental handedness distribution will produce an offspring who has a similar position in the offspring handedness distribution (if shared additive genetic variation is contributing to the trait formation). Rather than dealing with inheritance patterns as the all-or-nothing transmission of a discrete trait, the polygentic approach interprets genetic causation from similarities in distributional placement (degree of covariance) between related individuals. This approach requires that lateral preferences vary in side and in strength. For this reason, the most common statistical methodology used in tests of polygenetic hypothesis is correlation and regression, where the degree of genetic involvement is inferred from patterns of correlations between related pairs. Statistically, the size of the correlation between two relatives should be equal to the amount of genetic material that they share, if the expression of the particular trait depends solely on genetic factors. Thus, the correlation between parents and offspring, or between two siblings, should be .5 (since they share 50% of their genetic complement). The correlation between MZ twins should, theoretically, be 1.00, while that between DZ twins should be the same as that of any other sibling pair, namely .5.

The actual obtained correlations between relatives is seldom equal to that predicted theoretically. A number of factors can inflate the correlations, such as environmental similarities or similar life histories. Conversely incomplete genetic dominance or contravening environmental dissimilarities can deflate the obtained correlations. Therefore, one must be careful in interpreting the *absolute* magnitudes of familial correlations. Rather, one expects that if polygenetic mechanisms are involved in the formation of a phenotype, all of the correlations between pairs of first-degree relatives should be of approximately the *same* magnitude, since full siblings and parents and offspring are assumed to share the same degree of genetic similarity.

To exemplify this approach, we compiled Table 5-4 to show the correlational outcomes from a number of family studies exploring the handedness phenotype. As can be seen, most of the correlations between related pairs are rather weak, and only a few reach statistical significance. In addition, the magnitude of the

Table 5-4: Polygenetic Analysis of Handedness Patterns in Families as Reported in a Number of Studies Using Correlational Techniques

Study	Parent-offspring correlations				Sibling correlations		
	F-S	F-D	M-S	M-D	S-D	S-S	D-D
Bryden (1977)	–	$.095^a$	–	$.148^b$	–	–	–
Annett (1978a)[†]	.08	-.19	.17	$.28^b$	.08	.21	-.01
Bryden (1979)	.087	-.134	-.062	.007	–	–	–
Bryden (1979)[†]	$.277^a$	.079	.065	-.016	–	–	–
Porac & Coren (1979a)	.12	-.01	$.20^a$	$.24^b$	–	–	–
Coren & Porac (1980b)	-.04	-.01	.02	$.12^a$	-.05	-.04	.03

Note. F means father; M, mother; S, son; D, daughter.

[†] Based on speed of peg moving or tapping rather than on unimanual preference.

[a] $p < .05$.

[b] $p < .01$.

obtained values fluctuates across pairs of relatives. The most consistent pattern found across these studies is the degree of handedness resemblance between mothers and daughters. However, since the father-offspring and full sibling similarities are weak, it is difficult to relate the mother-daughter similarity to a genetic cause. In fact, Table 5-4 shows one of the major difficulties with the polygenetic approaches to the study of genetic involvement in handedness: family members, and especially full siblings, do not consistently resemble each other. This lack of uniformity across related pairs has led some theorists to conclude that genetic mechanisms may give rise to differences between families but a number of nongenetic and even random factors contribute to the formation of handedness patterns within families (Annett, 1978a; Corballis, 1980a). If this is the case, then knowledge about the handedness of one family member will not help you to predict accurately the handedness of another member of the same family.

We have reviewed briefly both the single-gene and the polygenetic approaches in the context of their application to the study of the handedness phenotype. However, we are also concerned with the other types of lateral preference. Since human populations tend to be predominantly right sided, not only right handed, it seems reasonable to search for possible genetic causation as a determinant of foot, eye, and ear preference. With this brief background on the two basic genetic approaches, we can turn our attention to the study of genetic mechanisms in the formation of all four types of lateral preference.

Genetic Explanations for Sidedness Formation

Research into the similarities between related individuals in eye, foot, and ear preference has been relatively sparse. Parsons (1924) claimed that the general incidence of right- and left-eyedness (70% versus 30%, respectively) is indicative of the operation of a pure dominant-recessive mode of single-gene transmission. He asserted that this would be the population distribution of right- and left-handedness in the absence of existing social pressures fostering the use of the right hand. The worked examples demonstrating the single-gene approach in the appendix indicate that the value of .70 right-sidedness is close to the estimated gene frequency of the *RR* homozygote for handedness. Parson's assertion that eye preference is a manifestation of a pure single-gene transmission pattern did elicit some studies of eyedness in related individuals (Merrell, 1957; Porac & Coren, 1979a; Zoccolotti, 1978). These few studies have provided somewhat conflicting results concerning eye preference. With single-gene procedures. Merrell (1957) and Zoccolotti (1978) have argued for genetic involvement in the formation of eyedness, while Porac and Coren (1979a), using polygenetic procedures, found no evidence of familial resemblances. Only Porac and Coren (1979a) have provided any familial data on foot and ear preference. They find no evidence of familial resemblances for foot preference, but indicate possible parent-offspring resemblance patterns in earedness.

In our previous discussion, we demonstrated that the particular set of assumptions that one adopts concerning the mode of genetic transmission interacts with the obtained results and with their interpretation. For example, single-gene approaches assume relatively discrete trait characteristics and often find relatively good fits between estimated and obtained values of gene frequency. Conversely, polygenetic approaches assume that a trait is graded in character, and this approach, as Table 5-4 illustrates, has not provided strong evidence for genetic involvement in handedness. Because of these methodological complications, we felt it necessary to apply both types of analyses to the same set of familial data. This would allow an assessment of both the consistencies and discrepancies in resemblance patterns that may be due to differing underlying assumptions about and treatment of the data. We also wanted to obtain contemporary familial data, not only on handedness, but also on the other forms of lateral preference.

These considerations led to a study of familial patterns of lateral preference (Coren & Porac, 1980b). In order to obtain assessments of hand, eye, foot, and ear preference in a sample of families, we used the lateral preference self-report battery presented as Table 3-1. We contacted approximately 2,000 families throughout the Province of British Columbia, Canada. Families were selected for final analysis if we had received complete lateral preference inventories from both parents and from at least one biological offspring. This resulted in a sample of 459 family units, all of whom fulfilled these criteria. We also obtained data from 434 offspring pairs from the families in the sample that contained multiple offspring. This sample included some data where information was available from a number of offspring but from only one parent. We next analyzed the data from all four indexes of lateral preference along the lines suggested by the single-gene approach; afterward, we applied polygenetic analyses on the same familial data set. This allowed us to compare and contrast the results from the two approaches.

In following this line of investigation, we incorporated several features into our research procedure that have been ignored in other studies of familial handedness. First, we controlled for family size by randomly selecting one offspring in each family for the final analysis. This is important since differences in family size can influence the interpretation of the degree of familial resemblance, especially if random nongenetic influences intervene. Because no family is represented more than once in each analysis, statistical analyses are independent and can be simply interpreted.

Second, we studied only families where both the parents and the offspring completed their own lateral preference inventories. A number of previous family studies on handedness, for example, have relied on direct self-report information on the lateral preference of offspring but have used secondhand information, based on the offspring's recollection, to ascertain parental handedness. Such indirect assessments of parental preference patterns have been used often in the analysis of parent-offspring resemblance patterns (Annett, 1978a; Bryden, 1977; Chamberlain, 1928; Hicks & Kinsbourne, 1976; Ramaley, 1913). Both Annett (1973) and Ramaley (1913) have expressed concern that this indirect approach to parental handedness assessment could introduce a systematic bias into the resulting data, and this suspicion was confirmed by our own work. We asked a group of high school students to report on whether their mothers and their fathers were, generally, right or left handed. We then compared these offspring responses to the self-reports of handedness (items from Table 3-1) provided by the parents themselves. We found that the offspring tended to underestimate the proportion of left-handedness found in the parental population by approximately 50% (Porac & Coren, 1979c). This indicates that family members are insensitive to each other's lateral preference behavior patterns. Thus direct assessment of both parental and offspring behaviors seems to be the only justifiable methodological approach to the study of familial lateral preference. Finally, we attempted to take into account individual difference variables that affect incidence rates in lateral preference. As we indicated in Chapter 3, and will discuss more fully in Chapter 6, gender and age both affect manifestations of hand, eye, foot, and ear preference, and these factors must be considered in familial analyses.

We first considered our data in a manner similar to that used by single-gene theorists. We dichotomized parents, offspring, and siblings into right- and left-sided individuals on each lateral preference index and considered incidence rates as a function of parental mating combinations. As you may recall from the previous discussion, most investigators in the single-gene tradition predict that the incidence of right-sidedness will drop in offspring of left-left mating pairs or even in the offspring of pairs where only one of the parents is left handed. This expectation is based on one of two assumptions. The first is that left-sidedness is a recessive trait that tends to be dominated by the gene for right-sidedness (Chamberlain, 1928; Jordan, 1911; Levy & Nagylaki, 1972; Ramaley, 1913; Trankell, 1955). A second possible assumption is that the tendency toward right-sidedness is inherited and left-sidedness indicates the absence of such a genetic endowment (Annett, 1972, 1978a,b). Regardless of which specific position one adopts, the incidence of right-sidedness should vary as a function of the lateral preferences of different parental mating combinations.

Table 5-5 shows the results of our analysis of the incidence of right-sidedness in offspring of various parental mating combinations. The percentage of dextrals is given for all offspring and for male and female offspring separately. The comparisons of immediate interest are those between the incidence rates of offspring

Table 5-5: Percentage of Right-Sided Offspring as a Function of Parental Lateral Preference Mating Combinations

Lateral preference type	Mother	Father	All offspring (N=459)	Female offspring (N=237)	Male offspring (N=222)
Hand	Right	Right	82.4 (384)	83.7 (196)	80.3 (188)
	Right	Left	86.4 (37)	82.6 (23)	92.9 (14)
	Left	Right	69.4 (36)	64.7 (17)	73.7 (19)
	Left	Left	* (2)	* (1)	* (1)
	Any left	Parent	78.9 (75)	76.0 (41)	82.4 (34)
Foot	Right	Right	80.4 (319)[a]	82.6 (161)	78.5 (158)[a]
	Right	Left	71.4 (83)	80.4 (46)	59.5 (37)
	Left	Right	65.9 (44)	65.2 (23)	66.7 (21)
	Left	Left	85.7 (13)	85.7 (7)	83.3 (6)
	Any left	Parent	71.1 (140)[a]	76.3 (76)	64.1 (64)[a]
Eye	Right	Right	64.7 (247)	62.3 (130)	66.7 (117)
	Right	Left	57.3 (81)	59.0 (39)	54.8 (42)
	Left	Right	66.3 (82)	55.0 (40)	78.6 (42)
	Left	Left	70.6 (49)	60.7 (28)	85.7 (21)
	Any left	Parent	63.9 (212)	61.5 (107)	70.5 (105)
Ear	Right	Right	59.2 (149)	64.9 (77)[a]	52.8 (72)
	Right	Left	54.7 (105)	54.7 (53)	53.8 (52)
	Left	Right	61.4 (82)	66.0 (47)	54.3 (35)
	Left	Left	52.0 (123)	45.0 (60)	58.7 (63)
	Any left	Parent	55.4 (310)	54.4 (160)[a]	56.0 (150)

Note. Numbers in parentheses indicate sample size. Based on Coren & Porac (1980b).

* Sample too small for meaningful computation.

[a] Items in same column differ significantly, $p < .05$.

of right-right matings and those of offspring of any mating pair that contains a left-sided partner. Only one of 16 possible comparisons of this type is significant when all offspring are considered, and two of 32 comparisons are statistically significant when males and females are analyzed separately (female ear preference and male foot preference). Thus, significant changes in the right-sidedness of offspring as a function of parental mating combination are seen in only 6% of all of the comparisons made, a result that does not deviate from chance expectations based on the presumption of no genetic involvement.

Although a number of previous studies have found decreases in the incidence of right-handedness in families with one left-handed parent (Annett, 1974, 1978a; Chamberlain, 1928; Falek, 1959; Merrell, 1957; Porac & Coren, 1979a; Wilson & Sanders, 1978), we did not find significant decreases in our present sample. However, the analysis in Table 5-5 does reveal a 13% decrease in the incidence of right-handedness when the mother is the left-handed parent. Although not statistically reliable in the analysis shown in Table 5-5, this trend is consistent with other reports of mother-offspring similarities and maternal effects in familial handedness patterns (Annett, 1973, 1974, 1978a; Chamberlain, 1928; Falek, 1959; Hicks & Kinsbourne, 1976; Porac & Coren, 1979a; Wilson & Sanders, 1978). For this reason, we decided to consider separately the effects of each parent's lateral preference on the incidence rates of right-sidedness in the offspring. This re-analysis is shown in Table 5-6. Here, there is a clear effect of maternal left-handedness. The presence of a left-handed mother reduces the incidence of right-handedness in offspring by approximately 14%.

Together, Tables 5-5 and 5-6 indicate that there are some familial effects in hand, eye, foot, and ear preference. Generally, they are gender specific (being found only in male or female offspring or as a function of a male or female parent), but overall the effect of parental mating combinations is not large. In fact, the maternal effect on the eye preference of male offspring is in the direction opposite to that predicted, with the percentage of right-eyed offspring increasing when the mother is left eyed. The analysis of preference patterns in offspring as a function of parental mating combinations does not offer much support for systematic familial or genetic effects in the formation of lateral preference. Even in handedness, which has formed the basis for most of the previous genetic analyses, the effects are not large and seem to be confined to increased sinistrality of offspring given the presence of a left-handed mother. This result could be indicative of modeling or training influences, as opposed to strictly genetic ones.

An alternate analysis, suggested by the polygenetic approach, is begun by looking at the pattern of correlations that exists among family members. In order to accomplish this analysis, the dichotomized scores were recorded numerically so that each individual classified as left sided on a particular index received a score of 1 and each individual classified as right sided received a score of 2. Correlation coefficients were then computed on each group of familial pairings. This form of data representation allows a number of advantages. For example, one can compare the relative magnitudes of any obtained relationships, both to the theoretically expected values and to each other. In addition, this mode of analy-

Table 5-6: Percentage of Right-Sided Offspring as a Function of Parental Lateral Preference for Mothers and Fathers Considered Separately

		All offspring (N=459)	Right-sided offspring (%)	
			Female (N=237)	Male (N=222)
Hand	Mother			
	Right	82.8[a]	83.6	81.2
	Left	69.2[a]	66.7	75.0
	Father			
	Right	81.3	82.2	79.7
	Left	85.4	83.3	93.3
Foot	Mother			
	Right	78.5	82.1	74.9
	Left	70.7	70.0	70.4
	Father			
	Right	78.6	80.4	77.1
	Left	73.5	81.1	62.8
Eye	Mother			
	Right	62.9	61.5	63.5[a]
	Left	67.9	57.4	81.0a
	Father			
	Right	65.1	60.6	69.8
	Left	62.4	59.7	65.1
Ear	Mother			
	Right	57.4	60.8	53.2
	Left	55.7	54.2	57.1
	Father			
	Right	60.0	65.3[b]	53.3
	Left	53.2	49.6[b]	56.5

Note. Based on Coren & Porac (1980b).
[a] Significantly differ, $p < .05$.
[b] Significantly differ, $p < .01$.

sis allows one to remove potential confounding individual difference variables, such as age, which are associated with changes in the relative dextrality observed in the population. Age effects are easily removed by the use of partial correlation coefficients. The resulting matrix of age-controlled familial correlation coefficients is shown in Table 5-7.

The data in Table 5-7 confirm the previous results, although some new information is apparent. The maternal effect on handedness emerges again, but now it seems to be predominantly carried by the relationship between mothers

Table 5-7: Correlations between Family Members for the Side of Lateral Preference

Familial pair	Hand	Foot	Eye	Ear	N
Mother-offspring	.08[a]	.06	-.05	.02	459
Mother-daughter	.12[a]	.12[a]	.05	.06	237
Mother-son	.02	.02	-.17[b]	.04	222
Father-offspring	-.02	.05	.02	.07	459
Father-daughter	-.01	.02	.00	.16[b]	237
Father-son	-.04	.14[a]	.05	-.03	222
Siblings	.02	.05	-.05	.17[b]	422
Sisters	.03	.10	-.05	.22[b]	124
Brothers	-.04	-.10	-.09	.03	70
Brother-sister	-.05	.02	-.04	.14[b]	228
Mother-father	.05	.03	.14[b]	.19[b]	459

Note. These are partial correlations with the effect of the age of the respondents removed. Based on Coren & Porac (1980b).
[a] Significantly different from 0, $p < .05$.
[b] Significantly different from 0, $p < .01$.

and daughters. There is also a mother-daughter relationship for footedness. The puzzling negative relationship between mothers and sons in eye preference is again apparent. Paternal effects emerge in a significant father-son relationship for footedness, and in a father-daughter relationship for ear preference. The only significant sibling correlations are found for earedness. Overall, the only index of lateral preference that shows several familial relationships seems to be ear preference; once again, however, the pattern is incomplete.

Of the 96 parent-offspring comparisons in Tables 5-5, 5-6, and 5-7, only 11 reach statistical significance, and of these 11, eight are gender specific. It seems that the pattern of familial similarities in the sidedness of lateral preference does not conform to a simple genetic model or even to a simple polygenetic model of determination. Of those relationships that emerge, environmental influences cannot be discounted. Mother-offspring correlations, in the absence of sibling correlations, could indicate behavioral modeling. Also, the significant mother-father correlations for eye and ear preference are suggestive of nonrandom mating patterns. With nongenetic similarity already present in the family as a result of biases in mate selection (thought to be an environmental biasing factor), it is difficult to interpret additional familial resemblances. For example, the presence of parental similarity may account partially for the patterns of sibling resemblance found in ear preference. Sibling resemblances in the absence of parent-offspring similarities often are used to suggest such environmental influences. We cannot formulate a convincing case for a genetic involvement in the determination of the side of lateral preference based on these data.

Strength versus Side

The overall picture obtained from the existing family studies and our data shows only weak, and predominantly negative, evidence for the genetic transmission of sidedness. The strongest case can be made for ear preference, and the only other consistent finding is a maternal influence on handedness. None of the resulting data patterns resemble those expected if sidedness is transmitted genetically. However, we may be looking at the wrong variable when we simply consider right versus left side in our familial analyses.

A number of investigators suggest that it is inappropriate to look for genetic influences in the side of lateral preference; rather, one might expect that genes contain information encoding the degree or consistency of the expression of a given lateral preference. It has even been suggested that genes may be left-right *agnosic,* producing asymmetries of degree rather than of direction of lateralization and lateral preference (Bryden, 1979; Collins, 1977; Levy, 1977; Morgan, 1977). These views are compatible with the polygenetic tradition that we discussed previously. When there are many genes of small effect, such as those thought to be responsible for determining characteristics such as height, one usually finds that the trait varies continuously in degree of manifestation and is distributed normally. In the present context, there are suggestions that some aspects of handedness, for example, may be polygenetic, since differences between the hands in strength (Woo & Pearson, 1927) and in skill (Annett, 1970, 1978a; Annett & Turner, 1974) manifest themselves as a continuous, unimodal, and approximately normal distribution. This is similar to most common polygenetic traits, which vary in the strength or consistency of appearance rather than segregating individuals into discrete classes (such as right versus left). Perhaps the degree of lateral preference expression is encoded genetically while the right-left directional shift is caused by environmental factors.

Such a theoretical position predicts that family members should resemble each other in the degree of consistency of lateral preference, rather than its direction. Bryden (1979) has provided familial handedness data in humans to support this prediction. Using a skill measure (speed of tapping), he found parent-offspring resemblances when he considered the absolute scores obtained, regardless of the hand used. When side was the criterion, however, relationships were minimal. These data are suggestive, although unimanual preference was not the variable under study. However, we re-analyzed the data in Table 5-7 to explore familial patterns in the strength of preference.

We rescored the self-report items in Table 3-1 by assigning a +1 value to each right response, a 0 to each both response, and a -1 to each left response. An algebraic sum of these scores for each index is a composite with both direction and consistency encoded. In essence, our first familial analysis (Table 5-7) used only the sign of this score, dichotomously indicating side of preference. In our re-analysis we used the absolute value of the score, which is an index of the consistency or strength of preference, regardless of the preferred side. An individual who is completely right handed (with a score of +4) and an individual who is completely left handed (with a score of -4) have identical consistency scores of 4. A score of 0 indicates complete ambi-sidedness, which is interpreted here as the weakest form of preference. Since the scores operate over a range of values, we applied standard correlation procedures to the data.

Table 5-8 shows the correlations for all parent-offspring and sibling pairs. As in Table 5-7, the age effect has been removed through the use of partial correlation coefficients. Of the 40 correlations (excluding that of mother-father), 15 are significant. Thus, when considering the degree of expressed preference, 38% of the family resemblances exceed chance expectations, as compared to the 23% seen when side of preference is examined in this way (the figure is actually 11% if one considers all of the side comparisons in Tables 5-5, 5-6, and 5-7). The greatest increase in the proportion of statistically significant values is in handedness and footedness. This finding replicates that of Bryden (1979), who reported greater degrees of handedness resemblance when the strength of the expressed preference was cross correlated among family members. Computations using the side of the preference as the dependent variable produced lesser degrees of similarity.

Regardless of the sex of the offspring, both the mother-offspring and the father-offspring correlations for the consistency of hand preference are significant. In addition, the sibling correlation is also significant. When a parent-offspring analysis is done (separating offspring into males and females), the strongest handedness relationship is found between parents and male offspring, where both the mother-son and the father-son correlations are significant. Foot preference differs slightly from hand preference. Here there is evidence for strong maternal effects, with offspring resembling their mother in the consistency of

Table 5-8: Correlations between Family Members for the Strength of Lateral Preference

Familial pair	Hand	Foot	Eye	Ear	N
Mother-offspring	$.11^b$	$.10^a$	.02	$.08^a$	459
Mother-daughter	.04	$.11^a$	.06	.09	237
Mother-son	$.13^a$	$.12^a$	-.02	.07	222
Father-offspring	$.09^a$	.04	$.08^a$	.04	459
Father-daughter	.01	.06	-.02	.06	237
Father-son	$.11^a$	.01	$.14^a$	.03	222
Siblings	$.10^a$	$.11^a$	.06	$.17^b$	422
Sisters	.08	$.20^a$	-.02	.13	124
Brothers	.03	.11	.03	.08	70
Brother-sister	.01	.00	.05	$.14^a$	228
Mother-father	.03	.07	$.19^b$	$.12^b$	459

Note. These are partial correlations with the age of the respondents removed. Based on Coren & Porac (1980b).

[a] Significantly different from 0, $p < .05$.

[b] Significantly different from 0, $p < .01$.

foot preference, regardless of the sex of the offspring. There are also significant sibling correlations, although only the sister-sister relationship remains significant when the siblings are subdivided by sex. There is no paternal effect on the footedness of offspring for either sons or daughters. The consistency of ear preference shows a significant mother-offspring correlation. The sibling correlation is also significant for ear, but no paternal effects are manifest. Perhaps the weakest effects are found for eye preference, where only father-offspring correlations are significant.

The size of the familial correlations and the relative consistency of the observed resemblance patterns are more striking in Table 5-8 than in Table 5-7. Thus, while the measures based on the direction or side of lateralization shown in Table 5-7 provide little suggestion of a familial component, the strength measures present a different picture, and show familial patterns of resemblance for three of the four preference indexes. In fact, the handedness correlations in Table 5-8 start to approach the full range of familial similarities required for a polygenetic interpretation. There are parent-offspring as well as sibling resemblances in the degree of manifest handedness.

The results of our combined analyses provide a new viewpoint on lateral preference. Investigators interested in genetic influences on handedness or other forms of lateral preference have to date relied on directional or sidedness measures. These procedures have usually provided only ambiguous evidence for the role of genetic or even familial factors in these behaviors, as the previous discussions and data have shown. However, there is stronger support for this interpretation when comparisons of the strength of the displayed preference are made among familial pairs.

The present finding has important theoretical consequences. It supports notions such as those of Bryden (1979), Collins (1977), and Morgan (1977), who contend that there is no directional code available in genetic material. They argue that genes act to encode the strength of asymmetry, rather than to determine the direction of preference. Since in most polygenetic systems genetic influence is expressed in quantitative rather than qualitative differences in a particular trait (McClearn & DeFries, 1973), the present results are consistent with the assumption of a polygenetic inheritance mode for hand, foot, and ear preference.

The genetic approaches to lateral preference are based on the assumption that all human organisms will display some type of functional asymmetry and that these asymmetries are encoded genetically. This notion can account for the fact that human populations are predominantly right sided. Whether or not genetic factors can account for individual differences (deviations from the dextral norm) is less clear. The simpler approaches associated with Mendelian genetics and single-gene explanations do not adequately explain familial patterns in sidedness, but neither does the polygenetic approach. The prediction of individual left- versus right-sidedness based on the knowledge of the lateral preferences of family members does not appear to be a successful approach. The one aspect of lateral preference that shows familial resemblances is the strength or consistency of these behaviors. These resemblances could indicate a genetic component for strength of hand, foot, and ear preference. However, if genetic factors cannot explain sidedness adequately, one must consider other variables. Some of these will be discussed in the following two chapters.

Appendix

Single-gene analysis of handedness patterns in families. This procedure is derived from the Hardy-Weinberg theorem to estimate the frequency of the three handedness genotypes (based on Cavalli-Sforza & Bodmer, 1971). First the binomial expansion is used to estimate the frequencies of the *RR, RL,* and *LL* genotypes. If *r* is the frequency of allele *R* and *l* is the frequency of allele *L*, the basic formula is

$$(r + l)^2 = 1 \tag{1}$$

which expands to

$$r^2 + 2rl + l^2 = 1 \tag{2}$$

For convenience we will designate r^2 as a, $2rl$ as b, and l^2 as c. Now the general computational process is shown in Tables 5A and 5B, while Table 5C shows a worked example based on the incidence of handedness reported in Chapter 3.

Table 5A: Procedure for Calculating the Frequency of Certain Mating Combinations in the Parental Generation

		Genotype of mother		
		RR	*RL*	*LL*
	f	*a*	*b*	*c*
Genotype of father *RR*	*a*	a^2	*ab**	*ac**
RL	*b*	*ba**	b^2	*bc**
LL	*c*	*ca**	*cb**	c^2

Note. For simplicity, the frequencies (*f*) from formula (2) are symbolized as *a, b,* and *c* as noted above. In the final computation of frequencies of mating types, the starred values are used once and doubled since the mating combination of father (*RR*) X mother (*LL*) is treated as equivalent to the combination of mother (*RR*) X father (*LL*).

Table 5B: Expected Frequencies of the Three Handedness Genotypes in the Offspring Generation as a Function of the Various Parental Genotypic Mating Combinations

Parental genotype mating combinations			Expected proportion of each genotype in offspring*		
Father	Mother	Frequency	RR	RL	LL
RR X RR		a^2	All	—	—
RR X RL		$2ab$	.50	.50	—
RL X RL		b^2	.25	.50	.25
RR X LL		$2ac$	—	All	—
RL X LL		$2bc$	—	.50	.50
LL X LL		c^2	—	—	All

*These proportions can be directly tested by formulating tables such as Table 5-1.

Table 5C: Single-gene Analysis of Handedness Patterns in Families
A worked example using normative data from Chapter 3 and the procedure illustrated in Table 5a.

I.

.87 = frequency of allele R (total % of all right-handers observed)
.13 = frequency of allele L (total % of left-handers and ambidextrous individuals observed)

$$(r+l)^2 = (.87 + .13)^2$$
$$= (.87)^2 + 2[(.87)(.13)] + (.13)^2$$
$$= .7569 + .2262 + .0169 = 1.0$$

II.

			Genotype of mother		
		Frequency	RR	RL	LL
			.7569	.2262	.0169
Genotype of father	RR	.7569	$(.7569)^2$	(.7569)(.2262)	(.7569)(.0169)
			.5729	.1712	.0128
	RL	.2262	(.2262)(.7569)	$(.2262)^2$	(.2262)(.0169)
			.1712	.0512	.0038
	LL	.0169	(.0169)(.7569)	(.0169)(.2262)	$(.0169)^2$
			.0128	.0038	.0003

Table 5C (cont.)

III. One can compute the expected numbers of parental mating combinations and the expected numbers of offspring of each genotype in a hypothetical population of 1,000 pairs with one offspring from each pair.

Parental genotype mating combinations			Expected number of pairs (*N*=1,000)	Number of offspring of each genotype (assuming one off-spring from each pair)		
Father		Mother	Frequency		*RR*	*RL*	*LL*
RR	X	*RR*	.5729	572.9	572.9	–	–
RR	X	*RL*	.3424	342.4	171.2	171.2	–
RL	X	*RL*	.0512	51.2	12.8	25.6	12.8
RR	X	*LL*	.0256	25.6	–	25.6	–
RL	X	*LL*	.0076	7.6	–	3.8	3.8
LL	X	*LL*	.0003	.3	–	–	.3

Assumption 1. Phenotypic right-handers = total *RR* + total *RL*
                                       =   .76 +   .23 = .99

Assumption 2. Phenotypic right-handers = total *RR* + .5*RL*
                                       =   .76 +   .11 = .87

6

Social and Cultural Environment

Meggie's worst sin was being left-handed. When she gingerly picked up her slate pencil to embark on her first writing lesson, Sister Agatha descended on her like Caesar on the Gauls. . . .

Thus began a battle royal. Meggie was incurably and hopelessly left-handed. When Sister Agatha forcibly bent the fingers of Meggie's right hand correctly around the pencil and poised it above the slate, Meggie sat there with her head reeling and no idea in the world how to make the afflicted limb do what Sister Agatha insisted it could. She became mentally deaf, dumb and blind; that useless appendage her right hand was no more linked to her thought processes than her toes. She dribbled a line clear off the edge of the slate because she could not make it bend. . . . nothing Sister Agatha could do would make Meggie's right hand form an A. Then surreptitiously Meggie would transfer her pencil to her left hand, and with her arm curled awkwardly around three sides of the slate she would make a row of beautiful copperplate A's.

Sister Agatha won the battle. On morning line-up she tied Meggie's left arm against her body with rope, and would not undo it until the dismissal bell rang at three in the afternoon. Even at lunchtime she had to eat, walk around and play games with her left side firmly immobilized. It took three months, but eventually she learned to write correctly according to the tenets of Sister Agatha, although the formation of her letters was never good. To make sure she would never revert back to using it, her left arm was kept tied to her body for a further two months; then Sister Agatha made the whole school assemble to say a rosary of thanks to Almighty God for His wisdom in making Meggie see the error of her ways. God's children were all right-handed; left-handed children were the spawn of the Devil. (Colleen McCullough, *The Thornbirds*, 1977, p. 37)

The confrontation between young Meggie and Sister Agatha occurred in a rural New Zealand school between 1915 and 1917. In a rather extreme fashion, it conveys the essence of the approach discussed in this chapter, namely, that the incidence of right-handedness (-sidedness) varies as a function of both the amount of pressure that an environment places upon the individual to conform to the dextral norm and the susceptibility of the individual to succumb to that pressure. This viewpoint is derived from a theory that maintains that lateral preferences, particularly handedness, result from some form of learning process. This learning process is supported by social pressure and biases built into the culture and the environment. However, the evidence for learning as a basis of lateral preference formation has always been somewhat inferential. The greater prevalence of right-handedness in older individuals, or the fact that some parents attempt to teach children right-handed use of eating utensils or pencils, has been sufficient evidence for psychologists of the stature of J. B. Watson (1919, 1925) to offer rather elaborate learning theories of lateral preference.

In some respects, the learning hypothesis for the development of lateral preferences is a sort of a fallback position based on the failure of purely physiological or genetic explanations to account fully for sidedness behaviors (see Chapters 4 and 5). It also results from common observations on attempts to train deliberately one side or the other. The most often cited evidence for a learning viewpoint is that, at least for specific tasks, individuals *can* be trained to use their nonpreferred hand. Of course, almost all of the reported instances of this successful training involve switching left-handers to right-handedness; there are, however, scattered reports of switches toward sinistrality. Most of these represent cases where injury to the preferred right hand necessitated left-hand use. For example, Carlyle (1884) recorded in his 1871 diaries his progress in shifting to left-handedness after a stroke had paralyzed his right arm. Other incidents involve consciously learned sidedness for sports activities, such as when the baseball player Mickey Mantle trained himself to be a switch-hitter. Shaw (1902) has provided the only experimental attempt to switch normal right-handed infants to left-hand use. He persistently placed articles in the left hands of two infants, who soon became quite proficient in left-handed use. He reports that he was later able to switch them back to dextrality, although he suggests that they were never able to develop as great a proficiency with the right hand as they had enjoyed with the left.

Eyedness is the only other index of lateral preference where training effects have been investigated. At the anecdotal level, microscopists usually are trained to view through their instruments with the right eye, regardless of natural eye preference. Also, experimental evidence shows that with intensive training over a short period and separation of the images to the two eyes, visual asymmetries related to eye dominance are weakened (Porac, 1974; Porac & Coren, 1975b). There are also reports that with extended practice over periods of days or months, eye dominance can be shifted to the contralateral eye (Berner & Berner, 1953; Hamburger, 1943).

In some respects, this notion is rather speculative. That handedness *can* be learned indicates only that it maintains a certain degree of plasticity, not that hand preference originally emanates from a learning process. One can easily imagine that some apparently innate behaviors can be modified by later learning, or that some early learned behaviors may well be relatively immutable in later life. Thus, we only have data permitting us to say that handedness is modified by learning processes, not that it initially arose as a learned skill. Regardless of whether the initial disposition of side preference was determined by some form of learning or due to a genetic or physiological mechanism, that it can be modified through experience means that the final distribution of lateral preferences observed in any population may be affected by factors unique to a particular environment, culture, or form of socialization. These factors can exert influence on sidedness simply because the majority of the population is dextral, and to the extent that this majority has arranged the world for their own convenience, one would expect the world to exhibit a bias in favor of right-side use.

There are subtle pressures toward dextrality exerted by the existence of a right-sided environment, in addition to overt pressure by various socializing agents (such as parents, teachers, and Sister Agatha), that increase the frequency of right-sidedness as left-sided individuals are forced to change their natural tendencies. Most of the research attention surrounding this approach to lateral preference formation has focused on handedness, since pressures to ensure that the right hand is used in writing, eating, and other socially relevant activities are the most obvious and widespread.

Pressure toward the right pervades the environment. For instance, many tools and implements are shaped for the convenient use of the right hand. Such everyday implements as scissors, gearshifts, ice-cream scoops, rulers, can openers, pencil sharpeners, and vegetable peelers, as well as the location of the winding stem on a wristwatch, are biased toward right-sided usage. Many musical instruments, such as violins, guitars, banjos, and saxophones, are designed for right-handed players. Sporting gear, including fishing reels, rifles, and even bowling balls carry a right-handed bias. The direction in which the threading of screws is angled favors the dextral individual on the power (forward) movement, thus resulting in biasing many other implements, such as corkscrews and wrenches, against the sinistral person. Sometimes, when confronting our technological environment, the left-hander must feel incredibly frustrated by the fact that voting machines, slot machines, time card punches, and even candy and soft drink dispensers all have levers oriented for the ease of right-hand use. To survive in this right-sided world, left-handers soon learn to do with the right hand many things that the right-hander could never and will never do with the left. The end result is a degree of ambidexterity, and a lessening of the consistency with which left-handed coordinations are emitted. More simply, the left-hander must become more right handed.

The other lateral preferences have been virtually ignored by proponents of the social pressure theories, probably because it is difficult to see how, or why, one would be influenced to change foot, ear, and eye preference. Yet subtle sidedness biases exist even for these indexes. For instance, automatic transmission cars are meant to be controlled solely with the right foot, as are many industrial machines. Pressure to the right also exists for the eye. For example, recently a major line of optical micrometers was marketed with the sight situated so that only the right eye could be used. However, since the population is not biased as strongly toward the right for foot, eye, and ear as it is for hand use, the world does not show so strong an environmental bias for these indexes. If, however, one assumes that handedness is the primary influence in the formation of all lateral preferences (an issue that was discussed in Chapter 4), one could argue that influences acting to change handedness patterns would also affect the other indexes of preference and the relationships among them.

The effect of a biased, right-sided world is apt to be quite subtle, and it should accumulate over time. Whether such environmental biases can influence side preference is difficult to evaluate in humans, since one would need a control group of humans brought up in an unbiased world to provide a comparative baseline. It is not known if any such environments exist. Humans always seem to alter the environment for their convenience, which implies a dextral bias. However, full environmental control can be achieved through the use of nonhuman subjects.

Many animals, including monkeys, chimpanzees, cats, rats, and mice (Collins, 1968; Finch, 1941; Warren, 1958), show the equivalent of handedness in the preferential use of one paw in specific activities, such as manipulation and prehension. Animals differ from humans in that they show no population bias toward dextrality or sinistrality. Although any individual animal has a dominant paw, there is an equal likelihood that it is the right or the left paw. As in humans, though, direct training can be used to alter or shift paw preference (Chorazyne, 1976). For example, to show the effect of a biased world on paw preference in mice, Collins (1975) placed mice in an apparatus where food could be obtained more conveniently with one paw. This type of exposure shifted the distribution of paw preference in the direction of the bias in the world. The learned paw preference was maintained, even if the world was shifted so that the other paw became the more convenient one. However, the strength of the paw preference seemed to be weakened in this anti-biased world. If one can extrapolate this work to human populations, it suggests that a sidedness bias in an environment can profoundly affect lateral preferences and may alter or weaken preexisting preference patterns. If environmental pressures modify human sidedness, one expects lateral preference incidence rates to vary as a function of the degree to which the world is overtly or covertly right biased, and as a function of an individual's exposure time to the enviroment. It may also vary as a function of the individual's general susceptibility to change.

The Right-Sided World Hypothesis

Our normative data in Chapter 3 contain significant age trends and gender differences that alter the incidence rates for the various manifestations of lateral preference in the population. The right-sided world hypothesis has been used to explain these individual variations in sidedness. We will use our own data to test some of the tenets of this hypothesis and to ascertain how well they predict the patterns of both age and sex differences that we have observed.

Age Differences

The right-sided world hypothesis argues that the cumulative effect of living in a world biased for the convenience of the right-handed majority is an increase in the amount of observed right-handedness over that caused by any right-biasing physiological mechanism. For this reason, the study of infants and young children was particularly relevant to the early cultural conditioning theories of handedness formation (Harris, 1980). It was argued that if handedness patterns are nurtured by a right-biased culture, young infants should begin life as ambi-handed with no strong hand preference. They should become gradually more right handed with increasing age as a function of accumulated pressures from the environment to use the right side of the body. As a consequence of the assumption that increased exposure to a right-sided world fosters increased right-sidedness, one can predict rightward age trends in handedness and perhaps in the other preference indexes.

Over the last 100 years, investigators such as Charles Darwin (1877), James Mark Baldwin (1890), G. Stanley Hall (1891), and John Watson (1925) have been interested in the problem of the development of handedness. These early studies, along with later observations, indicate that there is a developmental trend in the establishment of handedness patterns. Although infants appear to exhibit rudimentary hand preferences at an early age, these asymmetries increase in consistency with a gradual shift toward habitual right-hand use with increasing age (Bethe, 1925; Cernacek & Podivinsky, 1971; Coryell & Michel, 1978; Gesell & Ames, 1947; Giesecke, 1936; Hildreth, 1949, 1950; Ingram, 1975; Jones, 1931; Ramsey, 1979; Ramsey, Campos & Fenson, 1979; Roos, 1935; Seth, 1973; Woolley, 1910). Our data (Porac, Coren, & Duncan, 1980b; Figure 3-2) have shown that there are developmental trends in the incidence of handedness, with the population becoming gradually more right handed over the life span. We found similar trends for footedness; eye preference, however, shows only a weak developmental change, and ear preference shifts toward the left. The observed rightward shift in hand and foot preferences might be evidence for the influence of environmental pressures on limb use. The environment does not show the same clear pattern of increasing degrees of dextral bias for eye and ear use; hence, these indexes may be uninfluenced by such pressures.

Although our previous data show increased dextrality in limb use, they do not give as clear a picture as we would like. The major problem is that the youngest age we tested was eight years. By this age, social and environmental pressures would have been applied, and one could argue that the adult pattern of lateral preference would already have been determined. Therefore, we wanted to test younger individuals, preferably of preschool age, where the influence of formal school training in skills such as writing would not as yet have had an opportunity to influence manifest lateral preference.

Our target sample was children between three and five years of age. We wanted to compare their lateral preference patterns with those of young adults, which we did in a study by Coren, Porac, and Duncan (1981). To conduct this research, we devised an inventory that behaviorally tested each type of lateral preference (hand, foot, eye, and ear). We selected measures suitable for administration to very young children and also to older groups in an identical format. We were able to demonstrate experimentally that these behavioral measures have a high classification concordance with our self-report battery (Table 3-1); thus, we can compare with confidence the results of our behavioral testing to the data collected by means of the questionnaire. The behavioral inventory that we used is shown in Table 6-1. It is based on procedures employed in a number of previous studies (Clark, 1957; Coren & Kaplan, 1973; Coren & Porac, 1978; Harris, 1957; Koch, 1933; Kovac & Horkovic, 1970; Porac & Coren, 1975a; Raczkowski, Kalat, & Nebes, 1974), and we designed it for individual behavioral administration.

The inventory in Table 6-1 was administered to 384 preschool children, 202 males and 182 females, ranging in age from three to five years. A young adult comparison group, composed of 171 high school students (76 males and 95 females), was also tested. The comparison group had a mean age of 16.3 years. We scored the preference data using the trichotomous classification procedure described in Chapters 2 and 3. Individuals were classified as consistent right, consistent left, or mixed. These data are shown in Table 6-2 for both the preschool and the young adult samples.

Between early childhood and young adulthood, there are significant shifts in the pattern of lateral preference for hand, eye, and ear. These indexes show a significant increase in right-sidedness and a decrease in left-sidedness. The age trend for footedness, while in the same direction, does not reach statistical significance. Although hand, foot, and ear show a reduction in the percentage of

Table 6-1: Behavioral Measures of Lateral Preference

	Behavioral measure
Hand preference	1. Picks up and throws ball to experimenter.
	2. Points to experimenter's nose.
	3. Picks up crayon and draws a circle.
	4. Touches own nose with finger.
Foot preference	1. Kicks ball to experimenter.
	2. Stamps on replica of bug.
Eye preference	1. Looks through a telescope.
	2. Looks into opaque bottle resting on a table and reports its contents.
	3. Looks into a kaleidoscope.
	4. Looks through base of truncated cone at experimenter's nose (Miles ABC test, Miles, 1929).
Ear preference	1. A small box emitting a tone which varies in loudness is placed upon a table. The individual is asked to place an ear close to the box and to report when the tone can no longer be heard.
	2. The above task is repeated with a buzzing sound source.

individuals classified as mixed preferent, this shift toward more consistent lateral preference is only statistically significant for handedness.

The earedness result does not agree with the leftward life-span trend reported in Chapter 3. However, the present results are an earlier age-related change in ear preference, which may be a maturational effect that takes place during this formative period as the young child gradually comes to display the adult pattern of dextrality in earedness. Such an interpretation suggests that the adult leftward shift in ear preference is not a change toward sinistrality but rather a change away from dextrality. In other words, the leftward life-span trend is a regression toward an unbiased population where there is an equal distribution of right- and left-eared individuals. There is some support for this interpretation when we reconsider the data in Figure 3-2. If we take each age group separately, we find that the first three (individuals from 8 to 35 years old) show proportions of right-earedness that are significantly greater than the chance expectation of 50%. However, the proportion of right-earedness does not exceed chance levels for any of the remaining senior age categories. Combining the normative and the preschool data, we see that right-earedness seems to develop early in life; however, the population's dextral bias in ear preference diminishes during the adult years.

There is a dextral trend from early childhood to young adulthood in all preference indexes. The dextral trend continues for hand and foot preference from adolescence through the remainder of the life span. The trend for eyedness attenuates and is only weakly evident in later life, while the rightward trend in ear preference reverses and the early dextral bias disappears. These results replicate and extend the large numbers of studies that have shown dextral age trends in handedness throughout the childhood and adult years (Fleminger, Dalton, & Standage, 1977; Hildreth, 1949, 1950; McGee & Cozad, 1980; Porac, Coren, & Duncan, 1980b).

Table 6-2: Comparison of Preschool and Young Adult Samples on Behavioral Measures of Lateral Preference

Lateral preference	Preschool				Young adult			
	Consistent (%)			Mixed (%)	Consistent (%)			Mixed (%)
	Right	Left	Total		Right	Left	Total	
Hand[a]	68.3	6.2	74.5	25.5[b]	80.7	5.8	86.5	13.5[b]
Foot	76.9	10.6	87.5	12.5	81.9	7.6	89.5	10.5
Eye[b]	54.5	40.0	94.5	5.5	66.1	24.6	90.7	9.4
Ear[b]	52.7	40.0	92.7	7.3	70.2	25.1	95.3	4.7

Note. Mean age of preschool subjects was 4 years (N=384); mean age of young adults, 16.3 years (N=171).

[a] Overall age difference significant, $p < 0.05$.

[b] Overall age difference significant, $p < 0.01$.

The age differences conform, to some extent, to the predictions of the social pressure hypothesis, especially if we confine our discussion to the lateral preferences of the limbs. There is an increasing incidence of right-handedness in the older age groups, a finding that is consistent with the cumulative effect of living in a right-biased world. Before entertaining seriously the notion that the age trends in Table 6-2, and particularly in Figure 3-2, are a gradual accumulation of the effects of rightward-biasing mechanisms within the social and cultural environment, we must address ourselves to several other possibilities that arise as a result of the cross-sectional age sampling technique used in our research.

A likely hypothesis that maintains that these data are not true age trends is based on changing attitudes toward left-handedness over the years. For example, prior to about 1930, both psychologists and educators favored the practice of shifting a child's writing hand from the left to the right side. There was a very strong negative bias toward the use of the left hand for writing during this era (see Blau, 1946). In succeeding years, however, this attitude changed, and as a result there are reports that the incidence of left-handed writers has increased (Hildreth, 1949; Levy, 1976). Since the data in Figure 3-2 represent handedness responses from several generations, it is possible that the rise in the incidence of right-handedness that we observed over the life span reflects the changing pattern of social pressures on the training of the writing hand, which might then bias other hand preference behaviors.

One way to test this hypothesis is to consider a number of normative studies of adult hand preference that have been conducted over the span of years during which this shift in social pressure has taken place. If overt pressure on the selection of the writing hand plays a role in determining the handedness trend observed in Figure 3-2, the studies conducted earlier in this century should report higher proportions of dextral individuals than those conducted more recently. To assess this possible explanation for our age trends, we surveyed the reported incidence of right-hand use in a number of studies published over the last 65 years. We confined ourselves to a consideration of investigations conducted in North America and Western Europe that had used measures analogous to our own. We imposed this geographical restriction because cross-cultural differences in the incidence of handedness have been reported, as we will detail in a later portion of this chapter. We reasoned that if changing social pressure patterns accounted for the apparent age trend, the reported incidence of right-handedness within the population over this span of time should decrease in a manner that would be a mirror image of the handedness trend in Figure 3-2. Figure 6-1 shows the scatterplot from our literature search, based on 34 studies published between 1911 and 1978. Although the correlation between the year of publication and the percentage of reported right-handedness is negative (-.28), as predicted by the hypothesis that more contemporary generations display lesser degrees of dextrality, this correlation is not statistically significant. Furthermore, the slope of the observed decrease in reported right-handedness indicates a change of only .05% of the population per year. This is only 25% of the rate of the observed change in right-handedness that is revealed by the normative data in Figure 3-2.

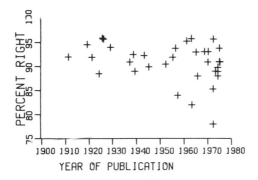

Figure 6-1. The percentages of right-handedness reported in 34 studies, plotted against the year of publication of each of the studies.

Thus the overt social pressure hypothesis can account for only a small portion of the observed change in handedness. There are no existing hypotheses that suggest that overt social pressure has been applied to foster certain types of foot, eye, and ear preference. Thus it seems even less likely that this hypothesis can account for the age trends obtained.

We must also consider the possibility that the reported rise in right-sidedness with advancing age is the result of the differential mortality rates of right- and left-sided individuals. In other words, left-siders do not live as long as right-siders, leading to their decreased frequency in the more senior age groups. In fact, one of the earliest theories of handedness actually depended on differential mortality of left-handers. The idea was based on primitive warfare. It was offered by Pyre-Smith (1871) as part of a theoretical treatise, and was mentioned by Carlyle (1884) in his 1871 diary. Both contended that the right-handed person holds a weapon in the preferred right hand, while the left side of the body is turned slightly away from the opponent and is protected by the shield carried in the left hand. This is important because the heart lies on the left side of the body. The left-hander, with a shield on the right side of the body, is more susceptible to fatal thrusts to the heart. The result is that right-handers had a distinct survival advantage over their sinistral companions when engaged in warfare. Right-handers survived to procreate and produce a right-handed population. Although this theory is rather imaginative, it probably has little relevance to our contemporary world, in which missiles, shells, bullets, bombs, and grenades afford little survival advantage to either dextral or sinistral soldiers.

The possibility of differential survival rates as a function of the side of the preferred hand was considered by Quinan (1921), who found higher frequencies of cardiac and cardiovascular disorders in left-handers. No readily apparent explanation for Quinan's results are available; however, there are environmental factors which might affect the survival of left-handers. One could argue that the technological incompatibilities that left-handers are exposed to are not only uncomfortable but also potentially dangerous. This might provide a rationale for suspecting that left-handers are more accident prone. For instance, most machine controls are set for right-handed operation. In a dangerous situation, left-handers are forced to make emergency responses with their nonpreferred right hand when operating power presses, lathes, and other complex pieces of machinery. These responses could be slower and less accurate. The results of such occurrences, accumulated across large samples and numerous incidents, might cause a difference in accident rates for left- and right-handers, and as a secondary consequence, cause a difference in mortality rates.

We tested 688 adults on the lateral preference inventory shown in Table 3-1. They were also queried about home or occupational accidents that had occurred within the previous three years of sufficient serverity to warrant medical attention. We found that left-handers were significantly more likely to have suffered from such accidents. Of course, it is a tenuous practice to extrapolate from accident rates to mortality rates on the basis of these data. However, since some percentage of all accidents are apt to be fatal, this differential accident susceptibility may be a crude index of mortality rates. Perhaps the age trend toward dextrality observed in Figure 3-2 rests somewhat on the differential mortality of sinistral individuals. This could be one explanation, although speculative, for the fact that we have no consistent left-handers in our normative sample over the age of 65 years.

Cultural pressure and differential mortality are two nondevelopmental hypotheses that we have entertained given the cross-sectional nature of our life span sample. However, neither one of them seems able to explain the magnitude of the age changes in handedness (data on differential mortality are too sketchy for this at present), nor can they explain the direction and magnitude of the age shifts in the other preference indexes. There is no evidence of differential accident rates as a function of foot, eye, or ear preference, and no overt social pressure seems to be brought to bear on them. Therefore, we must consider some developmental hypotheses that might account for the age changes.

First, let us consider the nonenvironmental hypothesis that these age trends are reflective of neural maturational processes that promote increasing degrees of right-sidedness as a secondary consequence of physiological changes. We have already reviewed data (in Chapter 4) that indicated that physiological asymmetries are more clearly manifest in adults than in children. In addition, there are some reports that indicate that neural developmental processes can continue into middle adulthood (Flechsig, 1920; Kaes, 1907; Yakovlev & Lecours, 1967). For example, handedness and footedness are the two forms of lateral preference assumed to have the closest neural association in terms of locus of neural control, and these are the two forms of lateral preference that show life-span age trends of the greatest similarity. This age trend may be the result of some as yet unknown developmental process that promotes increasing degrees of rightness in limb preference with increasing age. Such a hypothesis, however, would have difficulty explaining the contrary trend in earedness and the absence of a trend in eye preference. It also presumes but does not specify a physiological basis for lateral preference, and then adds the postulate that this mechanism must mature in order for dextrality to appear. As Chapter 4 showed, no simple neural mechanism, irrespective of its rate of maturity, has yet to be found to affect lateral preferences.

The second developmental hypothesis is simply a restatement of the right-sided world hypothesis. It maintains that the covert pressures on the individual due to biases in the environment accumulate as the individual ages and experiences new aspects of the world. The slight pressures toward dextrality build gradually, and the individual becomes more consistently dextral as a function of increasing chronological age. Several difficulties immediately come to mind with regard to this hypothesis. First, and most obvious, is that only hand and foot preference show marked shifts toward dextrality; eyedness shows no marked shift, and ear preference actually manifests more sinistrality with increasing age. Of course, one might counter by attempting to find a sinistral bias for ear preference as a secondary consequence of a right-sided bias to the world. A simple one might be the telephone, which is generally held against the left ear by dextral individuals in order to free their right hand for writing. With increased exposure to such a left-eared task, perhaps people become more left eared. Unfortunately, it does not make sense to ascribe whole shifts in a population to a single piece of apparatus. To return to handedness, for example, if one selected the typewriter as a key part of our civilization, one might predict a leftward shift in hand preference with age because the left hand makes more key strikes than the right. This fact has been used to explain the large number of left-handed world champion speed typists. The right-sided world hypothesis stands or falls on the existence of a multitude of dextral biases in the environment, and the cumulative effect of many encounters with these biases. Theoretically, it is unfortunate that all of the indexes do not show the expected rightward trend.

The maturational hypothesis and the right-sided world hypothesis make differential predictions if one considers the relative congruency of lateral preferences across indexes. Predictions from the maturational hypothesis presume that shifts in lateral preference with age represent the expression of physiological predispositions toward asymmetry, which simply become more manifest as the individual matures. Thus one might expect that with age, individuals predisposed toward dextrality will become dextral on all indexes of lateral preference, whereas natively sinistral individuals will become more congruently left preferent with age. The right-sided world hypothesis, of course, simply predicts that individuals will become more congruently right sided. Unfortunately, the existing data give little support to either position. Figure 6-2 shows the percentage of congruently left and right individuals as a function of age, based on the sample we introduced in Chapter 3. There are no noticeable age trends in congruency, whether we consider congruent dextrality, congruent sinistrality, or simply total congruency across the four indexes. Thus, an individual does not tend to become either right sided or one sided with advancing age.

Age trends in lateral preference present an equivocal picture. Unless we are willing to say that the right-sided world hypothesis is restricted to right-limb usage, it does not seem to be adequate. If we do single out the limbs, the data are consistent with a learned bias. The most salient competing hypothesis, if we

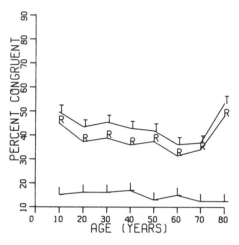

Figure 6-2. Percentage of individuals who are congruently sided on all four lateral preference indexes, plotted as a function of age (R is congruent right sidedness, L is congruent left sidedness, and T is total congruent sidedness).

restrict our argument to hand and foot alone, is a maturational one. However, it does not seem as cogent as the learning-based hypothesis, since the age trends manifest for limb preference in Figure 3-2 continue throughout the entire life span, including even the oldest age groups. Maturational processes that begin in the first decade and continue beyond the fourth decade of life are rare, and such a long physiological change, which could affect manifest handedness and footedness, has not as yet been isolated. At best, the data on limb preference are most consistent with an environmental hypothesis, although it is not conclusive.

Gender Differences

Numerous attempts have been made to assess whether there are sex differences in lateral preference behaviors. As usual, the principal focus has been on handedness. While there are many reports of no significant differences (probably due to restricted sample sizes), when differences are found, they always indicate greater proportions of right-handedness among females (Bryden, 1977; Clark, 1957; Dawson, 1972; Hardyck, Goldman, & Petrinovich, 1975; Harshman & Remington, 1975; Oldfield, 1971; Chapter 3). In addition, our evidence (Chapter 3) and that of Bryden (1977) indicate that females are more likely to be consistently right handed, whereas males show more mixed hand preference patterns.

This result is inconsistent with physiological theories of the etiology of lateral preferences. If lateral preferences arise as a result of cerebral asymmetries, as we discussed in Chapter 4, then the direction of the sex differences in lateral preference should predict that males will show less physiological asymmetry and less right-sided bias when cerebral structures and processes are examined. Males should show weaker patterns of localization of function and more bilateral cerebral organization. However, clinical and anatomical studies suggest the opposite, namely, that males are more strongly functionally lateralized than females (Bakan, 1971; Sherman, 1974). A number of sources of data support this conclusion. Wada (1974) physically measured the size of the temporal planum and frontal operculum. These are the areas that, as we noted in Chapter 4, usually contain the speech areas, at least in the left hemisphere. He found that the left and right hemispheres differed in bulk, an asymmetry that was interpreted as being indicative of lateralization of function in the brain. However, female brains showed significantly less asymmetry than male brains. Other neuroanatomical studies support this conclusion (Lansdell & Davie, 1972). Clinical reports lead to this same inference. Studies of unilaterally brain-lesioned patients indicate that adult males show greater and more selective impairments than do females, especially for verbal functions after left-hemispheric damage (Lansdell, 1961, 1973) and for nonverbal skills following right-hemispheric damage (Lansdell, 1962, 1968; McGlone & Kertesz, 1973). Again these results suggest greater degrees of functional specialization in males. If these processes are related to lateral preference formation, one should find more left-sidedness and mixed sidedness in females, not in males. The data in Chapter 3, however, indicate that females are more right sided in hand, foot, and ear preference, and more left sided only in eye preference. In all four indexes, however, they show more consistent sidedness than males.

Since a simple physiological notion does not explain these gender differences adequately, it is not surprising to find that some learning hypotheses have emerged. Basically these hypotheses presume that the right-sided world notion is true, but add that females are either more susceptible to environmental pressures or undergo more stringent socialization than do males (Dawson, 1977; Levy, 1976). Such hypotheses would be consistent with greater dextrality in females, especially for limb preference; however, no direct data have been brought to bear on this issue. Nevertheless, some secondary analyses are possible, based on the age trends that we discussed earlier and in Chapter 3.

If females are more susceptible to social and environmental pressures than males, and if the change that we observe in lateral preference over the life span reflect shifts due to environmental pressures, we might expect the rate of age change to differ for males and females. Using limb preference as an example (since it most clearly conforms to the notion of a right-biased world influencing preference formation), we would expect that both sexes would show a dextral shift over the life span; however, the greater susceptibility of females to environmental pressures ought to appear as a faster rightward trend. Statistically, there should be an interaction between age and sex in the percentage of the sample classified as right sided, but there are no such interactions. The difference between males and females remains relatively constant over the life span for all four indexes of lateral preference. This stability suggests that females are not responding more to environmental pressures on lateral preference than are males.

Collins (1977) has proposed a mechanism that may offer an explanation for gender differences and for the hypothesized differential responsiveness of males and females to environmental factors based on data concerning the formation of paw preference in mice (Collins, 1968, 1969, 1970, 1975, 1977, 1978). He argues that genetic codes may control the degree to which a functional asymmetry is expressed, rather than the sidedness or direction of the expression. We discussed this notion in Chapter 5 and provided empirical evidence that seems to support it for hand, foot, and ear (Coren & Porac, 1980b). Collins contends that female mice contain a genetic complement associated with stronger expressions of lateral preferences, whereas male mice have a genetic complement that promotes weaker preferences. Given this type of genetic mechanism, females always respond to a biased environment in a way that strengthens the degree of their native sidedness. Lateral preference expression operates in the opposite direction for males; their native lateral preference, regardless of its side, is weakened in a biased environment. If there are equal distributions of right- and left-sidedness in males and females, all of whom are living in a right-biased world, Collins (1977) predicts that the native right-handed females will be more right handed, the native left-handed females will be more left handed, and males will show lessened degrees of both right- and left-handedness.

Collins' viewpoint, applied to a human population, can partially explain some of the gender differences we have observed. For example, this approach predicts that females will show a greater tendency to fall within the response category showing consistent right-sidedness if we subdivide individuals into mixed versus completely consistent. This is the case for hand, foot, and ear preference where the gender difference favoring increased right-sidedness in females is greater for the consistently right-sided response class. This can be seen in Table 6-3, which re-analyzes the sample introduced in Chapter 3. Although more females also show consistent right-eyedness, the gender difference here is not significant. Except for eye preference, females are more right sided and more consistently right sided when compared to the male subsample. For left-sided response patterns, once again the Collins (1977) hypothesis would predict a higher percentage of females in the consistent response category. However, females do not show significantly more consistent leftness than males, except in eyedness, while males are significantly more left eared. An interesting fact emerges from Table 6-3. The gender difference is most pronounced when the total group of left-siders (rather than just the consistent responders) is considered. Apparently, the higher percentage of left-sidedness in males takes the form of a higher incidence of weaker, more mixed response patterns, while the increased right-sidedness in females takes the form of greater degrees of strong consistent responding.

This detailed analysis of the specific response patterns of males and females thus partially supports the genetic-environmental interaction hypothesis proposed by Collins (1977). Despite overall population gender differences in the incidence of right- and left-sidedness, there are additional gender differences in the degree to which the preference appears to be expressed. Females are more strongly right sided, while males display weaker right- and left-sided response patterns. Consistent left-sidedness shows an ambiguous pattern, favoring males on earedness and females on eyedness, with no sex difference apparent in hand

Table 6-3: Percentage Distribution of Lateral Preferences in Males and Females[a]

Lateral preference	Left-sided		Right-sided	
	Consistent	Total	Consistent	Total
Hand				
Females	4.9	9.8[b]	75.6[b]	90.2[b]
Males	5.8	13.4[b]	68.3[b]	86.8[b]
Foot				
Females	3.5	14.2[b]	54.2[b]	85.9[b]
Males	4.1	23.4[b]	37.8[b]	76.7[b]
Eye				
Females	17.2[b]	30.8[b]	55.4	69.2[b]
Males	12.3[b]	26.9[b]	53.2	73.1[b]
Ear				
Females	12.9[b]	35.5[b]	40.4[b]	64.3[b]
Males	16.8[b]	45.3[b]	29.7[b]	54.9[b]

[a] Sample comprised 2,391 females and 2,756 males.

[b] Significant sex difference, $p < .01$.

and foot preference. This ambiguity may indicate that gender-related factors in lateral preference formation based on genetic-environmental interactions have their greatest influence in the determination of right-sidedness, at least in a right-biased world. The determination of strong left-sidedness in a right-biased world may involve other mechanisms unrelated to gender. As usual, however, the hypothesis cannot be directly tested in humans, since it seems to require a population from both an unbiased and a left-biased world to serve as control groups. Unfortunately, only one (presumably right-biased) world is presently available.

Cultural Influences

The right-sided world hypothesis contains two major components. The first deals with a world arranged for the convenience of dextral individuals exerting a covert, but constant, pressure on sinistral individuals, thus bringing about conformity in dextral usage. The second aspect, to which we have also alluded in the preceding sections, deals with socialization of the individual. This refers not to the physical environment of tools and implements, but rather to social influences, both overt and covert, that cause persons to alter their pattern of lateral preferences to conform with the social expectations of others. These social pressures may arise in the immediate family environment or in the cultural milieu.

Traditionally, the right side is the side of honor and dignity, whereas the left side is associated with treachery and perjury. The right hands are clasped in marriage, and a marriage contracted with the left hand is held to be clandestine and irregular, and to generate only bastards (Hertz, 1973). The King or Queen of England wears the emblems of sovereignty on the right side, and places at his or her right side the people deemed most worthy. A similar practice prevailed in the physical layout of the prerevolutionary French National Assembly; it resulted in certain political labels (now often associated with political attitudes) that are still used today. The aristocrats were the government's "right wing," and the then not too respectable, politically upstart capitalists were its "left wing." These are but a few examples of how a culture places values on the two sides, values that permeate a society and are often reflected in a child's upbringing. These values, and their attendant pressures to conform, may alter an individual's manifest lateral preference behaviors.

The Role of Parents

Perhaps the most pervasive, and certainly the earliest, cultural and environmental influence on the developing child is the immediate family. Parents convey basic patterns of behavior to children, teaching them to use their first tools, such as spoons, knives, and pencils; they also serve as models that the child imitates in the process of learning complex activities. Unfortunately, very little study has been directed toward the role of the family environment in determining lateral preferences. The data are sparse, and often inferential. An example of this is the observation by John B. Watson (1919, 1925) that very young infants do not show systematic use of their right hand, while older children and adults show the usual dextral bias as a population. On the basis of this observation, Watson (1925) offered a theoretical structure to explain handedness that involved pressure and learning processes:

> Our whole group of results in handedness leads us to believe that there is no fixed differentiation of response in either hand until social usage begins to establish handedness. Society soon thereafter steps in and says "Thou shalt use thy right hand, Willy." We hold the infant so that it will wave "bye-bye" with the right hand. *We force it to eat with the right hand. This in itself is a potent enough conditioning factor to account for handedness.* (p. 101)

One of the first socialization and teaching tasks engaged in by parents, perhaps even before the overt teaching of language, is instruction in basic personal care and cleanliness. Even in the most primitive societies the notions of clean and unclean are established quickly. In this context, the left hand is often called the unclean hand (Wile, 1934). This designation probably arises from observation of several tendencies associated with toilet activities. Right-handers tend to clean themselves after a bowel movement (or, for a male, holding the genitals during urination) with the left hand. This same act usually is performed by the right hand of a sinistral person. Kovac and Horkovic (1970) refer to the hand used in the toilet act as one of the most reliable indicators of handedness. This fact has been observed and noted in many cultures (Hertz, 1973). In the English language, it appears in the form "cack-handed", an uncomplimentary epithet used to designate left-handers in many parts of England. Many cultural taboos and traditions arose from such humble observations. Eating with the left hand is considered not only a sign of improper breeding, but in many Arab countries it is also a sign of disrespect for the others in the room. In tribes of the lower Niger, for this same reason, women are forbidden to use their left hands when cooking, for fear of being accused of contaminating or poisoning the food. Such attitudes are bound to have an effect on an impressionable child. Hertz (1973, p. 5) notes that as recently as the early 20th century in Europe, one could state, "One of the signs which distinguish a well-brought up child is that its left hand has become incapable of any independent action."

One might expect parental pressure toward the use of the right rather than the left hand to take the form of conscious or unconscious training of offspring. Eating utensils would be placed in the right hand, drawing implements would be forcibly switched from the left to the right hand, and so forth. The parental pressure would be gentle but pervasive. In some cultures, however, intervention is even more extreme than that of Sister Agatha described in our opening passage. Kidd (1906) reports that there are a group of African tribes who set about to cure left-handedness in a rather drastic way:

> If a child should seem to be naturally left-handed the people pour boiling water into a hole in the earth, and place the child's left hand in the hole, ramming the earth down around it; by this means, the left hand becomes so scalded that the child is bound to use the right hand. (p. 296)

In contemporary Western cultures, there are a number of more subtle influences on a child's lateral preferences. Sometimes the simple act of watching parents will suffice. In Chapter 5 we presented data from a number of family studies when discussing possible genetic contributions to lateral prefernce. We noted that one of the most common findings, both in the existing literature and in our data, is the resemblance between mothers and children in hand preference (Annett, 1973, 1974, 1978a; Chamberlain, 1928; Coren & Porac, 1980b; Falek, 1959; Hicks & Kinsbourne, 1976; Porac & Coren, 1979a; Wilson & Sanders, 1978). Such a family resemblance, in the absence of strong similarities between father and offspring or among siblings, does not provide cogent support for a common model of the genetic transmission of sidedness. It is possible, however, that the mother-offspring similarity has arisen from the child's tendency to model the mother's behavior. The father is not modeled because in the Western samples tested, it is the mother who tends to be the primary caretaker. To the extent that the modeling of the mother's behavior occurs, one might expect that the strongest similarity would be between mother and daughter, and this is the relationship that is most frequently reported. This same line of reasoning could be applied as an explanation for the apparent familial similarities in the strength or consistency of lateral preferences (Coren & Porac, 1980b; Chapter 5). If the parents are ambilateral, consistent limb use would not tend to be modeled by the growing child.

Only one study has addressed itself to the issue of social-psychological factors in the family environment that might contribute to the formation of handedness. Falek (1959) found that right-handed parents are rarely familiar with the problems faced by left-handers in a right-handed world. This insensitivity of right-handers to handedness patterns has also been documented by other investigators (Etaugh & Brausam, 1978; Porac & Coren, 1979c). This indifference, Falek (1959) argues, leads to a lack of concern about the hand preferences of their children, most of whom are right handed anyway. In addition, he maintains that there is a higher frequency of left-handedness in offspring when the father is right handed and the mother is left handed (a finding that is replicated and discussed in Chapter 5). Ostensibly this arises for two reasons: first, there is a genetic propensity for a higher incidence of left-handedness in these families and, second, the left-handed mothers do not exert pressure to switch handedness, while the right-handed fathers remain indifferent to the behavior. Falek (1959) found that left-handed fathers, who may have experienced some discomfort and social pressure in their professional or occupational settings, strongly favor right-handedness and exert pressure to change any emerging left-handedness in offspring. Thus, one finds a lower incidence of left-handedness (increased right-handedness) in families where the father is left handed. This could offset any genetic effect that might increase the incidence of left-handedness in these families. Falek (1959) also reported that the left-handed fathers in his sample who were laborers or semiskilled workers were the most determined to change handedness patterns away from the left side. Presumably this was because this group of fathers had suffered the greatest disadvantage in job placement as a result of right-handed design of most tools. This finding suggests additional socioeconomic factors that might influence manifestations of handedness.

Falek (1959) has proposed an interesting familial influence system. Left-handed fathers attempt to exert pressure to change handedness, and their spouses, whether right or left handed, cooperate in these efforts. Totally right-handed parental matings are indifferent to handedness patterns, while left-handed mothers with right-handed husbands offer a family environment most conducive to the expression of left-handedness. Falek (1959) used this system to explain the increased incidence of left-handedness in mating pairs where the mother alone was left handed and the relatively equal incidence of left-handedness in offspring of the other mating combinations. This is the only study to collect data on how the family social environment can affect the expression of handedness. No investigations of this type have concerned foot, eye, or ear preference.

Parental effects may be quite subtle, and may well appear in disguised forms. For example, in Chapter 7 we shall discuss data that suggest that increased left-handedness is found in offspring of older mothers, especially when the offspring are second or later born (Coren & Porac, 1980a). Although the interpretation that we will consider there deals with the possible intervention of physiological trauma, it may also be the case that older mothers are more apt to be relaxed, and somewhat less attentive, in the upbringing of children. A natively sinistral child of such a mother could be subjected to little or no pressure to use the right hand and thus be more likely to express left-handedness.

During the latter part of the 19th century, suggestions were made that the way in which a mother held a child could influence the child's handedness. If mothers carried their children on the right arm, the child's right arm would be free to move and possibly develop more strength and agility. Unfortunately, the majority of mothers carry their children on their left arm; hence, the theory was abandoned. Salk (1962) revived this notion by suggesting that human infants are imprinted in the uterus to the sound of the mother's heartbeat, and that they exhibit a relative freedom from anxiety when they are in the presence of this imprinted stimulus. Since approximately 80% of both right- and left-handed mothers hold a newborn infant on the left side, close to the heart (Salk, 1962, 1973; Weiland, 1964; Weiland & Sperber, 1970), other investigators have argued that this practice calms the child and gives a survival advantage to right-handed mothers and their children (Huheey, 1977; Margoshes & Collins, 1965). For example, Huheey (1977) claims that in early hominid evolution, tool use and manual efficiency became predominant factors, and strong selective pressures existed for dextral mothers, who, while holding their infant in their left arm, could perform complex tasks with the free right hand. Left-handed mothers were not as fit from a survival point of view, since they had to hold their infant next to the heart with the preferred hand. This left them with a greater degree of ineptitude when compared to the performance of their right-handed counterparts. Of course, this survival-of-the-fittest notion seems to carry with it an implicit presumption of genetic transmission of handedness, which, as noted in Chapter 5, is contentious.

Cross-Cultural Studies

Although no society or culture has been found where the majority of individuals are left sided, attitudes concerning the right and the left, particularly pertaining to hand use, vary across cultural groups. Attitudes associated with hand use cover a broad range. Thus, the Bakitara tribe of the Victoria Nyanza in Africa openly hate left-handed people (Roscoe, 1923). The tribes of the Lower Niger, such as Ija, will not permit a woman to touch her husband's face with the left hand (Leonard, 1906). The Maori seem to attend to left and right only for ritualistic behaviors, where the left is bad and the right is good, a concept that appears frequently in anthropological reports (Hertz, 1973). The Chinese, while honoring the right side, are quite tolerant of left-handed people (Granet, 1973). Although the right hand tends to be the proper hand for most activities, contemporary Western societies tolerate or ignore the left-hander. However, the Meru of Kenya actually treat the left hand as the blessed hand (Needham, 1973). Given this diversity, one would expect to find many differences in the amount of pressure that diverse cultural groups place on individuals to conform to a dextral norm. This in turn could alter the distribution of dextrality observed in their respective populations. Thus, cross-cultural comparisons can test the limits of environmental and societal influences on lateral preferences.

Dawson (1977) attempted to analyze patterns of societal pressures on lateral preferences. He proposed that traditional hunting and fishing populations value independence, and therefore have extremely permissive socialization practices;

as a result, lower degrees of conformity, and consequently lower degrees of right-handedness, are expected. Agricultural societies have firmer socialization and more stringent requirements for conformity. This atmosphere leads to greater degrees of right-handedness. This suggests that the incidence of right-handedness across cultures will vary as a function of the degree of conformity pressure, ranging from extreme in agricultural societies to virtually none in hunting and fishing peoples.

In Chapter 1, we discussed the method used by Coren and Porac (1977b) to study the distribution of handedness across a historical period of approximately 5,000 years. They observed the hand depicted as active in unimanual activities in artworks of various eras. We can use a similar procedure to obtain an estimate of the distribution of handedness across regions of the world by analyzing these same data as a function of the geographical origins of the pieces of art. Table 6-4 presents such an analysis. The results are given in order of increasing incidence rates, and as can be seen, the population percentages of depicted right-handedness vary from 88 to 96%. Although Coren and Porac (1977b) reported that there was no overall statistically significant geographical difference, consideration of the extreme values (Mediterranean Europe and the Middle East versus the Americas and Africa) leads to some statistically reliable comparisons. This result is suggestive of, although not strong support for, geographical differences in lateral preference. However, we explored this issue further and conducted a literature search for contemporary reports of distributions of lateral preference from a variety of different geographical regions.

Table 6-5 presents a number of studies published since 1950 that have looked at various aspects of lateral preference. We surveyed all aspects of lateral preference, rather than restricting ourselves to handedness, because although encountered less frequently, there are also social traditions associated with the right and the left foot, eye, and ear. For instance, it is considered disrespectful to enter a church starting with the left foot in several South American cultures (Wile, 1934). In a similar fashion, in Bali, a woman must enter a granary with the right foot (Elworthy, 1895), and the Egyptians used the left foot to enter

Table 6-4: Geographical Distribution of Handedness as Sampled from Artworks Spanning 5,000 Years

Region	Right-handedness (%)
The Americas	88.0
Africa	90.0
Far East	91.0
Central Asia	92.0
Central Europe	93.0
Mediterranean Europe	95.0
Middle East	96.0

Note. Based on Coren and Porac (1977b). Sample included 1,180 works of art.

Table 6-5: Cross-Cultural Comparisons of the Incidence of Right-Sidedness in Lateral Preference

Study	Country	Age group	Right (%)
Hand Preference			
Clark (1957)	Scotland	Children and adults	86.0
Sutton (1963)	Australia	Young adults	88.0
Porac & Coren (Ch. 3, this volume)	Canada and United States	Children and adults	88.2
Dawson (1977)	United States (Eskimos)	Adults	88.7
Dawson (1972)	Australia	Adults	89.5
Pelecanos (1969)	Greece	Children	89.7
Hardyck et al. (1975)	United States	Children	90.0
Dawson (1972)	Hong Kong	Adults	90.6
Sutton (1963)	Rarotonga	Young adults	91.0
Teng et al. (1979)	Taiwan	Children and adults	94.0
Beckman & Elston (1962)	Sweden	Adults	94.6
Dawson (1972)	Sierra Leone	Adults	96.6
Hatta & Nakatsuka (1975)	Japan	Adults	96.9
Rhoades & Damon (1973)	Solomon Islands	Children and adults	97.2
Dawson (1972)	Hong Kong	Adults	98.5
Verhaegen & Ntumba (1964)	Congo	Children	99.5
Foot preference			
Clark (1957)	Scotland	Children	72.0
Porac & Coren (Ch. 3, this volume)	Canada and United States	Children and adults	81.0
Teng et al. (1979)	Taiwan	Children and adults	87.0
Eye preference			
Clark (1957)	Scotland	Children	61.0
Dawson (1972)	Australia	Adults	61.6
Spong (1962)	Australia	Children	65.0
Nagamata (1951)	Japan	Children	65.0
Dawson (1972)	Sierra Leone	Adults	66.3
Teng et al. (1979)	Taiwan	Children and adults	68.5
Porac & Coren (Ch. 3, this volume)	Canada and United States	Children and adults	71.1
Hughes (1953)	Great Britain	Adults	82.0

Table 6.5 (continued)

Study	Country	Age group	Right (%)
Ear Preference			
Porac & Coren (Ch. 3, this volume)	Canada and United States	Children and adults	59.4
Sinclair (1968)	United States	Children	70.3
Clark (1957)	Scotland	Children	71.0

evil places (Westermarck, 1926). However, both the left eye and the left ear held the positions of honor for the Chinese (Granet, 1973).

Table 6-5 shows each index separately, and the entries are arranged in order of the increasing incidence of right-sidedness. There are differences in the distributions of dextrality among the various studies. The values fluctuate, with handedness and footedness showing cross-cultural variations of approximately 13-15%, eyedness 21%, and earedness 11%. These variations in dextrality rates could indicate that social pressure specific to a given culture alter the observed distributions of lateral preferences.

Unfortunately, a specific meaningful pattern does not emerge from the data in Table 6-5. The data do not confirm Dawson's (1977) agricultural-hunting social dichotomy hypothesis. However, the three reports of the lowest incidence rates of dextrality are from English-speaking countries that share common historical and cultural traditions. In these countries (Scotland, Australia, Canada, and the United States), there is no cultural stigma attached to left-handedness; no moral strictures or religious or cultural taboos have been applied to sinistral individuals. If it is noticed at all, left-handedness is looked upon as a bit of an annoyance. Cultures that show the greatest degree of dextrality in handedness, however, do not seem to have a clearly distinguishing characteristic related to lateral preference formation.

The data in Table 6-5 also could be used to provide evidence for the involvement of genetic and physiological variables. There may be systematic genetic differences among various geographical regions and cultural traditions, the most obvious of which are differences in racial characteristics, since these samples differ racially as well as culturally. For example, the hand preference section of Table 6-5 shows support for an interesting speculation. With an incidence rate of 90% right-handedness as a division point, one finds that six of the seven samples with incidence rates equal to or below this level are Caucasian, while eight of the nine samples with incidence rates greater than 90% are non-Caucasian. This finding may indicate a racially based biological mechanism affecting handedness that differs cross-culturally, rather than one that is environmentally based. This suggestion is only a speculation, since within-culture racial differences in handedness incidence rates have not been found (Thompson & Marsh, 1976); however, it does propose an interesting alternative viewpoint.

This chapter has focused on a number of individual difference variables, such as age, sex, family, and cultural environment. All of them affect the degrees of manifest right- and left-sidedness. Some of these individual differences may be the result of pressures placed on the individual in the form of overt or covert reinforcement contingencies that alter manifest right- and left-sidedness. While many of the data are consistent with the assumption that reinforcement and learning can affect manifest lateral preferences, and most obviously handedness, many of these data are inferential in nature. We cannot substantiate an assertion that the *only* determinant of lateral preference is the pressure of a right-sided environment and right-sided societal norms on the basis of the data available. If this were so, somewhere, at some locale, we would have found a predominantly left-sided culture, but no such culture has ever been reported. Rather, we must look at environmental factors, and learning, as variables that alter the distributions of manifest right- or left-sidedness in some groups of individuals, as a function of their life history and societal membership.

7

Birth Stress

Chapters 4, 5, and 6 addressed themselves to the major classes of theories that have attempted to explain why populations of humans are predominantly right sided. These explanations included physiological and neurological predispositions, genetic factors, and environmental and sociocultural pressures. Although each approach could muster fairly cogent arguments for the population's dextral bias, each had problems when attempting to explain the small but persistently recurring population of left-sided individuals. Left-siders are not clearly physiologically different; often they are born into families of right-sided parents, even where many previous generations have been right sided, and they are exposed to the same sociocultural and environmental pressures toward right-sidedness as dextrals. Yet they manifest sinistral tendencies, a fact that has puzzled many investigators. Somehow, despite the presence of the theoretically relevant factors, these individuals do not become right sided. Thus, it is not surprising that hypotheses were offered which explained sinistrality as an abnormal condition. In essence, these approaches are derived from the notion that the theories proposing universal right-sidedness are correct, and those individuals who do not conform to these theories are pathological. The particular mechanism of this inferred pathology and the nature of its action have varied from one theoretical position to another.

The contention that left-sidedness represents some form of physiological, neurological, or behavioral aberration has a long history, and it will manifest itself in a variety of different forms in the discussions in Chapters 8, 9, and 10. Some of the theoretical positions that we will discuss in these chapters will be rather extreme, associating sinistrality with almost every imaginable behavioral malady from slow reading to clumsiness and bed-wetting, and finally to retardation and criminality. The rationales that link each of these behaviors to left-sidedness differ, but they all begin with the presumption that left-sidedness must be explained in pathological terms. Several observations and assumptions are characteristic of pathological approaches to left-sidedness. Most assume that physiological and/or genetic factors render all typical individuals right sided.

The general mechanism presumed to mediate this right-sidedness is some form of left hemisphere dominance or control, expressed in the form of one of the theoretical positions discussed in Chapter 4. Left-sidedness emerges as a consequence of some physiological trauma or insult that disrupts the normal processes that result in dextrality.

Since most left-sided individuals do not manifest obvious evidence of neuropathy, the argument maintains that the hypothesized damage was relatively slight or subtle, or that it must have occurred early enough in the individual's life so that the normally plastic developmental processes partially compensated for the damage. If one does not include this theoretical modification, one is left with the necessity of accounting for the large numbers of sinistrals who have risen to prominence in the arts, sciences, politics, and sports. For instance, Leonardo da Vinci was left handed, as were, according to tradition, Julius Caesar, Alexander the Great, and Charlemagne. Three Presidents of the United States, Harry Truman, Gerald Ford, and Ronald Reagan, numerous musicians such as Cole Porter, and two of the Beatles, Paul McCartney and Ringo Starr, as well as many actors such as Charlie Chaplin, Harpo Marx, and Rock Hudson, have been and are left handed. The list also includes artists (Pablo Picasso and Paul Klee), sportsmen (Ted Williams and Babe Ruth), and even Queen Victoria. All were unusual but not abnormal. The two presumptions of a physiological basis for dextrality and a subtle pathology that must be inferred are characteristics of most pathological theories of sinistrality.

The position that we will consider in this chapter has been explicated by Bakan and his associates. They maintain that left-sidedness results from physiological trauma occurring during stressful births. Bakan (1971b, 1977, 1978) specifically suggests a relationship between left-handedness and brain damage resulting from birth trauma. He contends that oxygen deprivation to the brain is associated with some forms of birth trauma, such as breech birth, prolonged labor, multiple births, or Rh incompatibilities. This oxygen deficit can have an adverse effect on pyramidal system cells in the left motor cortex and he provides evidence that such hypoxia is more frequent in difficult births. In addition, there is evidence that the left hemisphere is more vulnerable to the effects of hypoxia than the right hemisphere. For example, some investigators suggest that focal lesions are more likely to appear in the left cerebral hemisphere (Geschwind & Levitsky, 1968; McRae, Branch, & Milner, 1968). Even with an equal likelihood for damage to both hemispheres, evidence that the functions of the right hemisphere are represented more diffusely than those of the left hemisphere (DeRenzi & Faglioni, 1967; Semmes, 1968) has led to the conclusion that shifts in cerebral function from the left hemisphere to the right are more likely than shifts in the opposite direction (Schonblum, 1977). If there is any undetected or undetectable cerebral pathology, then it is more likely to affect the left hemisphere, causing a shift toward right hemisphere functional control. Since Bakan accepts the notion of right-handedness because of left-brainedness, one concomitant of such a shift is tendency toward sinistrality in unilateral behaviors. This type of pathological left-handedness would not be associated with the appearance of gross pathology. Although pyramidal lesions may cause an initial contralateral motor weakness or paralysis, the overt symptoms are transient, and these types of behavioral manifestations might be overlooked in a very young infant. Thus, the change in hand preference (or side preference) may be the only residual effect of the birth trauma and hypoxia. A research strategy associated with such reasoning involves the separation of individuals into groups according to risk factors that could be associated with an increased likelihood of undetected pathology. One then ascertains whether these risk factors are predictive of differences in patterns of lateral preference. Some direct evidence has resulted from this approach but much of it is also inferential.

Bakan (1978) has suggested several indirect variables that designate groups at high risk for birth stress. An example of conditions that could increase the probability of birth difficulty is the presence in the womb of another fetus, as in the case of twin and other multiple births. Thus Bakan (1978) predicts the existence of a higher incidence of left-handedness in twin pairs than is found in the general population. Investigators generally believe that twin pairs show more sinistrality of hand preference (see Springer & Deutsch, 1981; Springer & Searleman, 1980); however, the supportive data are ambiguous. Table 7-1 presents the incidence of observed left-handedness in groups of monozygotic (MZ) and dizygotic (DZ) twins reported in a number of studies. Since the Bakan hypothesis does not predict greater birth risk for one type of twin, we have summed across the MZ and DZ twin groups. The mean reported incidence of left-handedness in these studies is 14%, an average value that is consistent with three other reports that undertook a similar literature analysis (Carter-Saltzman, Scarr-Salapatek, Barker, & Katz, 1976; McManus, 1980; Springer & Searleman, 1980). The contemporary population incidence figures for left-handedness are approxi-

Table 7-1: Observed Incidence of Left-Handedness in MZ and DZ Twins as Reported in Published Studies from 1920 to the Present

Study	Left-handedness reported (%)
Gordon (1921)	12
Siemens (1924)	22
Lauterbach (1925)	11
Dahlberg (1926)	11
Verschuer (1927)	15
Newman (1928)	12
Wilson & Jones (1932)	11
Stocks (1933)	10
Newman, Freeman, & Holzinger (1937)	17
Rife (1939)	13
Carter-Saltzman et al. (1976)	19
Springer & Searleman (1980)	17
McManus (1980)	15
Mean	14

mately 13% (see Chapter 3); thus, the average incidence in twin pairs is equivalent to that found in the general population. The notion that left-handedness occurs more frequently in twins is often supported by specific comparisons to single births (see Springer & Searleman, 1980). However, if one re-analyzes the familial handedness data presented in Table 5-3 and computes the incidence of left-handedness in the data of the singleton offspring reported there, one finds that it is approximately 18%. Once again, this value is similar to the incidence rates reported in several of the twin studies listed in Table 7-1. Thus, contemporary estimates of the incidence of left-handedness in the general population and in groups of single-born offspring do not differ from those reported in twin populations. The earlier reports of increased sinistrality in twin samples may have been confounded by the existence of age-related trends in lateral preference (see Chapters 3 and 6). A report by Teng, Lee, Yang, and Chang (1976) supports this contention. They found that twins showed greater sinistrality than nontwins when elementary school-aged groups were compared. There was, however, no difference when twin and nontwin college students were studied. In the present context, it seems that this form of birth stress does not produce the marked increase in sinistrality expected and predicted by Bakan (1978).

In an effort to establish an empirical link between birth stress and sinistrality, Bakan (1971b) attempted to demonstrate a relationship between the incidence of left-handedness and birth order. He contended that firstborn children, or children born in the fourth or later positions, were more likely to suffer from birth stresses of some type, such as prolonged labor or instrument deliveries. In support of this notion, medical statistics show that birth order is related to such factors as fetal growth rate and birth weight, as well as to the risk of stillbirth (Montagu, 1962). Bakan (1971b) measured handedness in college students and found the expected increase in left-handedness as a function of birth order. Although there has been one report that replicates this result (Leviton & Kilty, 1976) and another partial replication (Bakan, 1977), the overall pattern of data on this relationship has been negative. Other investigators have failed to find any association between birth order and left-handedness (Hicks, Evans, & Pellegrini, 1978; Hicks, Pellegrini, & Evans, 1978; Hicks, Pellegrini, Evans, & Moore, 1979; Hubbard, 1971; Schwartz, 1977; Teng, Lee, Yang, & Chang, 1976).

We felt that this issue needed further study to clarify some of the inconsistencies in the available data. Larger samples and data collected with a common measurement instrument might uncover a relationship between birth order and handedness. From a theoretical viewpoint, data on the occurrence of foot, eye, and ear preference would also be useful in this context if one extends the arguments to predict a relationship between birth trauma and any manifestation of left-sidedness. With the inclusion of all types of lateral preference, one can evaluate how birth process variables affect the incidence of congruent-sidedness (all indexes aligned on the right or on the left side). This aspect of the investigation could be enlightening, since several theories postulate that deviations from completely right-sided preference patterns represent the influence of some sort of pathological disruption (Critchley, 1970; Delacato, 1963; Orton, 1937; Zangwill, 1960).

We obtained responses from 2,761 individuals using the behaviorally validated questionnaire shown in Table 3-1. The subjects ranged in age from 15 to 40 years of age. They also indicated their birth order as well as their lateral preferences. Figure 7-1 shows the data that we obtained. The percentage of the sample classified as right sided (according to the criteria described in Chapter 3) for the various birth positions is shown for the four lateral preference indexes (Coren & Porac, 1980a). There is no systematic relationship between birth order and the appearance of left-sidedness for any of the indexes. If we replot the figure in terms of overall right- versus left-sidedness, we again find no systematic shift in the number of individuals who are congruently right sided across all four indexes as a function of birth order (Figure 7-2).

We explored the relationship between birth order and patterns of sidedness further by grouping the data according to the premise that first- and fourth- or later-born offspring are at higher risk for difficulties than those in the middle positions (Bakan, 1971b, 1978). Table 7-2 shows the incidence of right-sidedness and congruent-sidedness when the data are grouped in this way. None of the comparisons between the high and the low risk birth positions differ significantly. Our analyses suggests that birth order by itself does not predict the appearance of sinistrality on any of the indexes of lateral preference, nor does it predict cross-index congruency.

Both maternal and paternal age have also been shown to be factors that might affect the risk of prenatal and perinatal birth trauma. Lesinski (1975) reviewed 22 studies on birth risk and concluded that mothers 30 years of age or older were above the median risk of having stillbirths, offspring with congenital malformations, and prolonged labor. The data showed a steady trend in the likelihood of such birth problems with increases in the mother's age. Broman, Nichols, and Kennedy (1975) measured 168 variables and 26,760 children and concluded that the optimal age at the time of birth is between 20 and 29 years for Caucasian mothers, with older mothers showing a much higher percentage of delivery problems. Parental age is also relevant to genetic hypotheses, since studies have

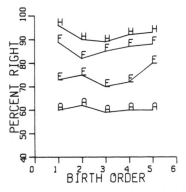

Figure 7-1. Percentage of right-sided subjects as a function of birth order position for four indexes of lateral preference (H is hand; F, foot; E, eye; A, ear).

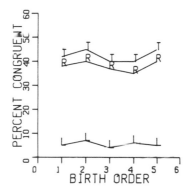

Figure 7-2. Percentage of congruently right- or left-sided subjects as a function of birth order position (R is congruently right sided; L, congruently left sided; T, total percentage of sample that is congruent).

shown that there is a significant correlation between aging and chromosomal changes in normal individuals of both sexes (Court-Brown, Jacobs, & Tough, 1967; Court-Brown, Jacobs, Buckton, Tough, Kuenssberg, & Knox, 1966). As a consequence, abnormalities in offspring based on chromosomal factors increase as a function of advancing parental age (Levitan & Montagu, 1971; Matsunaga, 1973; Polednak, 1976; Selvin & Garfinkel, 1972). Variations in the lateral preference of an offspring as a function of maternal age may arise from increased risk of birth stress due to an older mother, or from chromosomal changes, while

Table 7-2: Percentage of Right-Sidedness, Congruent-Sidedness, and Crossed-Sidedness as a Function of Birth Risk

	Total sample (%)		Males (%)		Females (%)	
	High risk[a]	Low risk[b]	High risk	Low risk	High risk	Low risk
Hand	89.4	88.8	89.0	88.1	89.8	89.3
Foot	81.8	79.5	81.8	79.0	82.3	80.0
Eye	73.1	73.4	73.3	73.0	72.8	73.6
Ear	60.3	60.1	59.9	59.9	60.3	60.5
All Indexes						
Congruent	42.9	44.4	41.5	42.6	44.6	45.8
Right	37.8	38.9	37.0	37.0	39.0	40.5
Left	5.1	5.5	4.6	5.6	5.6	5.4
Crossed	57.2	55.6	58.5	57.4	55.4	54.2

Note. No differences as a function of birth risk are statistically significant; $N =$ 2,761.

[a] High risk for birth stress is defined as first- or fourth- and later-born offspring.
[b] Low risk for birth stress is defined as second- and third-born offspring.

covariations of lateral preference with paternal age would most likely arise from chromosomal factors.

If maternal age is an index of birth stress risk and hence potential pathology, there is a suggestion of a relationship between birth stress and lateral preference. For example, Bakan, Dibb, and Reed (1973) reported that 17% of left-handers and ambilaterals in their sample were firstborn offspring of mothers over 30 years of age, while only 8% of the right-handers were included in this category. Although the report of Smart, Jeffery, and Richards (1980) generally supports this finding, other investigators have failed to confirm a relationship between maternal age and lateral preference (Hicks et al., 1979; Teng et al., 1976). Again, the equivocal nature of the data seemed to warrant further study.

Using the lateral preference inventory shown in Table 3-1, 506 individuals indicated hand, foot, eye, and ear preference, their own age, and the age of their mother and father (from which we computed parental age at the time of the subjects' birth). Father's age had no effect on manifestations either of right- and left-sidedness within each index, or of congruency of sidedness across indexes. However, as Table 7-3 shows, the picture is slightly different when considering maternal age. The data in Table 7-3 are again based on those presented by Coren and Porac (1980a) and show that mothers of left-handers are slightly older at the time of birth than mothers of right handers, with a strong relationship for male offspring in both hand and foot preference. Left-eyed individuals seem also to be born of older mothers, and another relationship emerges when the pattern across indexes is considered. Congruently left-sided individuals have mothers who were significantly older at the time of birth than congruently right-sided respondents. Thus, the maternal age birth risk factor seems to be affecting the incidence of leftness in hand and eye preference and in the congruency

Table 7-3: Mean Maternal Age in Years at Time of Birth for Left- and Right-Sided and for Congruent- and Crossed-Sided Offspring

	Total sample (N=506)		Males (N=269)		Females (N=237)	
	Right	Left	Right	Left	Right	Left
Hand	28.4[a]	30.1[a]	27.4[a]	30.6[a]	29.3	29.7
Foot	28.6	29.3	27.9[a]	29.8[a]	29.2	29.0
Eye	28.2[a]	30.1[a]	27.8	29.9	28.6	30.4
Ear	29.5	29.0	27.8	27.8	29.2	29.3

All Indexes

	Total sample (N=506)	Males (N=269)	Females (N=237)
Congruent	28.3	27.7	28.8
Right	27.8[b]	27.0	28.4
Left	31.5[b]	31.4	31.6
Crossed	29.0	28.6	29.4

[a] Right versus left difference significant, $p < .05$.
[b] Right versus left difference significant, $p < .01$.

across the four indexes for the total sample as well as the incidence of leftness in hand and foot preference for the male subsample.

The size of the sample allowed us to divide the group by birth order position as well as maternal age at the time of birth, and this analysis is shown in Table 7-4. Once again, first- and fourth- or later-born individuals are classified as high risk, while second- and third-born offspring are called low risk. The age of the mother at the time of birth is dichotomized into two categories, 29 years or less and 30 years or older. This maternal age dichotomy is based on research showing that the optimal maternal age for minimal birth risk is between 20 and 29 years, with the risk of birth difficulties increasing after the age of 30 (Broman, Nichols, & Kennedy, 1975; Lesinski, 1975). The entries in Table 7-4 indicate the observed percentage of right-sidedness, congruent-sidedness, and crossed sidedness among the respondents as a function of both birth order position and maternal age at birth. It seems that these two birth risk factors do interact; older mothers have fewer right-handed or right-eyed offspring, although this effect is limited to the second and third birth order positions (low risk positions). The effect is repeated in the male and the female groups, although it is found in only one index for each, and again is limited to those positions defined as low risk. There seems to be no effect on or interaction between these two variables that alters the incidence of congruent-sidedness and crossed sidedness.

These data support the notion that parental age and birth order are birth risk factors that affect incidences of right- and left-sidedness. However, this statement must be qualified considerably in light of these findings. For example, birth order produces fluctuations in the incidence of left-sidedness only when maternal age at birth is taken into account. Also, only handedness and eyedness seem to be affected; the other indexes are not altered. The values presented in Tables 7-2, 7-3, and 7-4 indicate that maternal age at birth is the most significant birth stress variable that we have studied, but its relationship to lateral preference incidence rates is very specific. In addition, it does not interact with the birth order variable in a manner predicted from Bakan et al. (1973); instead, we found an increased incidence of left-handedness and left-eyedness exhibited in offspring of older mothers in the low risk birth positions.

Bakan, Dibb, and Reed (1973) took a somewhat more direct approach in order to assess the relationship between birth trauma and handedness. They asked college students to report whether or not they knew of any difficulty (premature birth, prolonged labor, Caesarean delivery, breech birth, and so forth) associated with their own birth in addition to reporting on their handedness behaviors. The results indicated that left-handed and ambilateral university students were more likely to report birth stress for themselves or for other family members than were right-handed individuals. This seemed to confirm some relationship between birth stress and sinistrality. Additional evidence for the involvement of birth factors in the formation of handedness comes from Churchill, Igna, and Senf (1962). They observed that children born with the less typical head positioning, where the right occipital portion of the head is forward, were more likely to be left handed than were children born in the more common posture with the left occipital portion of the skull forward.

Table 7-4: Percentage of Right-Sidedness, Congruent-Sidedness, and Crossed-Sidedness Shown by Birth Risk and Maternal Age

| | Total sample (%) | | | | Males (%) | | | | Females (%) | | | |
| | High risk | | Low risk | | High risk | | Low risk | | High risk | | Low risk | |
Maternal age (years)	≤29	≥30	≤29	≥30	≤29	≥30	≤29	≥30	≤29	≥30	≤29	≥30
Hand	84.9	89.4	86.7[a]	77.2[a]	82.7	88.1	88.5[a]	69.6[a]	86.4	90.4	84.9	82.9
Foot	86.7	88.3	77.6	79.7	86.8	79.1	72.1	78.1	86.2	96.1	81.6	80.6
Eye	68.3	73.7	74.8[a]	60.7[a]	78.6	76.7	72.1	62.1	58.5	71.2[a]	76.7[a]	58.8[a]
Ear	62.8	63.8	63.6	60.3	64.2	63.4	61.3	50.0	61.0	64.2	63.6	69.0
All Indexes												
Congruent	50.3	50.0	51.2	50.0	55.9	52.9	50.6	38.1	45.9	47.1	50.9	59.3
Right	45.8	47.1	43.9	37.5	50.0	52.9	41.4	23.8	42.4	41.2	44.7	48.1
Left	4.5	2.9	7.3	12.5	5.9	0.0	9.2	14.3	3.5	5.9	6.1	11.1
Crossed	49.7	50.0	48.8	50.0	44.2	47.0	49.4	61.9	54.1	53.0	49.1	40.7

Note. High risk for birth stress is defined as first- and fourth- or later-born offspring; low risk is second and third birth order positions; N = 506.

[a] Significant difference, p < 0.05.

Smart et al. (1980) report increased left-handedness in breech born children; however, Schwartz (1977) was unable to replicate the relationship between birth stress and left-handedness using measures of birth complications similar to those of Bakan et al. (1973).

Again, the pattern of data presents an equivocal picture. Some studies report relationships between birth stress and left-handedness (or at least find elevated percentages of sinistrality in groups that might be more susceptible to birth stress), while other studies do not. In addition, all of the existing studies have limited themselves methodologically by using somewhat indirect measures and by limiting the lateral preference measures to handedness. It is the indirectness of the measures of birth complications that is a bothersome aspect of these data. If we ask adults about their own births and complications associated with their births, we are dealing with secondhand retrospective reports by the very nature of the information required. One must be told, at a considerably later time, of any difficulties surrounding one's own birth. On the other hand, mothers themselves would be quite aware of the events surrounding the births of each offspring, especially if any were marked by unusual circumstances. The more direct method of acquiring data on this issue is to obtain maternal reports on the births of their various offspring, and direct offspring measures of lateral preference, which is what we did in our study (Coren & Porac, 1980a).

We contacted by mail approximately 4,000 families, and each mother was asked to answer a questionnaire containing items about various difficulties or complications involved in the births of each of her children. The birth stress factors that were listed were premature birth, prolonged labor, breech birth, blue baby or breathing difficulty at birth, low birth weight, Caesarian delivery, multiple births, RH incompatibility, and finally, instrument births or other medical difficulties. Mothers were asked to complete this questionnaire for each offspring. The children, who were available in the home or who were contacted at their university, were asked to complete the self-report battery shown in Table 3-1. This survey resulted in data on both lateral preferences and possible birth stress for 1,410 college-aged individuals, which is shown in Table 7-5. The only significant effect of birth stress is found in the incidence of handedness in males. There is a 7% increase in left-handedness in the male group where mothers have reported a stressful birth. There is no significant effect for any other index of lateral preference or for the relationship between the various indexes.

What can be said about the relationship between birth stress and the formation of sidedness behaviors? Systematic investigation of this association using the types of variables suggested by Bakan and others have not provided overwhelming evidence in favor of birth stress variables as a major influence in the determination of sidedness. Considering the number of comparisons that have been made, we have been able to derive only a significant effect of maternal age at birth (limited to handedness, eyedness, and congruent left-sidedness) and of direct assessments of birth stress (limited to handedness in males). If we can make any general statement, it is that the incidence of right-handedness in males is likely to be reduced when the predisposing variables of birth stress are present.

Table 7-5: Percentage of Offspring Classified as Right Sided, Congruent Sided, or Crossed Sided as a Function of Maternal Report of Birth Stress (N=1,410)

	Total sample (%)		Males (%)		Females (%)	
	Birth stress	No birth stress	Birth stress	No birth stress	Birth stress	No birth stress
Hand	87.7	89.5	81.8[a]	89.0[a]	91.5	89.7
Foot	82.1	83.8	76.4	80.4	86.6	87.1
Eye	71.6	73.4	70.1	75.6	59.3	65.7
Ear	58.7	61.9	58.3	58.3	58.6	64.9
All Indexes						
Congruent	38.3	40.1	38.4	37.6	38.8	42.4
Right	32.8	35.1	30.8	31.9	34.8	37.9
Left	5.4	5.0	7.6	5.7	4.0	4.5
Crossed	61.8	59.9	61.6	62.4	61.2	57.6

[a] Effect of birth stress significant, $p < .05$.

The overall pattern of evidence obtained when addressing a possible relationship between birth stress and lateral preference is similar to patterns that will be encountered in future chapters; hence, it warrants some general consideration in terms of its theoretical salience. Certainly some relationship between variables presumed to be indicators of potential birth traumas and variations in lateral preference has been shown. However, the pattern of data is scattered. Some of the variables (such as maternal age and direct reports of birth stress) produce shifts in the distribution of lateral preference, whereas other variables (e.g., birth order) show no effects. Furthermore, even when effects are found, they are limited in nature. For example, the effects seem to be confined predominantly to handedness, and even then they are often sex specific. Thus the results can only be considered as suggestive, neither directly proving nor refuting the theoretical position.

Such scattered patterns of evidence do not usually withstand the rigors of analysis at the theoretical level. Certainly it is difficult to use these data to substantiate Bakan's theory of a specific mechanism of causation, namely, that hypoxia-induced damage to the left hemisphere occurring during the birth process results in a change of handedness from right to left. We cannot adopt this position at present for several reasons. First, the discussion in Chapter 4 has shown that the relationship between a cerebral speech organization and the formation of handedness is far from a settled issue. In fact, Kimura (1976) has stated that cerebral localization for speech processing functions and handedness control may or may not reside in the same hemisphere. The notion that damage to a "dominant" hemisphere, resulting only in a switch in handedness with no other overt signs of impairment, requires that one assume a causal and a necessary connection between right-handedness and left-brainedness. At the minimum, such a theory requires a similar pattern of shifts toward left-footedness, since motor control of both hand and foot reside in the same hemisphere. Such a pattern simply does not manifest itself in the available data. Thus, the type of data that have been discussed here can only suggest possible relationships; they cannot pinpoint mechanisms of causation that would assist in our understanding of how sidedness behaviors do or do not develop normally.

The notion still persists that left-sidedness is atypical and represents an abnormality. It will appear in many forms in the following chapters. Therefore, it is important to look at the details of the argument to see if they can be substantiated in order to ascertain whether or not we are dealing with a correlational result in search of a mechanism. An example will help to clarify this point. Leviton and Kilty (1979) recently reported that the birth of left-handed females displays a seasonal trend. The peak incidence of the birth of left-handers seems to occur in November in their data. Within the tradition that sinistrality is a "soft sign" of abnormality, they quickly proposed a physiological trauma argument to explain this result. They speculate that there are seasonal variations in the exposure to infectious agents and to temperature extremes. These factors might affect the developing organism in a manner that contributes to the larger deviation from the dextral norm found in individuals born at this time of year. This speculation exemplifies some of the theorizing that has been and will be encountered in later chapters. The covariation of the birth of left-handers and the season of the year is an interesting finding; however, it simply does not provide adequate data to allow one to focus on a specific causal mechanism for lateral preference, and certainly not on one that postulates the role of physiological damage. One could as easily propose that a child born near the harvest season, where there is an increase in the availability of fresh fruits and nuts, is better nourished and healthier prior to birth. Thus, the more natural and healthy pattern of sinistrality is more likely to emerge. Neither position has much to recommend it, since one is faced only with the existence of a seasonal correlation. That the abnormality or stress hypothesis was the one offered, however, does indicate a pattern of thought frequently found to be most acceptable to researchers. Dextrality is the norm, hence sinistrality is abnormal. In the next chapter there are clearer examples of this line of reasoning.

8

Special Populations

The left hand is weak and awkward for the typical right-handed individual. When forced to do something with the left hand, a typical right-hander will almost invariably perform the task less adequately. Considerations such as these may have led the right-handed majority to look upon the left hand as inferior, or perhaps even evil. Such an attitude is reflected in many ways, as demonstrated in Chapter 6. The moral and religious encoding of this notion is particularly interesting. Christianity demonstrates its bias against the left in the Gospel according to St. Matthew (Chapter 25) in the parable of the sheep and the goats. In this vision of Judgment Day, God gathers before Him all of the people of the world, and He divides them into two groups, one on the right side and the other on the left. Then, according to the Bible, He designates the relative value of the two sides: "Then shall the King say unto them on His right, 'Come ye blessed of my Father, inherit the Kingdom prepared for you from the foundation of the world. . . .' Then shall He say unto them on the left hand, 'Depart from me, ye cursed, into everlasting fire, prepared for the Devil and his angels.'" This point of view is not confined to Christianity, since the Buddha made it clear that there were two roads through life. There is a left road, which is fraught with peril and is of ill omen, and an eightfold right path, which is of good omen. Perhaps it was such a context of religious antipathy toward the left that led to the opinion that the left-handed individual is also suspect. Left-handedness was referred to by a philosopher in 1686 as a "digression or aberration from that way which nature generally intendeth" (quoted in Wile, 1934, p. 92). This viewpoint indicates that left-handedness should be regarded as direct evidence for some pathology or abnormality.

The association between left-sidedness and pathology was introduced in Chapter 7, which discussed the nature of some of the birth stress hypotheses, their supposed relationships with incidence of sinistrality, and the neurological considerations that have guided research into the problem. Initial theorizing about the "pathological left-hander" tended to be emotional, and often seems somewhat extreme (if not bizarre) in light of contemporary knowledge. In the context of early research efforts, many prodextral or antisinistral statements were offered on the basis of very little data. One of the more dramatic examples is that of Lombroso (1903):

> To understand the exact significance of this research it is necessary to know that a greater tendency to asymmetry is seen in the animal species the nearer they approach man and the more perfect they are. . . . Therefore, as man advances in civilization and culture, he shows an always greater right sidedness as compared to savages.

He then presented some data that have served as the prototype for many later studies. He reported that the incidence of left-handedness is elevated in mentally defective and criminal populations. On this basis he concluded, "I do not dream at all that all left handed people are wicked, but that left-handedness, united to many other traits, may contribute to form one of the worst characteristics among the human species."

Given such an atmosphere, it is not surprising that many studies early in this century turned to comparisons of the relative distribution of lateral preference in normal and atypical or pathologically affected samples. The results of these studies tended to support the presumed association between the incidence of left-handedness and atypicalities of neural and behavioral development. In addition, it supported the contention that left-handedness (and other forms of left-sidedness) is the result of some type of damage to the organism. Although much contemporary work agrees with this conclusion, a number of restrictions and limitations have now been applied to this position.

Neurological Injury

If one makes two assumptions, that dextral preference is the norm and that lateral preference is primarily determined by cerebral and neurological asymmetries, one has a basis for expecting an increased incidence of sinistrality in neurologically impaired or brain-injured groups. Satz (1972, 1973) has offered a simple model to explain how such an increased incidence in atypical samples may occur. The Satz model, in a manner similar to the Bakan (1977, 1978) hypothesis discussed in Chapter 7, presupposes that various forms of neuropathy, pathology, or neurological insult can result in shifts in lateral preference behaviors. While Satz maintains that this resulting shift occurs because of some change in hemispheric dominance, such as that observed in recovery following infantile hemispherectomies (see Dennis & Whitaker, 1977; Witelson, 1977), he also offers a mathematical model that is independent of the actual physiological basis of lateral preferences. It is dependent only on the presumption that pathological interventions can alter the observed pattern of lateral preferences in an individual, and that the original population shows an initial asymmetrical distribution, predominantly dextral.

The Satz (1972, 1973) model works in the following way. Suppose, for example, that the population distribution of handedness is 90% right and 10% left. In addition, imagine that some pathological intervention involving the neural control mechanisms for handedness causes 10% of the population to switch to the side opposite their naturally physiologically determined side of preference. This process causes 10% of the natural right-handed group (9% of the total population) to switch to left-hand use and 10% of the natural left-handers (1% of the population total) to become right handed as a result of the neural pathology. This switching process is illustrated in Figure 8-1, where the circles represent individuals with naturally determined (nonpathological) preference and the squares represent the proportion of individuals in the pathologically determined preference group. In this example, we obtain a final population distribution of 82% right-handedness and 18% left-handedness. However, if we now look at the relative proportion of pathological and nonpathological individuals in the right- and the left-handed samples, 50% of the left-handers are displaying this behavior because of pathologically caused switches in sidedness, whereas only 1.2% of the right-handers are in this category. If this hypothetical population was divided on the basis of right- versus left-handedness, the probability of finding a pathological individual in the left-handed group would be approximately 42 times greater than the probability of finding one among the right-handers.

The Satz (1972, 1973) model depends strongly on two factors. The first is the relative asymmetry in lateral preferences as they appear in the initial population, and the second is the percentage of individuals who are shifted pathologically from a left to a right preference. Table 8-1 shows the effects of variations in these two variables. With an initial population of 90% dextral and 10% sinistral, with 10% undergoing a pathological shift, 1.2% of the final population of right-handers are pathologically determined, while 50% of the population of left-handers are sinistral because of pathology. This, of course, is the example that we described in the preceding paragraph. However, as the left-right asymmetry in

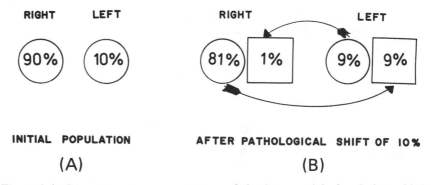

Figure 8-1. Diagrammatic representation of the Satz model of pathological left-sidedness, where circles represent percentages of normal individuals and squares represent pathologically affected individuals.

the initial population becomes less extreme, the difference in the percentage of pathological individuals among the left-versus the right-sided individuals becomes less pronounced. For example, a population of 70% right-siders and 30% left-siders produces a final population of right-siders of whom 4.5% are pathologically determined, and a population of left-siders of whom 20.6% are pathological. With a 90-10% split in the population, we are 42 times more likely to find a pathological left-sider than a pathological right-sider. With a 70-30% dichotomy, this proportional difference is reduced and now there is only a 4.6 times greater likelihood of finding a pathological left-sider as opposed to a pathological right-sider.

We have been considering a pathology that switches the sidedness of 10% of the population. This is, of course, an extremely high and rather unreasonable percentage of affected individuals; a more reasonable, yet still generous, estimate might be that 1% of the population would be affected in this way. When we reduced the likelihood of experiencing a pathological shift in sidedness, we increase the probability of finding a pathological left-sider as opposed to a pathological right-sider. This effect is illustrated in Table 8-1. With a 1% incidence of a pathological shift in preference and a 90-10% population dichotomy, 8.3% of the population of left-siders is pathologically determined, whereas only 0.1% of the population of right-siders is affected in this fashion. Although we have markedly decreased the likelihood that a pathological individual will be found, the ratio of pathological lefts to pathological rights is greatly increased. With a 10% switch factor we are 42 times more likely to find a pathological left-sider than a pathological right-sider; with a 1% switch factor, we are 83 times more likely to find a pathological left as opposed to a pathological right.

Satz (1972, 1973) restricted himself to explaining pathologically induced handedness; however, this type of analysis can be carried out for all of the indexes of lateral preference. For instance, Porac and Coren (1976) applied this

Table 8-1: Variations in the Predicted Distribution of Pathological Left- and Right-Sidedness as a Function of the Original Population Distribution of Sidedness and the Likelihood of Occurrence of a Pathologically Induced Switch in the Side of Preference

Initial population distribution (%)		10% likelihood of pathological switch			1% likelihood of pathological switch		
Right-siders (%)	Left-siders (%)	Pathological right-siders (%)	Pathological left-siders (%)	Ratio L/R	Pathological right-siders (%)	Pathological left-siders (%)	Ratio L/R
90	10	1.2	50.0	41.7	0.1	8.3	83.0
80	20	2.7	30.8	11.4	0.3	3.9	13.0
70	30	4.5	20.6	4.6	0.4	2.3	5.8
60	40	6.9	14.3	2.1	0.7	1.5	2.1

model to eyedness. Since the other indexes of lateral preference show a less pronounced asymmetry or dextral bias, it is likely that the relative proportion of pathological left-siders found in these indexes of preference will be less pronounced than that reported for handedness, as the statistical considerations in Table 8-1 indicate. The most important thing to recognize about applications of the Satz model to such situations (in order to explain the higher incidence of pathological left-sided individuals) is that this model works, regardless of the nature of the pathological intervention encountered and regardless of one's theory of the etiology of lateral preferences. All that is required is a skewed population distribution and some form of abnormality capable of causing a fixed percentage of the population to alter their lateral preferences. Thus it is actually a descriptive, rather than a theoretically based, model.

This type of reasoning does not brand all sinistrals as suffering from some sort of neural pathology or brain injury. It distinguishes between constitutionally left-preferent individuals (presumably born with natural left-sided tendencies) and pathologically left-preferent individuals (Jordan, 1922; Lattes, 1907; Satz, 1972, 1973). Also, it makes the implicit presumption that the pathological condition that caused the shift in lateral preference occurred at an early enough age for the plasticity in the neural system to allow the contralateral side to assume effective control. Furthermore, the injury would not be so great as to paralyze permanently or to deform the side that would have been preferred naturally. This notion was expressed earlier in this century by Brewster (1913), who maintained that

> An adult brain, wrecked on the educated side by accident or disease, commonly never learns to do its work on the other; the victim remains crippled for the rest of his days. But a child in whom the thinking area on the other side is still uncultivated, hurt on one side, can usually start over again with the other. A shift of this sort carries the body with it, and the child, instead of being permanently disabled, becomes left handed. (p. 179)

An early attempt to study the effect of obvious brain damage on handedness was by Sachs and Peterson (1890), who tabulated data from 156 hemiplegic patients. They reported that 48% of their sample was left handed. Later, Doll (1933) reported that 33% of a sample with cerebral lesions was left handed as compared to a 12% incidence of left-handedness in an institutional control group of similar age and intelligence. There are several early studies on laterality in epileptic populations that also show elevated sinistrality in groups of affected individuals. Redlich (1908, as cited in Bingley, 1958) reported that 17.5% of his epileptic patients were left handed as opposed to 8% in his control group. Similar data have been offered by Stier (1911, as cited in Hecaen & de Ajuriaguerra, 1964) and in a number of more contemporary reports (Bolin, 1953; Hecaen & Piercy, 1956; Roberts, 1955). Other suggestive evidence comes from Chayatte, Abern, Reddy, & Bottichelli (1979), who observed 64 patients with electro-encephalographic signs of brain pathology. They found that 53% of them were left handed, which is about five times the normal incidence of sinistrality.

Psychopathy, Emotional Instability, and Criminality

In the preceding section, we explored the possibility that left-sidedness might be more prevalent in individuals with certain forms of neurological insult. We were able to observe that sinistrality was, in fact, more frequent in some groups with severe forms of brain trauma, and we discussed a model that predicted such an association, although it did not actually specify a mechanism. There are many other conditions, however, where we can infer the existence of some sort of pathology, although we may not be able to isolate any particular neurological disruption. For example, if one considers groups of individuals who show various forms of cognitive and behavioral disruptions, including learning disabilities, mental retardation, or various forms of psychopathy, one might infer that some form of pathological intervention has been responsible for the observed abnormal cognitive and emotional functioning. Without isolating the particular abnormality involved (the model does not require this), one still may suggest that the same pathology that caused the cognitive malfunctioning may be of sufficient severity to alter the normal pattern of lateral preferences. If that is the case, then the Satz (1972, 1973) model is sufficient to predict that there will be a higher proportion of left-sided individuals who will fall into the pathological groups.

If there is some neurological insult that disrupts normal psychological functioning, a number of behavioral manifestations may become apparent. For heuristic purposes, we can separate these behavioral syndromes into two general classes. The first class involves affective dysfunctions, while the second involves cognitive malfunctions affecting the intellect. The affective dysfunctions are of the type often associated with neurotic behavior, psychopathy, sociopathy, violence, and a number of other factors that often bring individuals into conflict with societal norms or cause them to show general signs of emotional maladjustment. This affective cluster of disorders is predominantly emotional and is not necessarily associated with cognitive processes. If an individual's cognitive functioning is distorted, so that language and spatial skills as well as normal learning functions are altered, affective disorders also can result as a secondary consequence of the cognitive and intellective difficulties.

The body of research that deals with affective disorders and lateral preference patterns is small. The rationale behind linking preference patterns to affective disorders seems to have emerged from indications that there is cerebral lateralization or hemispheric localization of emotional processes. For example, Goldstein (1939) observed that patients with left hemisphere damage manifested what he called "catastrophic reactions" characterized by outbursts of anxiety and despair that did not seem to be exhibited by other patients. Conversely, Denny-Brown, Mayer, and Horenstein (1952) observed a pattern of reduced emotional response and indifference in patients with lesions of the right hemisphere. More systematic research of both left and right hemisphere-damaged patients showed that the left hemisphere lesion group exhibited more manic-depressive reactions (crying, cursing, and so forth), while the right hemisphere group frequently reacted with indifference or denial (Gainotti, 1972). Gasparrine, Satz, and Heilman (1978) reported that patients with left hemisphere damage showed higher scores on the MMPI depression scale than those with right hemisphere damage. Several studies using intact subjects also suggest cerebral lateralization of emotional response. Harman and Ray (1977) recorded EEG responses from both the left and right hemispheres, while inducing positive and negative emotional responses. They reported that the left hemisphere showed increased activity during strong negative affective states and reduced activity during strong positive ones. No significant changes were found in the right hemisphere activation. Tucker, Stenslie, Roth, and Shearer (1979) have replicated the main findings of greater left hemisphere involvement during the subjective experience of depression.

In an attempt to explain such findings, Bakan (1976) and Galin (1974) have hypothesized that there are interactions between the two hemispheres in the formation of the emotional response. It is assumed that the left hemisphere exerts an inhibitory influence on the more primary and emotional capacities of the right hemisphere. Extending the theory into the clinical realm, Bakan (1976) has suggested that some forms of affective psychoses may arise from a breakdown in the left hemisphere's inhibitory functions. For example, he theorizes that the usual inhibition of the right hemisphere is released in schizophrenia and its more dreamlike reality spills over into the waking life of the schizophrenic. Some support for this position comes from Flor-Henry (1969), who observed temporal lobe epileptics who had been classified as psychotic. He reported that focal epilepsy in the right temporal lobe is associated with manic-depressive disorders, whereas focal epilepsy of the left temporal lobe is associated with schizophrenia. In a later study, Flor-Henry (1976) compared a typical nonpsychotic control group to schizophrenics and affective psychotics (manics, depressives, and schizo-affectives). He reported that the schizophrenics were impaired relative to the controls on tests of left hemisphere functioning, while affectives were impaired on tests of right hemisphere functioning.

These types of data and theorizing lead to lateral preference behaviors in a circuitous manner. They begin with the recurrent presumption that functional specialization of the two cerebral hemispheres is responsible for lateral preference, particularly for handedness, as discussed in Chapter 4. If disruptions of normal emotional patterns, such as are found in psychopathy, depression, schizophrenia, or various forms of sociopathy, are associated with the alteration of and/or differences in the activation of the hemispheres, then the rationale for expecting some alterations in lateral preference patterns is established. This is a simple extension of the notion that the normally functioning left hemisphere holds the emotional right hemisphere in check and, of course, of the assumption that the normally functioning left hemisphere also controls the right hand. If there is left hemisphere malfunction in individuals suffering from psychopathy or emotional disorders, there might also be coincident deviations in normal lateral preference patterns, especially in handedness. This leads to the prediction that emotionally disturbed individuals should manifest more left-handedness and presumably left-footedness, since foot control is influenced by similar neural control mechanisms.

We have pointed out already in Chapters 4 and 7 that hemispheric differences in function might not suffice as an explanation of lateral preferences. However, a number of other theoretical routes also lead to the hypothesis that affective problems and altered lateral preference distributions might be associated. The simplest of these is again the Satz model (1972, 1973). With its application, one need only presume that the affective disorder arises from some pathological condition that is sufficiently general to alter lateral preferences. From this presumption, all of the previous reasoning leads to the prediction of a higher incidence of pathological left-sided individuals in these subsamples. An alternate position, which one also might assume, begins with left-handedness and then derives predispositions toward emotional instability and affective disorders from the very existence of the sinistral preference. Even without data suggesting hemispheric specialization of emotional response or any hidden or inferred pathology, sinistral individuals, particularly left-handers, are likely subject to stresses that are not experienced by right-handers. Historically, left-handedness has been viewed as shameful and equivalent to a physical, moral, or even a mental defect. As noted in Chapter 6, it is common for parents to compel the left-handed child to use the right hand, and for teachers to apply additional pressure by chastising left-handed use of drawing and writing implements. Conceivably, a left-hander could develop a self-image of abnormality, of being a misfit in a right-handed world. Since so many tools, instruments, games, and customs are oriented exclusively toward dextrality, the sinistral may act clumsily, reinforcing feelings of awkwardness or of being a misfit. Although this pressure is slight, it is continuous. A life history of continuous negative reinforcement, negative feedback, and frequent social blunders may adversely affect the quality of the left-hander's life, perhaps leading to an increase in levels of emotional tension. While most left-handers adjust to such pressures, those who already have a poor self-image or who lack good emotional adjustment could manifest overt psychological disorder due to this prevailing negative ambience associated with hand use. This environmental factor, independent of any neurological substrate toward emotional responsiveness, may lead to an association between increased incidence of sinistrality and emotional disturbance.

Cuff (1930b) empirically investigated the relationship between affective state and lateral preference by administering a questionnaire to measure symptoms of psychopathy or emotional instability and by behaviorally testing hand and eye preference in a sample of grade school children. A comparison of the psychopathy scores showed that there were more left-handed and left-eyed children in the 25% of the sample with the most extreme psychopathic scores when compared to the 25% of the sample who had received the lowest scores on the scale. Orme (1970) confirmed this observation with teenage girls by reporting more emotional instability in the left- as opposed to the right-handed group. Over the years, a raised incidence of left-handedness has been associated with a number of emotional and behavioral problems and syndromes, such as alcoholism, bedwetting, and neurotic behavior (Bakan, 1973; Blau, 1946; Burt, 1937; Chayatte, Chayatte, & Althoff, 1979).

Affective disorders also have been associated with altered patterns of lateral preference. For example, Mills (1925) found that emotional instability is most frequently associated with children who display crossed hand and eye preference. Chandler (1934) found more crossed hand-eye preference in a psychotic group, while Oddy and Lobstein (1972) found an elevated percentage of crossed preference in schizophrenics. Turner (1938) has reported that variations in side of preference and in cross-index congruency are associated with affective factors. Children ranging in age from 10 to 17 years were tested on a questionnaire designed to reveal the relative presence or absence of emotional instability. The group showing the highest degree of instability was then compared to a control group that showed the least evidence of emotional instability. She found that 77.2% of the children classified as emotionally stable had right hand, foot, and eye preference, as compared to 43.7% of the children categorized as emotionally unstable. In addition, 15.9% of the emotionally stable children had at least one noncongruent index, whereas 55.1% of the emotionally unstable children showed evidence of crossed preference pattern.

As previously noted, Lombroso (1903) reported a greater proportion of left-handers in criminal populations. Several years later, Smith (1917) obtained data on inmates of a reform school and found that the percentage of left-handedness was elevated in this population when compared to an equivalent noninstitutionalized group. Thus, there has been a long-established association between agressive and antisocial behavior, criminality, and the incidence of left-handedness. For example, Burt (1937) observed that "again and again in my case summaries the left-handed child is described by those who know him as stubborn and willful. At times he is visibly of an assertive type, domineering, overbearing, and openly rebellious against all the dictates of authority" (p. 317).

Since affective disorders, independent of criminality, may be associated with increases in sinistrality, one cannot determine whether criminal tendencies are related to increased percentages of left-handedness directly, or whether they are linked indirectly, with emotional instability or psychopathy as the mediating variable. An attempt to separate the effects of criminality from those of affective disorders was undertaken by Dr. Robert Hare of the University of British Columbia. Hare (1980) has developed a scale for the assessment of psychopathy in criminal populations. Based on the scores of this scale, he divided a sample of 166 inmates of a medium security prison. Individuals with low scores served as the nonpsychopathic criminal control group, while moderate to high scorers were designated as the psychopathic group (see Hare, 1979). In addition, each subject received the handedness portion of the lateral preference inventory (Table 3-1). He next determined the number of his subjects giving left-handed scores in a dichotomous classification scheme. The normative data in Chapter 3 for the 2,417 subjects equivalent in age to the criminal group show an incidence rate of 11.4% left-handedness. The two criminal subgroups studied by Hare show a 13.3% rate of left-handedness, which is approximately equal to the noncriminal incidence rate. Thus, the criminal group does not show a statistically significant higher percentage of sinistrality for hand use. However, when one considers the data according to the categories of psychopathy, an interesting pattern emerges. The nonpsychopathic criminal group shows an incidence of left-handedness of 8.3%, which does not differ from that found for an age-equivalent control group. For the moderate and high psychopathy criminals, the percentage of left-handedness is 17.8%. Thus the psychopathic criminal group shows an incidence of left-handedness that is more than twice that seen in the nonpsychopathic criminal group, which is statistically significant. These control group data clarify the relationship between criminality and handedness. The higher incidence of sinistrality found in previous criminal samples probably resulted from the greater incidence of psychopathy in inmate groups. Psychopathy, rather than criminality, seems to be associated with elevated levels of left-handedness. Nonpsychopathic criminals show no greater incidence of left-handedness than do normal populations of equivalent age.

There seems to be some association between affective disorders and patterns of lateral preference. Unfortunately only a few studies are available, so we must consider this a tentative, rather than a proven, link. However, studies of clinical populations suffering from cognitive, rather than affective, disorders have been more extensive, and clearer conclusions concerning variations in lateral preference patterns have emerged from them.

Cognitive Deficits

In his book *The Backward Child,* Burt (1937) devoted an entire chapter to the issue of left-handedness. His basic premise was that "if it is even safe to treat left-handedness as a sign or symptom, it should be regarded rather as a mark of an ill-organized nervous system" (p. 287). As the book title suggested, the specific type of abnormality under his consideration was cognitive deficit. The notion that sinistrality or ambilaterality is associated with subnormal cognitive functioning, perhaps as a result of unobservable neuropathy, neural immaturity, or disorganization, has produced an extensive body of research. In order to obtain the broadest possible range of cognitive functioning, one popular paradigm has involved the comparison of lateral preference behaviors in samples with normal intelligence to those observed in clinically affected groups, such as institutionalized mental retardates or samples of slow learners.

An early study by Smith (1917) is typical of this approach. She tested 200 children in a school for the mentally retarded and found that 9.8% showed manifest left-handedness as compared to an incidence rate of 5% left-handedness in a normal control sample. This finding is comparable to results reported by Burt (1937), who found a 4.8% occurrence of left-handedness in a group of 5,000 normal school children, 7.8% left-handedness among children classified by their teachers as being backward, and 11.9% left-handedness among mentally defective children. Gordon (1921) tested 3,298 normal children, ranging in age from 4 to 14 years, and compared their hand preference to that of 4,620 children in schools for the retarded. He reported a rate of left-handedness of 7.3% among the controls and of 18.2% among the retarded sample. Similar results showing a raised incidence of left-handedness in retarded samples have been reported by other investigators (Doll, 1933; Mintz, 1947; Wilson & Dolan, 1931; Zangwill, 1960). Left-handedness averages about 20% in retarded groups as compared to approximately 5-10% in the nonretarded. Hicks and Barton (1975) have even suggested that the frequency of left-handedness increases with the degree of retardation. They reported that 13% of their mildly and moderately retarded patients were left handed, as compared to 28% of their severely and profoundly retarded group.

The results of these studies are quite consistent. All show increases in sinistrality and ambilaterality in the mentally retarded as compared to nonretarded controls. Given this fact, it is unfortunate that most of the empirical studies have limited their measures to manual preference alone, with the occasional inclusion of eyedness. There is little systematic data assessing simultaneously all four indexes of lateral preference in a retarded sample. The advantage of measuring the four indexes of lateral preference on the same individuals is that one can assess the congruency of preference across indexes concurrently with the assessment of right- or left-sidedness within each index. Interest in the cross-index patterning of lateral preferences stems from the work of Orton (1937), who noted that crossed preference (specifically, of hand and eye) tends to be more frequent in clinical samples. This finding has been confirmed by recent reports based on data from neuropathic, learning disabled, and dyslexic populations. In general, one finds reports of an elevated incidence of crossed hand-eye preference in these groups (Critchley, 1970; Delacato, 1963; Harris, 1957; Hecaen & de Ajuriaguerra, 1964; Zangwill, 1962).

It seems reasonable to expect that a population of retardates could manifest patterns of lateral preference that differ from the nonretarded, both in the relative distribution of right-sidedness and in the relative agreement of lateral preferences across indexes. Since no study had ever looked at all four indexes of lateral preference in this type of group, we undertook this task (Porac, Coren, & Duncan, 1980a). Our clinical sample was a group of 138 retardates who were attending either a community-based school for the mentally retarded or a school located within an institution for the mentally retarded. Their mean age was 17 years. The severity of retardation was determined from recorded IQ scores and/or clinical diagnosis. None of the individuals was severely physically handicapped, deaf, or blind, nor did any one of them manifest unilateral sensory or motor incoordination. We could not simply compare the lateral preference of the retardates to a general, randomly selected group of individuals. A number of methodological safeguards had to be instituted if the obtained data were to be interpretable. Since there are systematic differences in the preference distributions as a function of chronological age (see Chapters 3 and 6), the inclusion of a control group equivalent in age to the retarded sample was appropriate. To assess the relationship between lateral preference formation and cognitive or sensorimotor stage, independent of chronological age, we used an additional control group. This was a sample matched to the retardates on the basis of mental age, a control procedure that has been used in other types of clinical studies (e.g., Dunn, 1954; Lipman, 1960). Therefore, we tested two comparison groups. The first was chosen to approximate the chronological age of the retardate sample; it was composed of 171 high school students, with a mean age of 16.8 years, all of whom were enrolled in public high schools. The second group was a control for the mental age and cognitive capacity of the retardate sample. Since the mean mental age of the retardates was approximately four years, we tested preschool children attending several community day care centers. These 384 subjects were 3-5 years old.

We measured lateral preference in the three groups by using the behavioral inventory described in Chapter 6 (Table 6-1). It contains 12 behavioral measures that ascertain hand, eye, foot, and ear preference. The presentation format of these items was designed to be suitable for administration to the retarded group, while still providing valid estimates of lateral preference behaviors in preschool and high school-aged groups. After the individuals were tested, the preference responses were scored for each index separately. We utilized the scoring procedure of $(R-L)/N$ where R is the number of right-sided responses, L the number of left-sided responses, and N the total number of responses made for a given index. The relative distribution of left- and right-sidedness in the retardates and their chronological and mental age groups was ascertained by dichotomously classifying each individual as either right or left sided on each index of lateral preference. Individuals with a score greater than zero on any index were scored as right sided for that index, whereas negative or zero scores were classified as left sided (see Chapter 3). Since preliminary analysis indicated that there were no within-group sex differences in these samples, all of the comparisons were collapsed across this variable.

Table 8-2 shows the percentage of right-sidedness for the four types of lateral preference for each group. Since we have already discussed the age differences between the two control groups in Chapter 6, we will note age differences only

Table 8-2: Percentage of Obtained Right-Sidedness in Retardate, Cognitive Control (Preschool), and Chronological Control (High School) Groups

	Right-sidedness (%)			
	Hand	Foot	Eye	Ear
Retarded (N = 138)	60.9[b]	57.2[a,b]	50.0[b]	44.2[b]
Cognitive equivalent (N = 384)	94.3[b]	77.1[a]	61.3[b]	52.7
Chronological age equivalent (N = 171)	94.7[b]	81.9[b]	75.4[b]	70.2[b]

[a] Significantly different when compared to retarded group, $p < .05$.

[b] Significantly different when compared to retarded group, $p < .01$.

where they are relevant to the comparisons against the retarded group. The retardates show significantly more left-sidedness than either their chronological peers or their cognitive peers for seven of the eight comparisons. The results for handedness confirm the general pattern found in the existing literature. The retarded sample manifests a higher incidence of left-handedness than that found in the unaffected groups. In addition, these data demonstrate that the retardates also show increased left-sidedness on the remaining three indexes of lateral preference. Thus, there is a general sinistral shift in the retarded sample relative to their age-mates, and that shift affects all four preference indexes.

Hildreth (1949, 1950) and Hecaen and de Ajuriaguerra (1964) have suggested that brain trauma or some type of physiological insult may affect not only the preferred side but also the degree to which a lateral preference can be established. Within the context of our data, this theory suggests that the retarded group might be expected to show lesser degrees of response consistency in their manifestations of lateral preference. We re-analyzed the data to explore this possibility. Individuals were classified as left or right sided only if all measurements taken within an index were consistently to that side. Any response patterns that contained both right and left scores were classified as mixed. The results of this trichotomous consistency analysis are shown in Table 8-3.

The retardates were found to be significantly different from both control groups on all four preference indexes. Individual pairwise comparisons revealed that the retarded sample shows a decrease in consistent right-sidedness for hand, foot, eye, and ear relative to either their age or cognitive peers. The retarded group also shows a greater frequency of occurrence of mixed preference patterns for hand, eye, and ear than either of the two control groups. Thus, the prediction of less consistent preference in the retarded group is confirmed for these three indexes. There is also a concomitant increase in the relative proportion of individuals showing consistent left-sidedness in the retardate sample. This is found for all of the indexes when compared to the chronological age control group, and it is a significant increase in consistent left-sidedness for hand and foot preference when compared to the mental age control group. As one moves from the high school to the preschool and then to the retardate group, there is a decreasing proportion of consistently dextral individuals for each of the four dimensions of lateral preference and an increase in both sinistrality and mixed preference. Regardless of the index considered, the retardates are most disparate from their chronological controls, with smaller, but nonetheless apparent, differences between the retardates and the cognitive control group.

As the literature has suggested, clinical and nonaffected populations may differ in the relative incidences of cross-index congruency. A higher rate of crossed preference patterns (where the right side is preferred for some indexes and the left for others) might be expected in atypical samples. We attempted to assess this possibility in our data by performing an across-index congruency analysis similar to that described in Chapters 3 and 7. Individuals who scored both right or both left on the two indexes of a given preference pair were classified as congruent, while those preferring opposite sides for a pair of indexes were called

Table 8-3: Percentage of Obtained Right-, Mixed, and Left-Sidedness in Retardate, Cognitive Control (Preschool), and Chronological Control (High School) Groups

	Percentage classified				
	Hand	Foot	Eye	Ear	Mean
Retarded (N = 138)					
Left	15.9^b	30.4^b	37.0^a	45.7^b	32.3
Mixed	44.2^b	13.0	24.6^b	$13.0^{a,b}$	23.7
Right	39.9^b	56.5^b	38.4^b	$41.3^{a,b}$	44.0
Cognitive equivalent (N = 384)					
Left	6.2^b	10.6^b	40.0	40.0	24.2
Mixed	25.5^b	12.5	5.5^b	7.3^a	12.7
Right	68.3^b	76.9^b	54.5^b	52.7^a	63.1
Chronological age equivalent (N = 171)					
Left	5.8^b	7.6^b	24.6^a	25.1^b	15.8
Mixed	13.5^b	10.5	9.4^b	4.7^b	9.5
Right	80.7^b	81.9^b	66.1^b	70.2^b	74.7

Note. Overall chi-square analyses show each control group to be significantly different from the retarded group ($p < .01$) for all indexes except when compared to ear preference for the preschool sample ($p < .05$).
[a] Significantly different from retarded sample, $p < .05$.
[b] Significantly different from retarded sample, $p < .01$.

crossed. The normative data in Chapter 3 showed that there is a rather high incidence of pairwise congruency but a rather low rate of total congruency in a general population. Therefore, in the present analysis we have confined ourselves to the pairwise comparisons, since this is where deviations from normal congruency patterns would be most apparent. Table 8-4 presents the results of the congruency analysis. In this instance, we have chosen to give the incidence of the crossed rather than the congruent pairs, since the issue of lack of congruency is a more salient one for comparisons involving a clinically affected group.

The retarded group shows higher rates of crossed preference for every pair of indexes when compared to their chronological peers. On average, the proportion of crossed preference is nearly twice as great in the retarded as in the high school sample. However, the preschool sample is similar to the retarded group in terms of the relative percentage of crossed versus congruent preference; only the hand-foot and the eye-ear pairing significantly differ for these two groups. The relatively low degrees of congruent lateral preference within the retardate sample can be illustrated by following the procedure that we outlined in Chapter 3. At

Table 8-4: Percentage of Crossed Lateral Preference Patterns in Retardates, Cognitive Controls (Preschool), and Chronological Age Controls (High School)

Lateral preference pairs	Retarded	Cognitive equivalent	Chronological age equivalent
Hand-foot	35.5^b	23.3^b	12.9^b
Hand-eye	47.1^b	38.7	20.5^b
Hand-ear	52.9^b	45.7	29.2^b
Foot-eye	43.5^b	39.7	28.7^b
Foot-ear	49.3^b	45.2	30.4^b
Eye-ear	47.8^b	33.5^b	27.5^b
Mean	46.0	37.5	24.9

^{b} Significantly different from retarded group, $p < .01$.

that time, we compared the observed incidence of pairwise congruency in the normative sample with theoretical values that were computed based on assumptions of the chance occurrence of congruency. The rationale for this type of analysis arises from an attempt to evaluate whether congruency rates are related solely to the rightward bias in population distributions of lateral preference, which in and of itself would produce high rates of right-sided congruency, or whether there are additional factors involved in fostering ipsilateral preference patterns. If congruency rates are greater than those expected assuming a random distribution of sidedness patterns, one can infer that additional factors are promoting congruency among the indexes of preference. In our previous analysis (Table 3-8) we used the incidence of right- and left-sidedness for each index found in the normative sample (Table 3-4) to compute the theoretical probabilities of congruent occurrence for each of the six pairs of lateral preference indexes. We used these values and applied a formula that is a modification of the computations of independent conditional probabilities (see Chapter 3).

We can adopt the same procedure for evaluating the incidence of pairwise congruency in the retarded group; in this instance, however we must use the incidence of right- and left-sidedness found for a typical retarded population as the basis of our computations of theoretical values. To do this, we assumed that the right-left incidence rates for the various preference types found in our sample (Table 8-2) represent those that would be found if any retarded sample was measured in a similar fashion, and used these values to compute the theoretically expected rates of congruency. The comparisons between the observed and the theoretically expected rates of congruency are shown in Table 8-5 for each pair of indexes. Only one pair of indexes, the hand-foot pair, shows greater observed congruency than that predicted on the basis of chance expectancy. The normative sample in Chapter 3 (Table 3-8) shows much greater congruency than expected based on assumptions of random assortment. This is the case for all six pairs of preference types. Thus, the retardates show much less cross-index congruency than the general population. If there are naturally occurring processes

Table 8-5: Percentage of Obtained Congruent Lateral Preference in the Retardate Sample as Compared to Theoretical Values Based on Random Assortment of Sidedness for Preference Pairs in That Population

Lateral preference pairs	Percentage congruent	
	Obtained	Theoretical
Hand-foot	64.5[b]	51.6[b]
Hand-eye	52.9	50.0
Hand-ear	47.1	48.7
Foot-eye	56.5	50.0
Foot-ear	50.7	49.2
Eye-ear	52.2	50.0

[b] Significant difference, $p < .01$.

that encourage increases in the degree of congruency between preference behaviors, they appear to be absent in lateral preference formation in retardates. In light of the discussion in Chapter 4, it is interesting that the only preference pair that shows the previous pattern of greater than chance congruency is the hand-foot pair. This seems to confirm the strong connection between these two forms of preference. Although the retarded group shows large deviations from generally expected congruency patterns, the sidedness association between limb preferences is maintained at a relatively high rate, even for this group.

Many researchers and clinical practitioners have treated sinistrality as a potential soft sign for neurological abnormality. In accordance with this assumption, we expected that we would find higher percentages of left-sidedness in our retarded sample, and our findings have supported this expectation. Tables 8-2 and 8-3 indicate that retarded individuals are less likely to be right sided than either their age or their cognitive peers. The retardate group shows a definite increase in the percentage of mixed and consistently left-sided individuals. While confirming earlier data that suggested a relationship between left-handedness and retardation, our findings also establish the empirical observation that a similar pattern exists for all four indexes of lateral preference. The retarded sample that we studied was symptomatically heterogeneous; hence, we cannot make statements about the specific abnormalities of brain and neurological development that exist within the group. However, these results tempt one to argue that the physiological assaults that retard the normal cognitive development in this sample are also responsible for the reduced likelihood that a subject will show consistent dextrality.

One theoretical approach that has been offered for mental retardation is the concept of *maturational arrest* or *maturational lag*. Such hypotheses assume that in retardation not caused by a specific injury, the course of cognitive development differs in its rate and final level, rather than in its qualitative nature (Achenbach, 1974). Thus, the retardate may manifest slower development (maturational lag) or may stop normal development at a stage below that expected of an adult (maturational arrest). Within this framework the stage of development may be indexed by an individual's mental age. Thus a 10 year old with a mental age of six and hence an IQ of 60 would be assumed to be equivalent to a six year old with a mental age of six and hence an IQ of 100. Evidence shows that the performance of mental age-matched normals and retardates differs little on standard measures of cognitive functioning (Achenbach, 1970) or Piagetian tasks (Gruen & Vore, 1972). One might extend this argument to suppose that most neurophysical processes will develop in synchrony. If there is some maturational disruption, it will manifest itself in sensorimotor activities as well as in the cognitive realm. Since lateral preference behaviors are subject to developmental trends, these considerations are relevant in the present context. Perhaps one can merge this notion of retardation with some of the developmental theories of lateral preference. For example, Corballis and Morgan (1978) and Morgan and Corballis (1978) (see Chapter 4) have argued that human laterality and lateral preference are under the influence of a maturational gradient that favors more rapid development on the left side of the human brain. Because of the contralateral neural control of limb motor function, this asymmetrical development gradient could result in an early emergent preference for the right side. Presumably this argument applies to sense organ preference as well, although the bilateral cerebral representation of ocular and auditory information somewhat weakens its relevance. Any abnormal physiological intervention that hinders this normal developmental gradient may result in preference patterns that deviate from the common right-sided human pattern. This deviation could manifest itself behaviorally in either reduced dextrality, lessened degrees of consistency of preference, or reduced congruency across preference indexes.

The Corballis and Morgan (1978) hypothesis rests upon assumptions of neurological maturation that occur during the prenatal or in the immediate postnatal portion of the life span. However, there is evidence that neural and cortical development continue beyond this portion of life. Studies by Yakovlev and Lecours (1967), which address themselves to the myelination of neurons, indicate that the brain continues to develop into adolescence if not beyond. Electrical recordings of brain activity confirm this finding. Thus, Eeg-Olofsson (1971a, b), Lindsley (1939), and Petersen and Eeg-Olofsson (1971) have found systematic changes in the frequency of alpha waves from infancy through adolescence, and similar age-related changes in event-contingent evoked cortical responses have also been reported (Beck & Dustman, 1975). Such changes often continue into the third or fourth decade of life. Perhaps the same process that caused the cognitive retardation has arrested the normal neural maturational process and has frozen lateral preferences at an earlier, less well-developed age. Alternatively, perhaps this process has fostered a lag within the maturational process, slowing the rate of change, so that the retarded group, after a longer period of time, has only reached a level equivalent to a much younger normally developing sample. If this is the case, it is not surprising to find the retarded group showing a pattern of lateral preference similar to that of chronologically younger subjects, namely, more inconsistency, less congruency, and greater sinistrality. Our data are not totally consistent with this hypothesis, since the retarded group shows even more sinistrality than does the sample selected as their mental age controls; however, the notion is suggestive.

There are alternatives to this maturational arrest hypothesis. One worth considering is based on a learning component. It is likely that subtle environmental pressures fostering dextrality operate over the life span (see Chapter 6). Hypothetically, these lead to the progressively higher percentages of right-sidedness in the population as individuals grow older as a consequence of living in the right-biased world. Since most of the retardates in the present study have spent the larger portion of their lives in an institutional setting, the higher incidence of observed left-sidedness could be enhanced by the lack of specific modeling and training of laterality patterns, especially for hand use, that seem to be part of some societal and family environments (Dawson, 1977; Falek, 1959; Teng, Lee, Yang, & Chang, 1976). The absence of the normal right-biased environment for the institutionalized retardate might result in the reduced consistency and increased sinistrality observed. Of course, one might argue that the lower cognitive capacity of retarded individuals would also lead to the same result. They simply may not have the capacity to modify their behaviors toward the dextral bias in the world, even when it is present.

Overall, the retardates more closely resemble their mental age peers (the preschool group) than they do their chronological age peers (the high school students). This is very evident when we collapse across all indexes and consider the relative proportions of sinistrality, mixed preference, and crossed lateral preference, as shown in Table 8-6. There seems to be some relationship between mental age, or cognitive level, and the manifest pattern of lateral preference.

The data presented and reviewed in this chapter indicate that the patterns of lateral preference observed in clinical samples, particularly of individuals suffering from neural assaults, disruptions of cognitive functioning, or affective disorders, differ from those of nonaffected populations. These effects are clearly statistical in nature. Certainly the presence of sinistrality does not automatically classify an individual as a member of a clinical subgroup, nor do all individuals

Table 8-6: Relative Lateral Preference Patterns for Retardates, Cognitive Controls (Preschool), and Chronological Age Controls (High School) Computed Across All Indexes and Pairs of Indexes

	Mean percentage		
	Within indexes		Across indexes
	Left sided	Mixed preferent	Crossed preferent
Retarded	44.2[b]	23.7[b]	46.0[b]
Cognitive equivalent	28.7[b]	12.7[b]	37.5
Chronological age equivalent	19.5[b]	9.5[b]	24.9[b]

[b] Significantly different from retarded, $p < .01$.

within such a clinical population show sinistrality. Rather there is an increased incidence of sinistrality and of mixed or inconsistent lateral preference patterns, and a lack of congruency across indexes. In this chapter, we have dealt mainly with data regarding groups with large functional deficits. Such deficits may be associated with undetected brain damage or other forms of disruption of neural control. However, these individuals also usually have atypical behavioral histories, and have often been subjected to atypical institutional environments for long periods of time. Any of these factors could, as a secondary consequence, result in some alterations in the observed pattern of lateral preference along with other behavioral changes.

The finding that the lateral preference pattern of clinical samples is dissimilar from that found in normal groups may not be of direct diagnostic value. It does not allow any means of differentiating, for instance, the pathological left-hander from the normal left-hander. However, it is of theoretical importance. It shows that a particular pattern of lateral preference (namely, a dextral bias, relative consistency within index, and relative congruency across pairs of indexes) is the norm, and that the mechanisms that maintain this norm can be altered or disrupted by physiological and/or environmental change. Atypical patterns of lateral preference seem to be characteristic of samples that show behavioral problems or deficits in cognitive functioning. Furthermore, if samples suffering from clinical problems associated with cognitive malfunctioning show unusual distributions of lateral preference, one might ask whether these findings can be generalized to other populations. For example, will groups who show performance deficits in such cognitive tasks as reading, mathematical reasoning and logical deduction, but remain within the normal range of ability, also manifest typical patterns of lateral preference? The next two chapters will address this issue.

9

Reading

In Chapter 8 we observed that groups suffering from brain and neurological damage, mental retardation, affective disorders, or psychopathy exhibit distributions of lateral preference behaviors that differ from those observed in the general population. Most of the empirical evidence suggests that these clinical groups display a higher incidence of left-sidedness, greater degrees of inconsistent sidedness, and higher incidences of crossed preference patterns. In our discussion of these findings, we encountered a number of theoretical positions that attempted to link such distributions of lateral preference, which differ from the norm, with observed or inferred pathological factors. These theoretical positions ranged from a rather mechanism-free statistical argument through notions of maturational lags, environmental factors, or disruptions of the patterns of hemispheric specialization. Although we cannot establish the most valid theoretical position, the data reviewed indicate that there is an association between certain classes of affective and cognitive abnormalities and the incidence of certain patterns of lateral preference. A number of investigators have posed the obvious reciprocal question and have explored whether or not specific patterns of lateral preference can be used to indicate some form of cognitive deficit.

Reading was one of the first cognitive dimensions connected to lateral preference patterns. As noted in Chapter 4, there is still a very strong presumption that the localization of language function in the left hemisphere and the dominance of the right hand in the majority of individuals are linked at the functional level. This position served as the stimulus for much of the ensuing research. Additional clinical observations, such as the apparent behavioral similarity between severely retarded readers and patients suffering from language deficits resulting from injuries to the language centers of the left hemisphere (Bryant & Patterson, 1962; Orton, 1937), also furthered this type of study. Methodological considerations (such as that indexes of lateral preference, especially handedness, are easily assessed, and that there are few *early* predictors of reading and learning problems) probably sustained the interest in establishing a connection between variations in lateral preference incidence rates and reading performance. Researchers wanted to develop a readily observable and measurable diagnostic instrument that would predict potential reading problems at a young age so that remediation could begin early in life.

Orton (1925, 1928, 1929, 1937) provided the first systematic data linking reading problems of the general class known as dyslexia to patterns of lateral preference. He studied hand and eye preference and observed that children with reading disabilities displayed different preference patterns than children with no reading problems. In a series of studies, Orton reported that poor readers showed an increased incidence of left-handedness, left-eyedness, and/or crossed hand-eye preference patterns. Although his criteria are ambiguous, he also indicated that poor readers are more likely to show mixed, rather than consistent, hand preference.

Following Orton's initial reports, over a hundred articles and chapters have appeared dealing with the relationship between lateral preference and reading. Most of the existing studies deal with the distribution of right- and left-handedness in groups of individuals with various levels of reading ability. These studies have replicated Orton's finding of an increased incidence of left-handedness among groups of poor readers (Allison, 1966; Clark, 1970; Dearborn, 1931; Fink, 1938; Granjon-Galifret & de Ajuriaguerra, 1951; Harris, 1957; Naidoo, 1966; Stephens, Cunningham, & Stigler, 1967; Wall, 1945). Other indexes of lateral preference have also been implicated. For instance, there are two reports that found an increased incidence of left-footedness in groups of impaired readers (Tinker, 1964; Wolf, 1967). In a similar fashion, there have been a number of reports of a higher incidence of left-eyedness in reading disabled samples (Fink, 1938; LaGrone & Holland, 1943; Macmeeken, 1939; Monroe, 1932; Orton, 1928, 1937). Thus a number of reports indicate that the incidence of left-handedness, -footedness, and -eyedness is elevated in samples of poor readers. While the studies reported above focused on the side of preference and its relationship to reading proficiency, others have looked at the strength or consistency of preference. The general finding is that a mixed response pattern (or a lack of consistency) is more characteristic of the slow rather than the average reader (Bender, 1968; Clements & Peters, 1962; Granjon-Galifret & de Ajuriaguerra, 1951; Harris, 1957; Ingram & Reid, 1956; Kucera, Matejcek, & Langmier, 1963; Zangwill, 1960). Granjon-Galifret and de Ajuriaguerra (1951) have summarized such results: "Dyslexics are not more often left-handed than normals, but are more often badly lateralized." Thus one is less apt to find consistent or strong right-handedness in populations of poor readers.

The relationship of cross-index congruency to reading proficiency has also received some experimental attention, prompted by Orton's (1928, 1937) original reports which found an increased incidence of crossed hand-eye preference in the reading retarded samples. Orton argued that any deviation from congruent preference patterns is a deviation from the normal pattern and thus places the individual in a clinically suspect category. Specifically, he contended that the normal pattern of lateral preference is congruent right-sidedness and that any deviation from either congruency or right-sidedness (in any index) is a potential sign of abnormality. In exploring this line of reasoning, a number of investigators have studied the congruency of lateral preference in reading groups of various ability levels. Most have confined themselves to measuring hand and eye preference, and some of them have replicated Orton's findings. They have found a greater incidence of crossed hand-eye preference in poor readers relative to readers experiencing no difficulties (Dearborn, 1931; Forness & Weil, 1970; Gilkey & Parr, 1944; Harris, 1957; Koos, 1964; Rengstorf, 1967; Teegarden, 1932; Vernon, 1957; Zangwill, 1962).

The previous paragraphs have emphasized those studies that reported a difference in lateral preference patterns when poor readers were compared to appropriate control groups. There are, however, numerous reports showing no apparent relationship between the side, consistency, or congruency of lateral preference and reading performance (Balow & Balow, 1964; Belmont & Birch, 1965; Colman & Deutsch, 1964; De Hirsch, Jansky, & Langford, 1966; Halgren, 1950; Imus, Rothney, & Bear, 1938; Satz & Friel, 1974; Shankweiler, 1963; Sparrow & Satz, 1970; Stephens, Cunningham, & Stigler, 1967; Stevenson & Robinson, 1953; Witty & Kopel, 1936; Zurif & Carson, 1970). Thus, a large body of literature contradicts the notion that indexes of lateral preference differentiate groups manifesting different reading abilities.

Given the number of both positive and negative findings, is there a coherent way to summarize the empirical relationship between lateral preference and reading performance? A close look at the studies reporting positive findings indicates results with a patchwork character. Some investigators report an increased incidence of left-sidedness in reading impaired groups but do not find, or do not report, increased incidence of inconsistent or crossed preference. Others report differences in the incidence of crossed preference patterns but no differences in the distributions or right- and left-sidedness. In addition, reports of differences in the incidence of mixed response patterns are occasionally accompanied by reports of greater degrees of crossed preference, while in other reports these two manifestations of lateral preference are not related. However, one general statement can be made; samples of poor readers are *never* found to be more dextral, more consistent, or more congruent in their lateral preference patterns than average or good readers. Thus, the literature suggests, although ambiguously, that shifts away from consistent and congruent dextrality can be associated with reading impairment.

The theoretical explanations suggested for these findings represent a recurrence of familiar themes, with most emphasizing hemispheric specialization. First, one finds the hypotheses that state that subtle damage to the left hemisphere simultaneously causes shifts in lateral preference and slight impairment of language-related cognitive skills. We have discussed these approaches extensively in Chapters 4, 7, and 8. The only slight alteration in their application to reading problems arises from the assumption that the brain damage causes only minor behavioral impairments. The shifts away from dextrality are both a byproduct of and a sign of some hemispheric damage. Second, there is the theoretical position most clearly identified with Orton (1928, 1937). He maintained that normally the language dominant, or left, hemisphere has preeminence. When the dominance of the left hemisphere is well established, inputs to and commands from the right hemisphere are suppressed. One may recall that the Corballis and Morgan (1978) theory, which we discussed in Chapter 4, also postulated such suppression of one hemisphere by the other. Orton maintained that when this asymmetrical relationship is not well established, a tendency exists to reverse the order of stimulus input. He called this problem *strephosymbolia,* or twisted symbols. He stated that it is the major component in reading problems since it results in letter reversals, scrambled perceptions of the orders of letters and words, and other similar confusions. The etiology of strephosymbolia resides in an alteration of the normal asymmetries in the left hemisphere-right hemisphere relationship. He asserted (without any direct empirical evidence) that sensory inputs are registered simultaneously in the two hemispheres but with opposite orientations. Incomplete dominance of the left hemisphere results in an inability to ignore the reversed representation registered in the right hemisphere. Disruptions in visual processing (especially visual reversals) and a breakdown of normal right-sided behavioral preferences are the by-products of a poorly established left-hemispheric superiority. The notion that the representations of visual inputs to the two hemispheres are mirror images of each other has been challenged on both empirical and theoretical grounds (see Corballis and Beale, 1976); however, the notion that incomplete hemispheric dominance might be responsible for both the observed reading difficulties and the observed variations in patterns of lateral preference has been echoed in the reasoning of a number of researchers (Brain, 1965; Critchley, 1964; Gooddy & Reinhold, 1961; Hecaen & de Ajuriaguerra, 1964; Travis & Lindsley, 1933; Zangwill, 1960).

These brain damage and incomplete hemispheric dominance theories have been used to explain variations in the incidence of right- and left-sidedness in poor as compared to average or good readers based on the underlying presumption of a left hemisphere-right preference connection. There is, however, another approach often applied to explain the higher incidence of mixed versus consistent response patterns and of crossed versus congruent preference in poor readers. It is the theory of maturational lag, mentioned briefly in Chapter 8. This hypothesis is based on the general observation that as individuals mature, lateral preference behaviors become more dextral, at least for limbs and eye. In addition, preferences become more consistent and somewhat more congruent across indexes of preference (see Chapters 3 and 6). Thus, an increased incidence of sinistrality, mixed response patterns, and crossed lateral preference could be said to characterize young as opposed to mature groups. Hypothetically, poor reading performance and weaker, less dextral manifestations of lateral preference coincide because of the neuropsychological immaturity of certain individuals. It is suggested that poor reading and language skills and "immature" patterns of lateral preferences arise jointly from disruptions (usually assumed to be cerebral or neural) of the normal maturational process. Critchley (1970) summarized this position: "Both ambilaterality and dyslexia are expressions of a common factor, namely immaturity of cerebral development."

Unfortunately, as indicated by the review of the evidence on the relationship between lateral preferences and reading ability, the current data are too ambiguous to establish the nature of the association, if one exists. There are many studies that report an association between reading performance and fluctuations in incidence rates of lateral preference, and there are also many studies that report a lack of association between these two variables. There are some methodological considerations that may explain the inconsistencies in the published literature. First, if the differences in lateral preference patterns between samples of good and poor readers are relatively small, they may not always be detected. We noted a similar problem when we explored the existence of gender differences in lateral preferences in Chapter 3. This problem becomes most crucial in clinical studies, where, typically, small numbers of cases are examined. If, for example, one studies an experimental group of 50 individuals and compares it to a control group of 50 individuals, selected independently, the lateral preference distributions must differ by approximately 20% for a statistically significant difference to emerge. This is a sizable percentage difference, much beyond the levels usually encountered. Second, most studies have limited themselves to the use of only one or two preference indexes and usually only report a composite index of reading skill. Perhaps lateral preference patterns are predictive of some classes of reading skills but not of others. A global analysis cannot permit such results to emerge. Third, there is a possibility that some of the existing studies included mildly retarded individuals. As shown in Chapter 8, manifest retardation alters patterns of lateral preference in exactly the same direction as the data reported for the slow reading groups. If some of the studies reporting positive findings included individuals who were mildly retarded, positive results could be produced for spurious reasons. Thus, when evaluating the literature, one must attend to these three specific problems, in addition to considering the general methodological problems of measurement differences among studies (see Chapter 2) that make it difficult to compare results across various investigations.

We decided to conduct a study on the relationship between reading performance and the incidence of right- and left-sidedness in a manner that takes many of these factors into account and rectifies a number of the methodological problems. We assessed a group of individuals who vary in reading ability, but who otherwise are not impaired behaviorally in any way. We tested their reading skills on a number of dimensions and measured all four forms of lateral preference. This allowed us to assess the relationship between sidedness and reading performance for specific indexes of lateral preference and for specific reading skills. The study was conducted in collaboration with Dr. Geraldine Schwartz of the University of British Columbia. It was part of a larger effort to assess the reading skills of incoming college and junior college students in selected institutions in the Province of Quebec, Canada. The sample consisted of 1,912 individuals, all of approximately the same age, socioeconomic status, and educational level. While this type of sample guaranteed that all of the individuals have intelligence within normal limits, it also, of course, simultaneously limits the overall range of reading skills within our sample. This limitation was mitigated somewhat by the fact that the sample was selected from incoming college students, who as a group manifest a broad range of reading abilities, with some individuals showing reading performances as low as sixth-grade levels. We assessed lateral preference by means of the behaviorally validated self-report inventory presented in Table 3-1; in this instance, however, in addition to the handedness and eyedness items, we used only questions 1 and 3 from the footedness and the earedness sections. The Diagnostic Reading Test (1966) was used to assess reading proficiency. This battery was selected because it allows separate scores to be obtained for reading speed, comprehension, and vocabulary skills.

Given the size of this sample, it was possible to divide the data in a way that maximized the likelihood of observing any differences in the lateral preference profiles of good and poor readers. This procedure involved separate scoring of reading proficiency along each of the three dimensions of reading speed, comprehension, and vocabulary. We computed the distribution of reading speed scores in terms of words per minute and the scores from the comprehension and vocabulary tests in terms of number correct. The 1,912 cases were rank ordered within each of the three divisions of reading ability separately, and the subjects scoring in the lowest and highest 25% were segregated for analysis. Those in the bottom quartile were designated as poor readers while those in the top 25% were designated as good readers. This was done for each dimension of reading ability. We reasoned that this procedure would increase the likelihood of detecting any existing systematic lateral preference differences as a function of reading proficiency.

The first analysis was designed to determine whether the percentage of individuals showing left- and right-sidedness on the four preference indexes differed between the good and the poor readers. Subjects were scored as right or left sided for each index by computing $(R-L)/N$ where R is the number of right-sided responses, L the number of left-sided responses, and N the total number of items for that index. Subjects were classified as right sided if the index was posi-

Table 9-1: Percentage of Left-Sidedness Observed in College Students with Scores in the Top and Bottom Quartiles on Tests of Reading Performance

	Measure of reading performance					
	Speed		Vocabulary		Comprehension	
	Bottom	Top	Bottom	Top	Bottom	Top
Hand	12.2[a]	8.1[a]	10.2	10.1	10.7	10.4
Foot	27.5[b]	18.3[b]	24.5	19.8	22.4	19.7
Eye	30.6	25.0	26.2	26.1	30.4	27.9
Ear	44.8	39.4	43.1	42.6	42.0	39.7
Any index left	67.6[b]	56.3[b]	65.6[a]	58.3[a]	61.4	60.3

Note. Sample comprised 1,912 students.

[a] Significant difference between top and bottom quartile, $p < .05$.

[b] Significant difference between top and bottom quartile, $p < .01$.

tive and left sided if the index was negative or zero. The distribution of right-versus left-sided individuals was tabulated for each lateral preference index and for each scale on the reading proficiency measures. These results are shown as Table 9-1. Because an increased incidence of left-sidedness is predicted within the poor reading group, Table 9-1 presents these results in terms of the percentage of sinistrality.

Table 9-1 shows some significant differences in the lateral preference patterns of good and poor readers. Most of these differences center on the speed aspect of reading performance. Slow readers show significantly more left-handedness and left-footedness than do the rapid readers. None of the other pairwise differences between the groups is statistically significant. However, there is a global aspect of this table that suggests increased sinistrality in the bottom quartile readers. Of the 12 possible pairwise comparisons between the groups, readers in the bottom quartile show more sinistrality in every instance (although in some of the comparisons these differences are quite small). The chance likelihood that the 12 comparisons would all show the same direction of differences is quite low ($p < .001$), indicating that there is an overall bias toward sinistrality in the readers in the bottom quartile. We also tabulated the percentage of individuals who showed any evidence of left-sidedness for either hand, foot, eye, or ear, as opposed to those individuals who are completely right sided on all four indexes. The results of this analysis for reading speed (bottom row of Table 9-1) reveals that the sample of slow readers contains more individuals who show some evidence of sinistrality on at least one lateral preference index than does the group of fast readers. This difference amounts to 11.3% and is statistically significant. We also find an increased likelihood that at least one index will be left sided in the sample of individuals scoring in the lowest quartile of the vocabulary test. This difference is somewhat smaller than that observed for speed, being only 7.3%.

Next we dealt with the response consistency within the indexes of preference. As in earlier chapters, an individual was classified as mixed preferent if some of the responses indicated a right and some a left preference within any index.

Table 9-2: Percentage of Mixed Lateral Preference for College Students with Scores in the Top and Bottom Quartiles on Tests of Reading Performance

	Measure of reading performance					
	Speed		Vocabulary		Comprehension	
	Bottom	Top	Bottom	Top	Bottom	Top
Hand	22.3	21.7	25.6	23.4	20.8	21.8
Foot	36.1[b]	20.7[b]	35.4[b]	22.5[b]	30.1[b]	21.3[b]
Eye	34.6	31.9	32.7	32.5	30.4	34.9
Ear	42.5	43.0	46.4	46.9	40.7	43.8

Note. Sample comprised 1,912 students.

[b] Significant difference between top and bottom quartile, $p < .01$.

Individuals who are completely right or left sided on all measures within an index were scored as consistent for that index. The data comparing the incidence of mixed lateral preference patterns in individuals scoring in the top and bottom quartiles on the three reading measures is shown in Table 9-2. This table does not show evidence of differences between the good and poor readers in terms of mixed versus consistent preference. The only index that shows association with reading performance is footedness. The lowest scorers on all three reading scales show higher percentages of mixed footedness (ranging from about 9% to over 15%). However, the poor readers show a greater incidence of mixed preference responses in only 7 of the 12 possible comparisons. This is the sort of distribution of differences one would expect on the basis of chance. It appears that mixed or weak lateral preference is not a very good indicator of variations in reading ability, except perhaps for foot.

In order to assess whether the incidence of crossed lateral preference is associated with different reading ability levels, each of the six possible pairs of lateral preference indexes were analyzed separately. As in previous chapters, individuals who were either right sided on both members of the pair or left sided on both indexes were classified as displaying congruent preference. Individuals who displayed right-sidedness on one index and left-sidedness on the other were called crossed preferent for that pair of indexes. This was done for those subjects scoring in the top 25% and the bottom 25% for each of the three reading measures considered separately. These data, presented in Table 9-3, indicate that for reading speed there are two index pairings where there is a greater incidence of crossed preference among the slower readers. The differences are in the hand-foot and foot-eye pairings. There is also an overall trend toward a higher

Table 9-3: Percentage of Crossed Lateral Preference for College Students with Scores in the Top and Bottom Quartiles on Tests of Reading Performance

	Measure of reading performance					
	Speed		Vocabulary		Comprehension	
	Bottom	Top	Bottom	Top	Bottom	Top
Hand-foot	21.1^a	15.2^a	22.1^b	14.4^b	18.2	15.1
Hand-eye	26.7	22.3	22.8	22.6	23.1	23.9
Hand-ear	37.4	35.8	39.2	36.4	34.6	36.3
Foot-eye	35.2^a	27.6^a	33.5^a	27.1^a	28.0	32.7
Foot-ear	37.3	34.9	39.3	35.8	34.7	37.6
Eye-ear	41.5	36.3	39.6	35.1	36.2	33.6
Any index crossed	63.1^b	53.3^b	62.3^b	53.5^b	56.2	56.6

Note. Sample comprised 1,912 students.

[a] Significant difference between top and bottom quartile, $p < .05$.

[b] Significant difference between top and bottom quartile, $p < .01$.

incidence of crossed preference among those in the lower end of the speed distribution. Of the six pairings, the slow reading group shows more crossed patterns on all of them. The chance likelihood that all six pairings would be in the same direction is quite low ($p < .05$), suggesting that there is an overall tendency toward more crossed preference among the readers in the bottom quartile of speed scores.

There is an almost identical pattern when we consider the vocabulary scores. The bottom quartile group shows more crossed hand-foot and foot-eye pairings. As in the case of the speed measure, all six of the individual pairings show more crossed preference in the low-scoring group. On the other hand, the comprehension measure shows no evidence of differences in cross-index congruency between the good and poor readers. In fact, the low scorers show more crossed preference on only two of the four comparisons. Although crossed preference patterns may be associated with slower reading and poorer vocabulary skills, this relationship is not maintained for overall reading comprehension.

As a final analysis, we considered individuals as a function of whether they were totally congruent (ipsilateral) as opposed to those who manifested a crossed pattern on at least one index. In other words, we separated those individuals who were completely right or left sided from those who had at least one preference index on the contralateral side. This analysis showed that slow readers are 9.8% more likely to have at least one index crossed than are the fast readers. When we consider the results from the vocabulary measure, those scoring in the lowest 25% are 8.8% more likely to have at least one index crossed as compared to those in the highest quartile. No significant differences in crossed versus congruent patterns emerge for the two groups on the reading comprehension scale. There is a similarity between these results and those shown in Table 9-1, where the composite index of sinistrality also showed significant difference between the high and low scorers for the speed and vocabulary scales, and did not show any effect when the sample was divided on the basis of the comprehension measure.

Our study suggests that there are some differences in the pattern of lateral preferences manifested by samples of slow versus fast and good versus poor readers. The statistically significant differences appear to be consistent with the overall tone of the data reported in the literature and reviewed in the first part of this chapter. There appears to be a general trend toward a higher incidence of left-sidedness and of crossed preference in groups that show poor performance on tests of reading skills. Mixed lateral preference response patterns do not seem to be as clearly related to reading ability. However, the relationship between lateral preference patterns and reading ability is task specific. For the three reading measures that we used, the strongest effects emerge in reading speed, followed by the vocabulary measures. Differences in lateral preference do not appear to be predictive of scores obtained on the comprehension scale. Such a pattern of results suggests that sinistrality and crossed preference are not simple indicators of an individual's level of global linguistic skill. Rather they may be indicators of performance proficiency in certain types of tasks associated with reading.

The strongest single predictors of variations in the measures of reading performance used in our study are the lateral preferences of hand and foot. Increased sinistrality in hand or foot is characteristic of the slowest reading group, as is mixed footedness, while a crossed hand-foot pairing appears to be the single most predictive measure of differences in both speed and vocabulary scores. Some theoretical considerations may lead one to expect that of the four indexes of lateral preference that we studied, limb preferences would be those most likely to be associated with aspects of reading performance. First, there are the statistical considerations that we discussed in Chapter 8. If there is a pathological condition that might be sufficient to cause poorer reading and also alter lateral preferences, it would be most evident in indexes where the dextral bias is strongest and the population is most asymmetrical. We noted this in our discussion of the Satz (1972, 1973) model and the process is demonstrated in Table 8-1. Since hand and foot show the most extreme bias in preference distributions, statistically it is easier to detect deviations in these distributions.

If shifts in lateral preference indicate an underlying neurological disruption that covaries with deficits in reading skill, the connection between reading and congruency of hand and foot preference is important. Because of the contralateral nature of motor control mechanisms to the limbs, one can assume that the limbs have control pathways emanating from the same cerebral hemisphere. We have postulated these anatomical facts as the basis for their close behavioral association, and certainly the normative data in Chapter 3 indicate that the most typical pattern is congruency between hand and foot preference, with both most often being right sided. Furthermore, handedness and footedness seem to share a common dimension as shown by the factor analysis described in Chapter 4. Thus crossed patterns between these two indexes may indicate disturbances of neural or cerebral control processes (or a combination of both). Disruptions in cognitive skills, such as reading performance, may be a by-product of a pathological condition, maturational anomaly, or processing disorganization arising from atypical neural-hemispheric factors and the altered preference patterns may be quite secondary. Footedness may be a slightly better indicator of these hypothetical disruptions than handedness because handedness is subject to social pressure that increases the use of the right side (see Chapter 6). Since there is no corresponding social pressure on foot use (this could mask natural sinistrality or ambilaterality in the hand), the foot may be a less contaminated indicator of the natural sidedness of limb preference and thus it may be more likely to demonstrate neuropathically induced changes in distributional properties.

Lateral preference patterns of typical young adults may covary with some aspects of cognitive ability, namely, reading speed and vocabulary skills. This result indicates that variations in lateral preference patterns may be related to very specific aspects of cognitive abilities. There is a long history of speculation that lateral preference, especially handedness, is an indicator of a variety of intellectual abilities. In the next chapter we will consider the relationships between lateral preference and a broad range of cognitive skills.

10

Cognitive Abilities

Chapters 8 and 9 explored possible associations between patterns of lateral preference and variations in cognitive abilities. We looked at various clinical groups, such as retardates, and we compared the top and the bottom of a distribution of typical cognitive abilities. Our emphasis was on observed or inferred pathologies, guided by the presumption that variations in the distribution of lateral preferences away from the dextral, consistent, and congruent norm are indicators of such pathological conditions. In this chapter we will explore the relationship between lateral preferences and a variety of cognitive skills within the average range of abilities. This is a natural next step, but it does involve a shift in emphasis. We are moving away from the pathological approach and into the realm of individual differences.

Why does one expect cognitive abilities to be related to any manifestation of lateral preference in typical nonclinical populations? In pathological groups, one could attribute the altered distributions of lateral preference to the particular neurological insult or developmental anomaly responsible for the observed disruptions in other functions. One cannot do this when a specific pathological condition does not exist. One could contend that lateral preferences are a secondary indication of functional integrity. If this is the case, then groups that differ in their general levels of cognitive functioning (e.g., retardates versus individuals of high intelligence) may also differ in their distributions of lateral preference behaviors. Traditionally, however, the impetus for such investigations has emanated from considerations of the functional specialization of the two cerebral hemispheres.

There is a huge body of research demonstrating that the two sides of the brain seem to be biased toward greater or lesser proficiency in certain cognitive tasks. A full review of this literature is beyond the scope of this book and it would take us far afield from the topic of lateral preferences. However, we can outline some of the general findings. Hecaen and Albert (1978) have presented a review of the empirical efforts supporting the notions of functional asymmetry in the hemispheres of the human brain. They have summarized the results of over 40 years of clinical research during which investigators have studied the patterns of cognitive deficits resulting from right or left hemisphere lesions. They report that the left hemisphere contains the neural substrate necessary for language and for nonverbal forms of communication, such as signs or gestures. It also deals with the analysis of perceptual stimuli that can be easily verbally labeled. The right hemisphere seems to be specialized for spatial orientation, some forms of pattern perception (including faces), and the perception and recall of nonverbal material or material containing a complex perceptual structure. Hecaen and Albert (1978) summarized this material as follows: "The following statement summarizes and serves as an initial approximation of the preceding observations; the left hemisphere is responsible essentially for verbal functions and abstracting ability; the right hemisphere, for nonverbal, perceptual, and spatial functions" (p. 410). This dichotomy is somewhat oversimplified and it cannot be maintained with strict clarity, since there is an overlap in hemispheric abilities. However, we can use this generalization to ask whether patterns of lateral preference covary with differences in cerebral organization under this simplified dichotomy of right versus left hemisphere function.

Several techniques, often involving clinical samples, have been used to study this relationship. By selectively incapacitating one cerebral hemisphere, either though electroconvulsive shock or the injection of sodium amytal (often done in connection with neurosurgery), one can study the impairment or lack of impairment of speech production and language production and processing when only the right or the left hemisphere is active. The results of a number of studies using these techniques in conjunction with the assessment of handedness patterns have produced fairly consistent results. In the samples of right-handers who have been studied in this manner, 1-4% display right hemisphere speech functions, while the remaining 96-99% show localization of speech in the left hemisphere (Milner, 1974; Milner, Branch, & Rasmussen, 1964; Pratt & Warrington, 1972; Rossi & Rosadini, 1967; Wada & Rasmussen, 1960; Warrington & Pratt, 1973). Results from similar procedures conducted on samples of left-handers show a much greater incidence of right hemisphere speech localization. In left-handers the incidence of right hemisphere speech has been shown to be 25%, which is six times greater than that found for right-handers (Warrington & Pratt, 1973). Another clinical procedure used extensively in studies of hemispheric localization of speech functioning is the observation of patterns of speech disorders in aphasic patients. Aphasia is a term that describes a variety of language disorders arising from injuries to the cerebral speech centers. If the hemispheric locus of the lesion is known, the resulting pattern of speech disorder (if any), its type, and the eventual recovery or lack of recovery from the posttrauma deficits can be taken as an indication of the primary localization of the speech centers. Observations of this type suggest that the occurrence of aphasias varies as a function of the side of the injured hemisphere and the handedness of the individual (Goodglass & Quadfasal, 1954; Hecaen & Sauget, 1971; Penfield & Roberts, 1959; Russell & Espir, 1961).

Based on the study of aphasias, several investigators have postulated an incomplete functional lateralization of speech in the vast majority of left-handers

(Gloning, Gloning, Haub, & Quatember, 1969; Hecaen & de Ajuriaguerra, 1964; Hecaen & Sauget, 1971; Zangwill, 1960), with a high probability that a large number of left-handed individuals may have bilateral representation of speech. Milner (1974) postulated three different types of hemispheric speech dominance in left-handers, a left-sided group (about 70%), a right-sided group (15%), and a bilateral group (15%). Satz (1980), after an extensive review of the literature, attempted to fit the existing data to several models of speech localization. His analysis reveals that right-handers as a population are best characterized as having a unilateral localization of speech function in the left hemisphere. Left-handers as a population, however, appear to be quite different. They seem to have both bilateral and variable unilateral organization of speech function. He contends that as many as 80% of left-handers probably have at least partial representation of speech in the left hemisphere, while some 40% may have bilateral representation of speech. This evidence suggests that a relationship exists between the side of the preferred hand and speech lateralization in the right or left hemisphere. However, the association is not perfect, as we pointed out in Chapter 4. For a given individual, knowledge of handedness alone does not predict perfectly the locus of cerebral speech functions. However, one can view populations of left-handers and right-handers as having different distributions of cerebral language and speech organization.

The prediction of variations in cognitive abilities in nonclinical samples as a function of lateral preference patterns is tied somewhat tenuously to the notion that different patterns of hemispheric specialization are preferable for certain cognitive skills. For instance, individuals with right-hemispheric speech centers seem to process sequential utterances more poorly and show poorer syntactic skills (Fromkin, Krashen, Curtiss, Rigler, & Rigler, 1974; Zaidel, 1973), and bilateral speech representation has been associated with language deficits (Marcel, Katz, & Smith, 1974; Satz, 1976; Witelson, 1976). This finding may be due to competition between the hemispheres during linguistic activity (see Moscovitch, 1977). Since left-handers are more likely to have bilateral or right-hemispheric speech representation, left-handers should, as a population, show poorer language skills than their right-handed cohorts, who almost exclusively display left-hemispheric unilateral speech control.

An interesting indirect piece of evidence related to this issue emerged in one of our studies. We determined, by means of the self-report inventory presented in Table 3-1, the lateral preference of 487 college students. Individuals were dichotomized into two groups for each of the indexes of lateral preference. The first contained those subjects who were consistently right sided, while the second contained those individuals who manifested mixed or left preference. The 497 students were subdivided on the basis of their major area of study into two academic groups; one comprised those in science, mathematics, and graphic arts, while the other contained students specializing in language and literature. We reasoned that students would specialize in areas that required cognitive abilities at which they were most adept and with which they were most comfortable. The resulting data are presented in Table 10-1. There is a relationship between expressed academic major and handedness. Those individuals whose majors are

Table 10-1: Percentage of Students with Consistent Right-Sided Preference

| | Academic major | |
	Science-graphic arts ($N = 225$)	Language-literature ($N = 262$)
Hand	69.2[a]	78.8[a]
Foot	65.2	60.8
Eye	63.0	65.0
Ear	40.1	46.0

[a] Significant difference, $p < .05$.

in the language and literature area show a 10% greater incidence of consistent right-handedness than individuals majoring in science and graphic arts. None of the other indexes of lateral preference show any relationship to area of major specialization. This is a rather informal measure, but it does replicate a similar observation by Koch (1933), who found that college students majoring in literature tended to be more strongly right handed, as a group, than students majoring in the sciences. Our results are weak support, then, for the notion that handedness behaviors covary with language abilities or linguistic interests.

An association between lateral preference and spatial abilities has also been suggested. For example, Levy (1969, 1974) contends that hemispheric specialization evolved so that each side of the brain could attain greater competence in its set of cognitive abilities. This neural segregation is presumably necessary because there is a basic incompatibility between language and analytic abilities and nonverbal visual-spatial processes. If there is greater bilateral representation in left-handed (-sided) individuals, so that verbal and spatial operations are performed in the same hemisphere, interference between them may result in a performance decrement in one ability or the other. Levy suggests that the verbal processes predominate in the presence of such a conflict. Thus, deficits in spatial cognitive activities are predicted for left-handers when they are compared to right-handers. Conversely, according to her reasoning, this dual representation could produce better language performance in sinistrals when compared to dextrals.

Levy's prediction that left-handers will show better language skills is, of course, in direct opposition to the view offered earlier. This highlights one of the recurrent theoretical problems in predicting cognitive skills from presumed hemispheric organization. Is dual representation an asset (as in two loci of control are better than one) or a deficit (because of potential competition)? For example, Herrmann and van Dyke (1978) and Dimond and Beaumont (1974) predict that bilateral language representation in the left-handed populations leads to better performance in spatial tasks than that found in populations of right-handers. If one assumes an association between the speech centers and decisional processes (see Corballis, 1980b), then right-handers must carry out perceptual-spatial analyses in the right hemisphere and transmit the results to the speech and decisionally dominant left hemisphere for response selection and emission. For the left-hander with bilateral or right hemisphere speech organization, perceptual processing takes place in the hemisphere that contains linguistic capabilities, removing the necessity of hemispheric transfer of information. Since hemispheric transmission consumes time, the perceptual response of left-handers should be faster than that of right-handers. Since there is a decreased probability of error because of neural "noise" or misrouting of information, left-handers should also be more efficient at spatial tasks than right-handers. Despite the conflicting conclusions, each of these positions begins with the same two postulates: Left-handers are more likely to have bilateral speech organization than are right-handers, and bilateral representation affects cognitive processing.

The two preceding chapters certainly provide some support for contentions that cognitive processing and lateral preferences are related. The data in Chapter 8 exhibited a relationship between lateral preference and cognitive deficit, at least in cognitively deficient populations. When we moved from extreme deficits to the low normal range and studied individuals with reading problems (Chapter 9), the relationship became less pronounced. However, some specific preference patterns, such as sinistrality, seem to be associated with the kinds of cognitive deficits that lead to reading problems. One must assume that any relationship between lateral preferences and cognitive skills will be even more subtle if one studies variations in other cognitive abilities in samples functioning within the normal range.

Most of the available literature on this topic has focused on the relationship between cognitive ability and handedness. Excluding those studies that deal with special or clinical populations and reading disabled groups (all of which have been reviewed in Chapters 8 and 9), a sample of 29 studies remains. These have looked at the relationship between some aspect of cognitive skills and handedness in typical subjects. These studies, summarized in Table 10-2, constitute a rather heterogeneous group in which a variety of different measures and reporting procedures have been employed. We have divided the reports along the two salient cognitive dimensions thought to convary with lateral performance, namely, verbal versus spatial cognitive ability. The verbal measures generally included vocabulary tests or the verbal subscales of various intelligence tests. Spatial tests included a variety of diverse tasks, including the performance scales of some of the standard intelligence tests, drawing, maze performance, mental rotation tests, and pattern memory tasks. Those reports listed in the "general" category in Table 10-2 are the ones that did not divide the results along verbal versus spatial lines, that employed numerical tests, or that used more global measures of cognitive efficiency, such as school achievement or composite intelligence scores.

This table reveals a mixed pattern of results. Eleven of the 29 studies (or 38%) show no relationship between any manifestation of hand preference and any cognitive ability. Of the 18 studies reporting the results of verbal tests (verbal column), only six (33%) found significant relationships between verbal skills and handedness. Four showed superior verbal ability in right-handers, one found left-handers to be better, and the last reported that individuals with mixed preference

Table 10-2: Relationship between Handedness and Cognitive Skills Measures Based on the Findings of 29 Published Reports

Study	Cognitive ability			Subjects	Comments
	Verbal	Spatial	General		
Flick (1966)	—	R+	R+	4-year-olds	Form copying, maze, and IQ
Fagan-Dubin (1974)	0	—	0	Kindergarteners	IQ scales
Annett and Turner (1974)	0	0	—	5- to 11-year-olds	Vocabulary, drawing, and maze
Hardyck et al. (1976)	0	0	0	First- to sixth-graders	Includes IQ, arithmetic, and vocabulary
Allison (1966)	—	—	0	Third- to fifth-graders	School achievement
Clark (1957)	—	—	M−	Grade 7	School achievement
Keller et al. (1973)	0	0	—	Third- to 12th-graders	IQ scales
Sabatino and Becker (1971)	0	0/L−	0	Primary school	IQ, academic achievement
Hillerich (1964)	—	—	0	Primary school	IQ scales
Annett (1970b)	0	—	—	Primary school	Vocabulary
Bannatyne (1971)	0	L+	—	Primary school	Auditory sequencing, form memory
Roberts and Engle (1974)	0	0	—	6- to 17-year-olds	IQ
Wilson and Dolan (1931)	—	—	0	Sixth-graders	Arithmetic and language skills
Calnan and Richardson (1976)	R+	—	R+/0	11-year-olds	General achievement/0 for arithmetic
Naidoo (1961)	M−	0	—	Primary school	IQ scales
Heim and Watts (1976)	R+	0	L+	9- to 20-year-olds	L+ on numerical test
Gilbert (1973)	—	0/L−*	0	High school	College entrance exam
Orme (1971)	0	0	—	14- to 17-year-olds	IQ scales
Wittenborn (1946)	R+	0	R+	College freshmen	Essay, arithmetic, and spatial tests
Nebes and Briggs (1974)	—	R+	—	College freshmen	Memory for patterns

Miller, E. (1971)	0	R+	—	College	IQ scales
Herrman and Van Dyke (1978)	—	L+	—	College	Speed of mental rotation
Hicks and Beveridge (1978)	0	—	R+	College	Vocabulary and IQ
James et al. (1967)	0	R+	—	College	IQ scale variants
Newcombe and Ratcliff (1977)	0	0	—	Adult	IQ scales
Milstein et al. (1979)	—	—	R+	Adult	Arithmetic
Nebes (1971a)	—	R+	—	College graduate	Part-whole test
Briggs, Nebes, and Kinsborne (1976)	R+	R+	—	Adult	IQ
Levy (1969)	L+	R+	—	Graduate students	IQ scales

Note. R means right handed; L, left handed; M, mixed; +, better; −, poorer; 0, no difference.

*Recomputation of Orme's statistics by Hicks and Beveridge (1978).

patterns showed the poorest performance on verbal tests. This review does not provide strong support for the position that handedness patterns are predictors of variations in verbal ability. Seven (47%) of the 15 studies listed in the general column showed evidence of an association between handedness and cognitive skills. The results are similar to those reported for verbal abilities. The majority of the studies (5) found right-handers to be superior, one reported left-handers to be superior on a numerical test, and one reported that mixed-handers were inferior in scholastic achievement. While pointing toward general superiority in right-handers, more than half of the studies found no differences. When one considers spatial skills (shown in the spatial column), the same picture emerges. Of the 21 studies that used spatial tests, 11 (52%) reported some significant association with handedness. Nine reported that right-handers perform better, while two reported superiority in left-handers. The pattern of results is similar for the three categories of cognitive skills. Approximately one-half of the studies have reported significant associations between handedness and cognitive skills, and the majority of significant findings have favored better performance in right-handers.

Table 10-2 has been arranged in a sequence as a function of the chronological age of the subjects tested within each study. As one looks at the table, one will notice that the majority of the negative findings are concentrated in the upper half of the table, where we have placed the studies that tested younger subjects. There are 15 studies that utilized primary school or preschool subjects, and of these, six (40%) reported at least one significant relationship between hand preference and cognitive ability. Of these, three reported superiority in right-handers, two reported that mixed-handers were inferior, and one reported that left-handers were superior. The child data, then, provide no evidence for a systematic relationship between handedness and cognitive ability. However, this conclusion changes when one considers the studies that tested adult subjects, including college students, graduate students, and the general adult population. There are 11 studies (starting with Wittenborn, 1946, in Table 10-2) in this category. Of these, 10 (91%) reported some relationship between handedness and cognitive ability. Of the 10 studies finding significant associations with handedness, 9 report that right-handers are superior on at least one scale, and 2 indicate that left-handers are superior on at least one scale. This aspect of the survey suggests that handedness and cognitive abilities may covary in adults.

The normative data in Chapters 3 and 6 showed that there are systematic changes in patterns of lateral preference as a function of age. As the population grows older, preference patterns, at least for hand and foot, become gradually more right sided. Patterns of lateral preference also become gradually more consistent with age; thus, adults are more likely to manifest consistent right-handedness than children. Of the 23 instances in Table 10-2 that found a significant relationship between hand preference and cognitive skills, 18 (78%) indicated superior performance in right-sided individuals and 2 showed superiority in individuals with consistent preference. Since both right-handedness and consistent handedness are associated with more mature individuals, the association between lateral preference and cognitive skills may emerge as a metaphenomenon related to an aspect of neurological or psychological maturity. In this context, immaturity is the predictor of poorer performance in cognitive tasks with lateral preference serving only as a secondary sign. This type of reasoning is consonant with the notion of maturational lag discussed in Chapters 8 and 9. There is an expected adult preference pattern characterized by dextrality and consistency (at least for hand preference), and deviations from this norm could be symptomatic of deviations from normal cognitive functioning.

The most appropriate population on which to test these conclusions derived from the literature survey is one that is postadolescent, preferably young adult or older. Since little is known about the relationship between foot, eye, and ear preference and cognitive skills, it would be useful to measure these variables as well. With these data, one could test a variety of hypotheses about the association between all forms of lateral preference and intellectual functioning in typical adults. Since data of this type are not currently available, we conducted a study to explore these variables. We used as subjects 1,283 students enrolled in an introductory psychology course, who completed the self-report lateral preference inventory in Table 3-1. All subjects were also tested on two measures of spatial ability. The first was a multiple-choice embedded figure test, which presents a set of five simple figures and requires the subject to indicate which of the five is hidden in a more complex design. A sample stimulus pattern is shown in Figure 10-1. This task is one of the subtests of the Comprehensive Ability Battery (CAB) developed by Hakstian and Cattell (1974, 1976), and it requires the ability to disembed a simple figure from a set of complex distracting elements. The second spatial test required that individuals mentally rotate objects. The subject was given a target form and a set of three alternative figures. One of the alternatives is the same three-dimensional shape as the target, but it is rotated

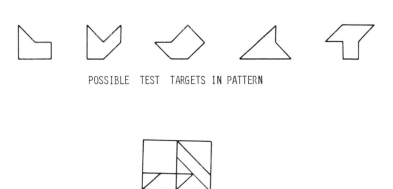

POSSIBLE   TEST   TARGETS   IN PATTERN

TEST PATTERN

Figure 10-1. Sample item from the embedded figures task: Subjects must determine which of the five test targets is hidden in the test pattern.

into a different orientation. The subject is required to find this form. An example of a typical test item from the mental rotation test is shown in Figure 10-2.

A subsample of 803 subjects also received three nonspatial cognitive abilities tests. The first was a speeded vocabulary test (the V scale of the CAB) in which the subject is given a test word and is required to select one of a set of five alternatives with a meaning identical to that of the test item. The second was a numerical abilities test (the N scale of the CAB); it involves arithmetic problems, such as addition, multiplication, and manipulation of fractions. The third involved inductive reasoning (the I scale of the CAB). Individuals are presented with five four-letter arrays and are required to select the array that violates the rule set by the other four. An example of an item from this test is the set

BBLJ   TTRU   FWZP   XXBK   MMEG

FWZP is the only item that does not contain a double letter, and therefore is the correct choice in this set.

We based our selection of these cognitive tests on several considerations. The two spatial tests assess different aspects of spatial ability; one involves two-dimensional and the other three-dimensional spatial visualization (see McGee, 1979). The remaining three tests are thought to explore both fluid and crystallized intelligence. These are concepts used by many psychometricians, including Cattell (1971) and Horn (1976), to differentiate types of cognitive abilities. *Crystallized intelligence* is defined as an awareness of acquired concepts, general terms, and techniques as measured in general information, mechanical aptitude, or vocabulary tests. It also includes knowledge of material found in a typical educational curriculum, such as mathematics and literature. *Fluid intelligence* is more analogous to reasoning ability, and is not dependent on education. It is often tested by using figural or nonword symbolic materials, mazes, figural classifications, letter series, analogies, matrices, or other general problem solving tasks. In our test battery, the vocabulary and numerical ability tests were measures of crystallized intelligence, and the inductive reasoning test was a measure of fluid intelligence.

We scored lateral preference responses with the dichotomous scoring procedure described in previous chapters (see Chapters 3, 8, and 9). Next, we

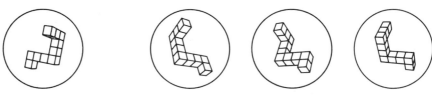

TARGET   ROTATED TEST ITEMS

Figure 10-2. Sample item from the mental rotation task: Subjects must determine which of the three test items is the same three-dimensional object as the target, rotated into a different orientation.

obtained the mean number correct on each test of cognitive skill for left- and right-sided individuals separately. Table 10-3 shows the results of this analysis for the four indexes of lateral preference and for the five cognitive tests.

Despite the large sample, handedness is related significantly to only mental rotation ability and inductive reasoning. The inductive reasoning test shows a significant superiority for right-handed individuals. Since the inductive reasoning test is a measure of fluid intelligence, these results replicate the findings of Hicks and Beveridge (1978), who also found that right-handers are superior in tests of fluid intelligence, but found no handedness effects in crystallized intelligence measures (also consistent with our results). When one considers the two spatial tasks, one finds that they do not act equivalently. Handedness does not interact with embedded figures performance; however, a clear difference favoring the left-handers emerges in the mental rotation test. Although this result is contrary to Levy's (1969) contention that left-handers are inferior in spatial tasks, it confirms a report by Herrmann and van Dyke (1978), who found that the speed of mental rotation, as measured by reaction time, was faster among left-handed individuals and another by Charman (1980), who found more accurate visuo-spatial recall in left-handed males. That the difference emerges in the mental rotation test and not in the embedded figures test supports the multidimensionality of not only spatial cognitive abilities (see McGee, 1979), but also the interaction between abilities and indexes of lateral preference. Eyedness and footedness are related only to the mental rotation test, and in both instances it is the left-preferent group that achieves the higher scores. Ear preference, however, is not related significantly to any aspect of cognitive skills tested by this battery.

We tried to obtain additional insights into the relationships between lateral preference and cognitive skills by using a more stringent definition of dextrality. We took the consistently right-sided group (with scores of +1) and compared their mean scores to those of the individuals in the remaining group of mixed dextrals, ambilaterals, and left-siders. This is a more stringent type of classification scheme than simple dichotomization. It is, however, the procedure that we used to obtain the significant association between handedness and academic major presented in Table 10-1. This scoring procedure changes the pattern of results. Table 10-4 reports the mean number correct on each test for the consistently dextral group as opposed to all of the others. Handedness is no longer predictive of either mental rotations or of fluid intelligence (as in the analysis of Table 10-3), but now relates to crystalline intelligence, with right-handers displaying better numerical and vocabulary skills. Individuals who are not consistently right-footed are better in mental rotations (as in the analysis of Table 10-3), and in this rescoring, they also do better in the inductive reasoning task. Non-right-eyed subjects continue to show superior performance on the mental rotation task, while right-eared subjects are better with the embedded figures task.

What accounts for the shift in the pattern of associations when we changed scoring procedures? In Chapter 2 we noted that many conflicting results in the literature may be due to differences in the categorization of individuals as left or right sided. Our reclassification into consistently right sided is not a pure

Table 10-3: Mean Number Correct on Five Tests of Cognitive Skills in a Sample of College Students as a Function of Right- or Left-Sidedness in Lateral Preference

| | Lateral preference type | | | | | | | |
| | Hand | | Foot | | Eye | | Ear | |
Cognitive test	Left	Right	Left	Right	Left	Right	Left	Right
Embedded figures ($N = 1{,}283$)	7.24	7.32	7.31	7.31	7.51	7.21	7.38	7.27
Mental rotation ($N = 1{,}283$)	10.30^a	9.62^a	10.29^b	9.55^b	9.94^a	9.60^a	9.90	9.59
Numerical ($N = 803$)	13.88	14.18	13.85	14.22	13.99	14.21	14.11	14.18
Vocabulary ($N = 803$)	10.54	10.57	10.52	10.58	10.55	10.57	10.57	10.57
Inductive reasoning ($N = 803$)	7.43^a	8.02^a	8.01	7.96	8.02	7.95	7.96	7.98

[a] Significant difference, $p < .05$.
[b] Significant difference, $p < .01$.

Table 10-4: Mean Number Correct on Five Tests of Cognitive Skills in a Group of College Students as a Function of the Strength of Right-Sided Behaviors

| | Lateral preference type | | | | | | | |
| | Hand | | Foot | | Eye | | Ear | |
Cognitive test	Mixed and left sided	Consistently right sided	Mixed and left sided	Consistently right sided	Mixed and left sided	Consistently right sided	Mixed and left sided	Consistently right sided
Embedded figures ($N = 1,283$)	7.21	7.50	7.36[b]	7.48[b]	7.46	7.41	7.24[a]	7.76[a]
Mental rotation ($N = 1,283$)	10.12	9.59	10.07[b]	9.27[b]	10.04[a]	9.52[a]	9.84	9.47
Numerical ($N = 803$)	13.70[a]	14.33[a]	14.23	14.09	14.04	14.29	14.03	14.39
Vocabulary ($N = 803$)	10.05[b]	10.80[b]	10.50	10.68	10.50	10.67	10.55	10.54
Inductive reasoning ($N = 803$)	7.77	8.05	8.15[a]	7.78[a]	8.03	7.99	8.02	7.91

[a] Significantly different, $p < .05$.
[b] Significantly different, $p < .01$.

measure in that it incorporates not only side but also consistency. The pattern of results in Table 10-4 actually reflects consistency more than side, as can be seen in Table 10-5. In this table we divided the sample on the basis of consistency of lateral preference. An individual was classified as consistent if all of the responses for a given index indicated the same side (either right or left), and individuals were designated as mixed if some responses on a given index were right sided and others left sided. After the division on the basis of preference consistency, the mean score on each test was computed. Nine of the 20 comparisons in Table 10-5 are statistically significant, as compared to only four based on side of preference (Table 10-3). In six of the nine comparisons, individuals with consistent response patterns produce better scores.

The consistency analysis in Table 10-5 produces a pattern of data similar to that in Table 10-4. Consistent handedness seems to predict greater facility for both of the crystallized intelligence measures (the numerical and the vocabulary tests). Consistency of foot preference seems to be associated with reduced scores in the mental rotation and the inductive reasoning tasks. Individuals with consistent eye preference have higher scores on the vocabulary test, while individuals with mixed eye preference show better mental rotation scores. The notion that the embedded figures test and the mental rotations test are different aspects of spatial ability is demonstrated again by the fact that individuals with consistent eye preference perform better at embedded figures while individuals with mixed eye preference are better at the mental rotations task. Ear preference also shows some association with cognitive skills, with consistent ear preference showing an association with better performance on the embedded figures and numerical tests.

These results are easier to interpret if we summarize them according to cognitive ability rather than according to preference index. The crystallized intelligence tasks (the numerical and vocabulary tests) show a significant association (when it is present) between better performance and consistent lateral preference. A similar pattern is present in the embedded figures test. When significant results are found for the mental rotation and the inductive reasoning tasks, they indicate that mixed preference is associated with superior performance. Comparison of Table 10-5 and Table 10-3 indicates that consistency is a better predictor of variations in cognitive skills than simple sidedness. Furthermore, the pattern of results in Table 10-4 likely reflects the effect of consistency rather than sidedness.

As a final analysis we explored cross-index congruency of preference and its relationship to these measures of cognitive ability. We classified individuals as congruent if their scores indicated the same side of preference for any pair of indexes as opposed to crossed if one index was right sided while the other was left. These data are shown in Table 10-6. Cross-index congruency does not appear to be related to any of the cognitive measures except the mental rotation test. Here, individuals who show crossed hand-foot, hand-ear, foot-eye, and eye-ear preference also show superior mental rotation scores when compared to those individuals who are congruent. The only other significant difference appears on the embedded figures test, where the individuals with crossed foot-

Table 10-5: Mean Number Correct on Tests of Cognitive Skills in a Group of College Students as a Function of Mixed versus Consistent Preference Response Patterns

	Lateral preference type							
	Hand		Foot		Eye		Ear	
Cognitive test	Mixed	Consistent	Mixed	Consistent	Mixed	Consistent	Mixed	Consistent
Embedded figures	7.30	7.34	7.31	7.31	7.21[a]	7.37[a]	7.20[b]	7.48[b]
Mental rotation	10.17	9.62	10.08[b]	9.31[b]	10.14[a]	9.59[a]	9.87	9.53
Numerical	13.58[a]	14.32[a]	14.25	14.07	14.11	14.22	13.96[a]	14.38[a]
Vocabulary	10.04[b]	10.76[b]	10.52	10.65	10.30[a]	10.66[a]	10.63	10.55
Inductive reasoning	7.81	8.02	8.17[a]	7.78[a]	8.06	7.98	8.07	7.89

[a] Significantly different, $p < .05$.
[b] Significantly different, $p < .01$.

Table 10-6: Mean Number Correct on Tests of Cognitive Skills in a Group of College Students as a Function of Across-Index Patterns of Lateral Preference

Cognitive test	Hand-foot		Hand-eye		Hand-ear		Foot-eye		Foot-ear		Eye-ear	
	Crossed	Congruent	Crossed	Congruent	Crossed	Congruent	Crossed	Congruent	Crossed	Congruent	Crossed	Congruent
Embedded figures	7.27	7.32	7.51	7.24	7.49	7.23	7.54^a	7.21^a	7.73	7.28	7.29	7.32
Mental rotation	10.34^b	9.59^b	9.93	9.62	9.99^a	9.56^a	10.20^b	9.47^b	9.70	9.69	9.97^a	9.53^a
Numerical	14.04	14.17	14.21	14.14	14.07	14.20	13.94	13.24	13.88	14.27	13.89	14.31
Vocabulary	10.66	10.55	10.45	10.64	10.55	10.58	10.62	10.55	10.54	10.58	10.52	10.60
Inductive reasoning	7.99	7.97	8.03	7.95	7.58	7.96	8.08	7.93	7.96	7.97	7.83	8.05

[a] Significantly different, $p < .05$.
[b] Significantly different, $p < .01$.

eye preference have higher scores. Total congruency in sidedness (all four indexes congruent) showed no relationship to variations in the cognitive measures.

There is no clear theoretical interpretation of these results. However, if we confine ourselves to a consideration of hand and foot preference, we may be able to achieve some explanation of these findings. The predominant adult pattern of hand and foot preference is right-sidedness coupled with consistent response patterns within these two indexes and relative congruency of sidedness between the two of them. It has been suggested that any deviation from this preference pattern reflects neurological immaturity, which in turn may be associated with lower degrees of cognitive efficiency. Thus, sinistral, mixed, and crossed-preferent hand-foot patterns may covary with poorer performance on cognitive skills tasks. We have observed this trend for the numerical vocabulary, and embedded figures tests. However, the mental rotation test produced data that are contrary to this expectation. Here, individuals with left-sided, mixed responses and crossed patterns in hand and foot preference outperform the other groups. This finding contradicts all of the others.

There is one speculative line of reasoning that would weave these results into a coherent theoretical tapestry. Although the higher mental rotation scores achieved by the left-, mixed-, or crossed-preferent individuals suggest greater spatial ability, this ability is specific to the mental rotations test. There is an argument that would predict this rotational superiority on the basis of the hypothesis that these preference patterns are manifestations of a general immaturity. As evidence we can turn to pattern discrimination errors characteristic of young children, involving mirror reversals and confusions. Children confuse lateral mirror image pairs, such as p and q or b and d. Such confusions seem to be quite common in young children, although they gradually decrease in frequency as the child ages (Davidson, 1935; Rudel & Teuber, 1963; Serpell, 1971). Indirect evidence suggests that this improvement is associated with the educational process, since the largest drop in mirror-imaging reversals is between the ages of 5.5 and 6.5 years, or at about the time that formal instruction in reading and writing begins. Furthermore, with appropriate training, kindergarden-aged children can learn to make these left-right discriminations more effectively (Clarke & Whitehurst, 1974). When such left-right confusions continue beyond early childhood, they can result in reading difficulties, and it is not uncommon to find dyslexic children showing confusions between targets of different orientation (Newland, 1972; Sidman & Kirk, 1974). These reversal errors suggest that children are relatively insensitive to the orientation of stimuli, but rather attend only to global shape. Adults seem to attend to both shape and orientation. For instance, consider a stimulus, such as a human face, that has a familiar orientation. When the face is inverted it seems to lose much of its facelike quality, and even familiar individuals are sometimes difficult to recognize when their photographs are inverted. Adult observers show much greater accuracy of identification when presented with faces that are upright rather than when the faces are presented upside down (Rock, 1974; Yin, 1970). However, the facial recognition performance of six-year-olds is not affected significantly by the orientation of the face. An inverted face is as easily recognized as an upright one.

By the age of 10, however, the child's facial recognition responses are like those of an adult; in other words, the recognition ability is disrupted when the faces are inverted (Carey & Diamond, 1977). Thus the adult pattern is to encode orientation as part of the identity of a given stimulus.

With this background we can make some interesting observations concerning performance on the mental rotation test. If an individual simply identified the shape of the object while performing this task, and did not separately encode the orientation as a component in the object's identity, this person would be more apt to accurately recognize the correct target stimulus in the test array. In other words, the more childlike response leads to better performance in this rotational task. If one argues that left, mixed, and crossed hand-foot preference patterns in adults reflect neural immaturity (and, by extension, relative cognitive immaturity), then one has explained our present pattern of data. In addition, this line of argument makes a number of predictions. We might expect left-handed and -footed individuals, or individuals with mixed preference on these indexes, to show a greater tendency to make left-right confusions if these patterns indicate some form of cognitive maturational delay. Data suggest that this is the case (Belmont & Birch, 1965). The association between left-handedness and spatial orientation confusions occurs even in intelligent adults (Harris, 1978). For example, Harris & Gitterman (1978) assessed the handedness of 364 university faculty members. They reported that left-handedness was associated with self-reports of frequent left-right confusions. We re-analyzed their data and found that only 17% of the right-handers reported such confusions "occasionally" to "all the time," while left-handers showed an incidence rate nearly three times as great (47%). Individuals who show left-right confusability are not encoding simultaneously the orientation and identify of an object, a fact that produces some directional confusions. However, in the mental rotation test, where the task is to select the object that is identical to the test object regardless of its orientation, the lack of encoded orientation is an advantage rather than a disadvantage. Once again, such failures to encode orientation are more typical of younger individuals, as are sinistrality and mixed and crossed preference of hand and foot.

Some relationship between cognitive skills and lateral preference in typical samples is suggested by our studies. Generally, right-sided and consistently sided individuals perform better in those instances where differences are found, with consistency of preference being the better indicator of the two. The only exception to this is the reversal observed in the mental rotation test. However, all of these effects are specific to certain preference indexes, and we can only derive a coherent explanation for the relationship between hand and foot patterns and these cognitive measures.

Chapters 8 and 9 also presented evidence for some association between lateral preference and cognitive abilities. The largest differences are found when we compare institutionalized clinical samples to normal control subjects. Such comparisons indicate an increase in the frequency of left-sidedness (particularly in limb preference), inconsistent lateral preference, and a lack of across-index congruency in the clinical populations. Thus, retardates differ from nonretarded controls not only cognitively, but also in terms of their manifest patterns of lateral preference. In Chapter 9 we considered a group of slow readers. Although they are below the population norm in the particular cognitive skills associated with this aspect of language processing, they are not so severely affected as to warrant clinical segregation. However, the same pattern found in the clinical groups reappeared. Although there are fewer significant differences between good and poor performers, when such differences occur, they indicate that sinistrality, mixed preference, or crossed lateral preference is more likely to be found in the poor performing groups. When we restrict our measures to typical adult samples and consider only variations within the normal range of cognitive abilities (as we did in this chapter), the number of significant relationships between lateral preference and cognitive performance again drops. However, the general pattern remains the same, with better performance associated with consistency of response and dextrality. The only exception to this is, of course, the mental rotation test.

At a theoretical level this pattern of results is susceptible to a variety of different interpretations. Perhaps a typical adult shows an expected pattern of proficiency in certain cognitive abilities and displays a typically dextral, consistent, and congruent pattern of lateral preference (at least for hand and foot preference). Any neurological or psychological disruption that is sufficient to disturb cognitive abilities also might alter this pattern of lateral preference. The more severe the neurological disruption, the more likely it will be that these secondary effects, such as shifts in lateral preference patterns, will occur. Unfortunately, this summary is purely descriptive and offers little explanation of the nature of the link between lateral preference and cognitive skills.

Another interpretation centers around a postulated theoretical link. This is a notion of neurological immaturity or incomplete neuropsychological development. In Chapters 3 and 6 we found that populations of young or immature individuals are less likely to manifest dextral preference for hand, foot, and eye relative to adults, and they tend also to show an inconsistent pattern of lateral preference behaviors, with some responses biased toward the right and others to the left. Sidedness becomes more consistent and more dextral (excluding ear preference) with age. The probability that across-index pairwise comparisons will be congruent also increases in mature populations. The patterns of lateral preference that are most typical of the adult tend also to be those typical of the more cognitively skilled individual. As shown in Table 10-2, the relationship between lateral preference (handedness) and cognitive ability is most evident in adult samples, where it is expected that neurological development has reached its completion. Perhaps the individual with more sinistral or inconsistent patterns of lateral preference is showing signs of neurological delay that manifests themselves as both a relative reduction in cognitive efficiency and a less adult pattern of lateral preference behaviors. If these speculations are correct, then sinistrality, inconsistent and crossed preference patterns, and reduced performance on cognitive measures arise from a common source, namely, the immaturity of neurological or neuropsychological development. These speculations are on the firmest ground when applied to hand and foot preference, with the relationship between sense organ preference and cognitive abilities remaining obscure at present.

11

Sensorimotor Coordination

There are four major manifestations of lateral preferences in humans. Two, handedness and footedness, deal with limb functions, while the other two, eyedness and earedness, deal with sensory functions. The limbs, of course, are the major effector organs upon which we rely to accomplish the majority of our interactions with the physical environment. The sense organs serve an input function, gathering information from the environment, and coordinating the movements of the limbs relative to the external conditions. This sort of sensorimotor coordination is taken for granted, as exemplified in the Spanish proverb, "What the eyes can see, the hands can grasp." However, the two hands are not used equally, nor are the two eyes. Thus one might be tempted to wonder whether our ability to grasp is affected by the eye used to guide the movement. More generally, one might ask whether specific patterns of lateral preference interact with sensorimotor abilities.

Hand-Eye Coordination

The most obvious sensorimotor pairing is the one highlighted in the proverb just quoted, hand and eye. This pair of preference indexes must coordinate with one another in order for a person to perform many activities, such as throwing a ball, aiming a weapon, or even simply picking objects up or putting them down again in a specific place. As a result, this index pair is the one that has been studied extensively in attempts to relate lateral preference behaviors to performance variables. Much of this research starts with the presumption that the preferred hand and the preferred eye are actually the better hand and the better eye, in the sense that they display greater dexterity, acuity, and so forth. As noted in Chapter 2, this idea does not withstand empirical assessment. However, it has been taken for granted by many of the researchers in this area, and instead of pursuing the truth or falsity of this postulate, they have debated whether one can find performance advantage for individuals who habitually display congruent versus crossed patterns of lateral preference across these indexes.

One of the first theorists to suggest that handedness and eyedness might affect sensorimotor coordination was Parsons (1924). His "primitive warfare" theory was encountered in Chapter 6 as an attempt to explain the predominance of right-handedness in the population. He also maintained that ipsilateral patterns of hand and eye preference offer a survival advantage. He proposed that the development of hand and eye preference was coincident with the emergence of tool and weapon use in the evolution of the human species. Eye preference emerged to meet the demands of sighting and aiming during hunting and battle activities, while hand preference arose because tools and weapons were handled more efficiently with one hand. He assumed that both the preferred hand and the preferred eye are superior to their partners, and then proceeded to argue that sidedness congruency between these two forms of preference allowed a warrior or hunter to place a weapon with greater accuracy, because the eye that aligned the weapon with the target and visually aimed it was on the same side of the body as the hand that threw it. This meant that the line of sight provided by the preferred eye was directionally compatible with the trajectory line of the thrown weapon, a situation that Parsons (1924) considered to be particularly advantageous from the standpoint of surviving an encounter with an armed opponent. The desirability of ipsilateral patterns of hand and eye preference is echoed in the following quotation from Mills (1925).

> Thought is conceived in the brain, formed by the eye and executed by the hand; and that perfect coordination of mind, eye and body which enters into the performance of all combined bodily movements, especially during games, would appear to make the placing and habitual fixing of control on one side of the body almost a necessity. (p. 934)

However, this doctrine has not been universally accepted. There is a long tradition that maintains that any forms of unilateral sidedness are disadvantageous. Some have contended that ambilaterality, where both sides of the body are used with equal facility, is preferable. This is an ancient argument that can be found even in the *Dialogues* of Plato (translation by Jowett, 1953, p. 362):

> In the same way that one who is perfectly skilled in the Pancratium or boxing or wrestling is not unable to fight from his left side, and does not limp and draggle in confusion when his opponent makes some change in his position, so in heavy armed fighting, and in all other things, if I am not mistaken, the like holds—He who has these double powers of attack and defense should not, in any case, leave them either unused or untrained if he can help it.

Proponents of ambi-sidedness have often captured both the popular mind and the fancy of educators. For example, John Jackson wrote several books supporting the notion that ambi-handedness was preferable to one-handedness, and his writings were sufficiently persuasive to allow him to found the Ambidextral Culture Society in Great Britain in 1903. This society drew the support of many well-known people, including Lord R. S. S. Baden-Powell, founder of the Boy Scout movement. He stated (quoted by Jackson, 1905):

I do not consider a man is a thoroughly trained soldier unless he can mount equally well on either side of his horse, use the sword, pistol, and lance, equally well with both hands, and shoot off the left shoulder as rapidly and accurately as from the right shoulder. (p. 12)

Given the history of debate over the relative advantages of strong unilateral hand-eye patterns versus ambi-sidedness, it is noteworthy that little experimental work has been done comparing the performance of individuals with crossed versus congruent hand-eye preference or looking at the performance of ambi-sided (crossed) versus unilateral (congruent) individuals. Much of the early research dealt with individual indexes, and simply tried to assess whether lateral preferences made any difference at all in various sensorimotor tasks. In addition, most of the reports treat lateral preferences as a secondary variable, and often the reports are based on casual observation rather than direct experimentation. The exploration of the relationship between hand and eye preference and shooting accuracy is an example of some of this informal research. Some reports have shown that accuracy in target shooting with a rifle is considerably better when individuals sight with their preferred eye (Banister, 1935; Crider, 1943; Doyne, 1915; Lebensohn, 1942). Most of these studies involved military personnel, and rifle proficiency was often based on ratings by superiors or trainers rather than on actual scores. Given the nature of the data it is not surprising to find that not all investigators have been able to verify the superiority of the preferred eye in this task (Simpson & Sommer, 1942). Recently, Landers (1980) reported that most Olympic shooters have ipsilateral hand and eye preference. However, other data suggest that the use of the preferred eye during shooting is more important than the use of the preferred hand (Brister, 1975; Daniels, 1981). For this reason some shooters utilize a device called the crossover stock. It permits one to press the stock of a rifle or shotgun against the shoulder on the side of the preferred hand, but its dog-leg bend places the barrel of the rifle beneath the contralateral eye. Thus, a right-handed left-eyed individual can handle the trigger of the weapon with the right hand, while sighting with the left eye.

Somewhat more formal investigative procedures appear in studies of athletic performance or gross motor behavior. For instance, Lund (1930) investigated the tendency to veer to the right or to the left in the absence of visual cues as a function of hand and eye preference. He reported that the observed directional errors did not covary with lateral preference for blindfolded individuals. Similar results were obtained by Sinclair and Smith (1957) and Luria (1979) when studying swimming. A group of studies involving more ballistic sport activities showed some interactions with hand and eye preference. Shick (1971) showed that the pattern of hand and eye preference interacted with the direction of errors in basketball shooting. These results were most evident in a nonselected sample, but were not significant for a more practiced group of individuals (Shick, 1974). Adams (1965) showed some interactions between hand and eye preference and baseball batting performance, although these were affected by postural and stance factors. Finally, Lavery (1943) presented evidence suggesting that children who have ipsilateral hand-eye preference perform better in general sports activities.

Few controlled laboratory studies have investigated sensorimotor coordination and patterns of lateral preference. One such study was conducted by Lund (1932). He used a target striking task (similar to dart throwing). His results indicated that subjects performed best when they utilized the preferred hand with the preferred eye. Shifting to either the nonpreferred hand or the nonpreferred eye reduced performance accuracy. A follow-up study by Freeman and Chapman (1935) used a pursuit task where subjects were required to keep a stylus on a moving target. Various combinations of hand and eye were tested. Their findings verified those of Lund (1932). The best performance was found for the preferred hand-eye combination, with both the preferred eye and preferred hand contributing separately to the accuracy of the pursuit skill. More recently, Ong and Rodman (1972), using a mirror tracing task, asked subjects to trace an optically inverted pattern. However, this study did not find any performance advantage conveyed by use of the preferred eye. These three studies were the only ones that we could find where the relationship between lateral preference and sensorimotor coordination was investigated systematically under laboratory conditions. Given the lack of data on the relationship between hand-eye preference in such activities, we decided to conduct some direct laboratory measurements.

We tested individuals on a task that required both speed and accuracy in sensorimotor guidance. Our apparatus was an inclined surface on which we projected mazelike patterns of dots. The starting point, or entrance to the maze, was indicated clearly by an arrow, and the subject's task was to move a hand as rapidly as possible along the maze, placing a dot in each target circle in order. The number of dots marked along the pathway within the fixed trial interval represented the subject's score. Targets varied in shape and starting point, but Figure 11-1 shows a typical one.

We separated the two eyes' inputs with anaglyphic goggles containing a red filter placed in front of one eye and a green filter in front of the other. By projecting the maze pathway through the appropriate filter, the pattern could be made visible to either the preferred eye (ascertained by the sighting tests listed in Chapter 2), the nonpreferred eye, or both eyes simultaneously. Subjects were tested using both their preferred and their nonpreferred hands (as determined by the questionnaire shown in Table 3-1). Each subject received eight trials, consisting of eight randomized mazes, under each combination of hand use and eye exposure. Each trial lasted 30 seconds, and the mean number of spots marked served as the subject's score under each condition. Our final sample was composed of 40 subjects, or 10 with each of the four possible hand-eye combinations (right hand-right eye, right hand-left eye, and so forth) as determined by our lateral preference testing.

We found no overall performance differences between the right- and the left-handers or the right- and left-eyed individuals. Also, there were no differences between the individuals who showed crossed as opposed to congruent sidedness patterns in their eye-hand preference behaviors. Therefore, we collapsed across these variables and conducted our analysis in terms of the preferred eye and the preferred hand, irrespective of its side or the congruency relationship. The mean

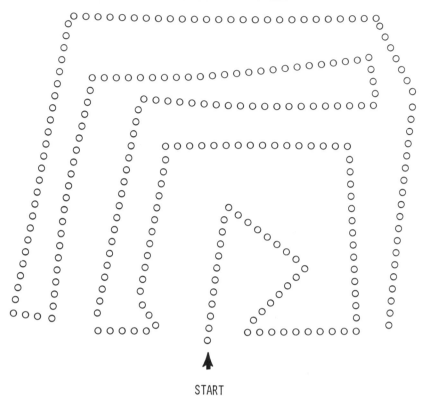

START

Figure 11-1. Typical maze pattern used in our study of hand-eye coordination. Subject begins at start, marking each circle in turn as rapidly as possible.

number of spots marked on the maze is graphed in Figure 11-2 as a function of the hand used and the visual exposure condition. There is a strong handedness effect, with the preferred hand performing significantly faster than the nonpreferred hand. There is also a systematic difference as a function of the visual exposure condition. Binocular exposure results in the best performance, followed by use of the preferred and the nonpreferred eyes in that order. These exposure effects also significantly differ from each other. If one considers only the comparison between the preferred and the nonpreferred eyes, one finds a significant difference favoring the preferred eye. Although this differential is small (a speed difference of between one and two marks in a 30-second period), it indicates greater sensorimotor efficiency when the preferred eye guides the hand, regardless of whether it is the preferred or nonpreferred hand. These data suggest that there are interactions between hand and eye preference and sensorimotor preformance. The use of the preferred eye and the preferred hand contribute, independently, to increase the efficiency of the task completion. However, neither patterns of crossed versus congruent preference nor the direction of sidedness behaviors (left versus right) interacts with performance.

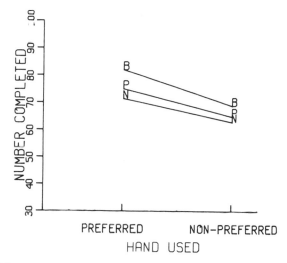

Figure 11-2. Mean number of circles marked for all eye-hand combinations (B is binocular; P, preferred eye; N, nonpreferred eye).

Sports Performance

Much of the interest in lateral preference and sensorimotor performance has emanated from the desire to improve the performance of athletes engaged in various sports, or to isolate variables that might predict the ultimate level of proficiency that can be attained. Within this context, the focus has usually been on a single sport, such as baseball or basketball, and lateral preferences have been assessed against a variety of limited performance indexes, such as performance at specific tasks during a practice session. Since these assessments are usually made within a single team, or sometimes within a physical education class, the range of abilities studied and the size of the samples are usually not very large. This makes it quite difficult to assess the effects of lateral preference patterns on the complex sensorimotor activities associated with many sports.

We decided to assess the interaction of lateral preference patterns and sports abilities over a wide variety of activities and proficiency levels. Furthermore, we used a common measure of lateral preference for all of our subjects and a common measure of attainment that could be applied to rate the level of proficiency in a variety of sports activities. With the assistance of Dr. Pam Duncan of the University of Victoria, we collected data from athletes engaged in a wide variety of different sports who varied over a wide range of proficiency levels (from novice to professional). To obtain these data, we contacted a selection of sporting federations, national athletic associations, college and university teams, and professional and semiprofessional teams in the United States and Canada. We obtained the names and addresses of individual athletes, and each of them was contacted by mail. Every potential subject was sent a copy of the self-report inventory presented in Table 3-1. In addition to eliciting lateral preference information, we also included items that asked about the individual's history of activity within the sport, the highest level of attainment in organized and official competitions, and any awards or honors received. Approximately 20,000 questionnaires were sent with an overall response rate of about 20%. We imposed further limitations on the sample for the purposes of analysis. Since there are age trends in lateral preference (Chapters 3 and 6), we restricted our investigation to individuals between 15 and 45 years of age. In addition, we included only those sports for which there were at least 75 respondents within the acceptable age range; thus, some sports were eliminated simply because an inadequate number of respondents made meaningful comparisons difficult. In some instances where sports were highly similar, such as softball and baseball, groups of athletes were combined. Our final sample consisted of 2,611 individuals from 15 sport groupings.

Because the purpose of this research was to explore the effects of lateral preferences on sports proficiency, as an indication of sensorimotor proficiency, we had to construct a general index of an individual's proficiency regardless of the sport category. We did this on the basis of actual competitive accomplishment in the sport. We assigned each subject a numerical proficiency score ranging from 2 to 10 that was based on the respondent's reported highest level of competition. Examples of the competitive levels represented by each proficiency score are shown in Table 11-1. In order to allow further gradation within these proficiency scores, index values were incremented if the team on which an individual played achieved recognition or honors beyond those typical of other teams in the same sport. For example, winning a league championship added one point to the proficiency score for an individual on the championship team. If the respondent

Table 11-1: Procedure Used to Code Levels of Sport Proficiency in the Study of Lateral Preference and Its Role in Sensorimotor Performance

Individual proficiency score	Competitive level
10	Professional, Olympic, international competition
8	National, AAA (minor league)
6	College varsity, state or provincial competition, Class A, semiprofessional
4	College junior varsity, Class B
2	Intramural, Class C, recreational
Added values	Team honors (i.e., championship) add +1 to score. Individual honors (i.e., Olympic gold medal, Outstanding Player award, etc.) add +2 to score.

achieved individual honors, for example, an Olympic gold medal, a league batting championship, or a Rookie of the Year award, two points were added to the individual's proficiency score. The maximum number of additions was two, with 12 being the highest possible score. This index allows comparison of individual performance within each sport, and at least crude comparison across sports.

We conducted a preliminary global analysis to explore the effects of lateral preference on sport proficiency by considering only the top one-third of all of the athletes, regardless of sport. These are the individuals with a proficiency score above 8—mostly athletes who compete at the national, international, and professional levels (as shown in Table 11-1). We selected a random control sample for comparison purposes from the normative sample discussed in Chapter 3. The control sample was unselected as far as athletic ability was concerned. however, each athlete was matched to an individual of the same age and sex to control for any variations in lateral preference because of these individual difference factors. These procedures resulted in two samples, each containing 1,084 individuals.

As in previous chapters, we analyzed the data in three ways. First, we computed the percentages of right-sidedness for the two groups, and then the percentages of consistent response patterns (regardless of side) within each index. Finally, we computed the percentages of congruency between the various preference types analyzed in pairs. The only difference between the present and previous analyses is the omission of a consideration of ear preference. Since we could not conceive of any relevance it might have for sensorimotor coordination or sport performance, and since it has never been studied in this context, we did not include it as part of the analysis. Table 11-2 shows the results of our first overall sport proficiency and lateral preference analysis. The only significant difference between the two groups is in the incidence of consistent handedness responses. Here, the top-performing athletes show a significantly lower incidence of consistent response patterns (either all right or left) in handedness. The group of athletes resembles the control group in every way except that it is more ambihanded.

This type of global analysis is probably too coarse to provide the specific data needed to illuminate the relationship between patterns of lateral preference and sensorimotor proficiency in sport performance. This comparison grouped a large number of individuals who have demonstrated high degrees of athletic ability for very different types of coordinations. An Olympic gymnast and an Olympic rifle marksman might both attain a proficiency score of 10; however, the superior level of proficiency within the two individuals' particular sports represents very disparate patterns of sensorimotor coordination. Therefore, we conducted a more specific analysis in which we considered the patterns of coordination within, not across, sport groupings. We subdivided our sample of athletes into 15 sport groupings and conducted the same three types of analyses as shown in Table 11-2, with one difference. We looked at the effect of sidedness on sport proficiency by dichotomizing the athletes in each sport into a right- and a left-sided group for the three indexes of preference. Then we computed the

Table 11-2: Percentage of Right-Sidedness, Consistent, and Congruent Sidedness for Athletes in the Top 33% of Rated Proficiency (Scores > 8) as Compared to a Matched Control Group

Lateral preference type	Athletes in top 33% of proficiency ratings ($N = 1{,}084$)	Unselected matched controls ($N = 1{,}084$)
	Right sided (%)	
Hand	88.3	88.4
Foot	79.2	78.9
Eye	71.7	70.2
	Consistently Sided (%)	
Hand	75.6[a]	80.1[a]
Foot	44.3	46.5
Eye	67.6	70.5
	Congruent (%)	
Hand-foot	81.6	82.1
Hand-eye	74.0	73.2
Foot-eye	69.1	67.2

[a] Significantly different with $p < .05$.

mean proficiency rating for the right- and the left-sided categories. In a similar fashion, we explored the effect of mixed (ambi-sidedness) versus consistent response patterns within each index by computing the mean proficiency score for these two groups in each sport category. Finally, we computed the mean proficiency rating for athletes classified as congruent versus crossed for the three pairs of lateral preference indexes of interest here, namely, hand-eye, hand-foot, and foot-eye.

Table 11-3 explores the notion that right- versus left-sidedness, in and of itself, will affect the level of proficiency in the performance of skilled sensorimotor co-ordinations in various sports. Anecdotal accounts in the literature often attribute remarkable degrees of clumsiness to left-handers (in our analyses, we can explore these notions relative to left-siders). Perhaps it was these observations that led to the theories in which left-handers have been considered to be inferior or damaged relative to right-handers. This is shown in the following quote from Burt (1937):

> Not infrequently the left-handed child shows widespread difficulties in almost every form of finer muscular coordination . . . they shuffle and shamble, they flounder about like seals out of water. Awkward in the house, and clumsy in their games, they are fumblers and bunglers at whatever they do. (p. 287)

Consider, for instance, the infamous clumsiness of former United States President Gerald Ford, who bumped his head, tumbled down airplane ramps, and col-

Table 11-3: Mean Sport Proficiency as a Function of Right- and Left-Sidedness

Sport group	N	Hand Left	Hand Right	Foot Left	Foot Right	Eye Left	Eye Right
Baseball	170	6.66	6.13	6.70	6.06	6.56	6.06
Basketball	260	5.21	5.48	5.17	5.51	5.92[b]	5.19[b]
Bowling	82	4.50	4.12	3.78	4.19	3.60[a]	4.46[a]
Boxing	84	9.38[a]	7.73[a]	8.91	7.85	8.36	7.83
Field Hockey	227	6.33	5.62	6.23	5.58	5.43	5.84
Figure skating	94	6.25	7.84	8.60	7.60	7.93	7.60
Football	327	6.68	7.05	7.06	6.99	6.66	7.14
Gymnastics	92	4.70	4.95	5.09	4.90	5.65[a]	4.56[a]
Ice hockey	129	6.14	5.95	6.36	5.85	5.41	6.19
Races	169	7.84	8.03	8.04	7.99	8.19	7.91
Racquet sports	299	5.77	6.08	5.82	6.10	5.76	6.14
Rifle, pistol, and archery	222	9.07	9.62	9.34	9.64	9.10	9.72
Soccer	123	6.70	6.66	7.19	6.40	6.52	6.72
Swimming	126	6.63	6.06	5.60	6.25	5.98	6.22
Volleyball	207	4.54	5.25	5.13	5.18	5.30	5.12

[a] Significant difference, $p < .05$.
[b] Significant difference, $p < .01$.

lided with his honor guards so often than his staff was prompted to put an election year embargo on official press releases and photos of such events. His problems and awkwardness were attributed by the popular press to his left-handedness (Bell, 1974). Athletes themselves seem to think that being right or left handed may affect their performance in a given sport. For example, the All England Women's Hockey Association *Handbook* is quoted as saying, "Any player using a left-handed stick would find it almost impossible to keep to the rules. They would find it difficult to receive the ball, or to get the ball away from other players" (Barsley, 1976, p. 224). However, the existence of many legendary left-handed sports figures, such as baseball's Babe Ruth or tennis's Rod Laver, seems to argue against a strict application of these notions to all sports.

As can be seen from Table 11-3, there appears to be very little effect of left or right preference across the 15 sport groupings. There is some suggestion that left-handedness conveys a certain advantage to boxers, since this group scores approximately two proficiency levels higher than the right-handed boxers. The advantage in this case may arise from the unfamiliarity of the sinistral boxer's stance, resulting in punches coming from directions and angles that differ from those used by the right-handed boxer. There is also a suggestion that eye preference may play a role in gymnastics, basketball, and bowling performance. These results are difficult to interpret, since left-eyedness appears to be associated with higher proficiency levels for gymnastics and basketball, whereas right-eyedness results in higher proficiency levels in bowling. However, given the 45 comparisons in Table 11-3, between one and four of the comparisons are expected to significantly differ on the basis of chance alone. Thus it is likely that left versus right preference for hand, foot, or eye does not interact with sensorimotor proficiency as manifested in athletic performance.

In our original global analysis (Table 11-2), we found that mixed handedness patterns were more prevalent in our most proficient group of athletes. The overall analysis did not allow us to ascertain if mixed lateral preference patterns are superior to consistent ones in individual sports activity. So we explored this possible effect with the data in Table 11-4. Each athlete was classified as consistent if all the responses within a given index indicate the same side preference, while individuals who showed right-sided preference for some behaviors and left for others were classified as mixed. As before, the mean sport proficiency ratings were obtained within each group.

The pattern of results observed in Table 11-2, which considers proficiency across all sports, indicates that mixed hand preference is associated with superior sports performance. Table 11-4, however, indicates that this superiority is not found across all sports groups. Only three sports classifications, ice hockey, field hockey, and basketball, show statistically significant differences in favor of ambi-handedness. Even if one ignores statistical significance and simply looks at the direction of the mean differences, only 9 out of 15 sport groupings favor

Table 11-4: Mean Sport Proficiency as a Function of Mixed versus Consistent Preference Patterns

Sport group	N	Hand		Foot		Eye	
		Mixed	Consistent	Mixed	Consistent	Mixed	Consistent
Baseball	170	6.41	6.16	6.54[a]	5.94[a]	6.37	6.16
Basketball	260	5.94[a]	5.29[a]	5.42	5.50	5.32	5.53
Bowling	82	4.92	3.96	4.07	4.19	3.42[a]	4.37[a]
Boxing	84	7.80	8.09	7.87	8.21	7.73	8.13
Field hockey	227	6.61[b]	5.40[b]	5.83	5.55	5.57	5.83
Figure skating	94	6.71	7.92	7.55	7.78	7.35	7.84
Football	327	7.30	6.92	7.14	6.88	7.26	6.85
Gymnastics	92	5.03	4.87	5.00	4.84	5.03	4.92
Ice hockey	129	6.88[a]	5.53[a]	6.03	5.87	6.05	5.98
Races	169	7.89	8.03	8.18	7.77	7.52	8.24
Racquet sports	299	5.56[a]	6.23[a]	6.20	5.86	5.79	6.12
Rifle, pistol, and archery	222	9.62	9.57	9.38	9.81	8.96[b]	9.91[b]
Soccer	123	6.30	6.77	6.93[a]	6.03[a]	6.59	6.71
Swimming	126	6.22	6.11	6.37	5.90	6.41	6.07
Volleyball	207	4.80	5.28	5.33	4.90	5.24	5.12

[a] Significant difference, $p < .05$.

[b] Significant difference, $p < .01$.

mixed handedness. There are certain commonalities among the three sports that show greater proficiency for mixed handers. All contain active body movement and all require rapid response to action on either side of the body. It is important to be able to dribble a basketball with either hand, and to receive or dispatch passes with either hand. In ice hockey, players must be able to respond to either side of the body, shifting one's grip on the stick rapidly, sometimes powering a shot from the right and at other times from the left side. Alternatively, in racquet sports, there is a significant advantage conveyed by consistent handedness. The racquet sports seems to have much in common with hockey, since both require the use of an implement to propel an object. The difference may lie in the fact that in the racquet sports the grip remains fixed; only the arm movements and the bodily stance change.

Only two sports show consistency effects for footedness. In one, soccer, the advantage of mixed footedness is apparent given the nature of the sport. Soccer players must be able to kick a ball with either foot. The only other sport manifesting a significant footedness effect is baseball, but the particular performance advantage conveyed by mixed footedness is not immediately apparent. Consistent eye preference is apparently an advantage in the shooting sports and in bowling. There is some theoretical commonality between bowling and the shooting sports, in that the same eye is doing the sighting in all instances. This fact could eliminate the common problems of cross firing in the shooting sports and cross-laned balls in bowling. Such errors could easily occur if an individual is ambi-eyed, since the right eye and the left eye could perform the alignment with the target area on different occasions. The two eyes have different lines of sight. Since individuals are not usually aware of the eye that is sighting (as detailed in the next chapter), should the coordination on a given shot begin with one eye and switch to the other this could result in a deviation from the originally intended trajectory.

Right- or left-sidedness alone does not seem to affect sports proficiency. Ambi-sidedness versus consistent preference is more predictive of ability. One might argue that such within-index considerations are not likely to be important because all of the sports under consideration involve the coordination of both sets of limbs and the eyes. Thus, one might expect that consideration of across-index patterns of preference congruency would produce more interesting results. Individuals were classified into congruent or crossed for each of the three possible pairings of indexes. If both indexes manifested the same side of preference, the individual was classified as congruently sided; if they manifested different preferred sides, individuals were classified as crossed. Within each sport group the mean proficiency score was computed separately for crossed versus congruent respondents. These results are shown as Table 11-5, which indicates that there are a number of significant differences in proficiency level as a function of crossed versus congruent preference patterns. However, whether increased or decreased proficiency is related to congruent preference depends on the particular sport and the particular pair of indexes under consideration. The largest number of significant findings are associated with the hand-eye combination. Two groups of sports, the shooting sports (including rifle, pistol, and archery) and the

Table 11-5: Mean Sport Proficiency as a Function of Crossed versus Congruent Preference Patterns

Sport group	N	Hand-foot		Hand-eye		Foot-eye	
		Crossed	Con-gruent	Crossed	Con-gruent	Crossed	Con-gruent
Baseball	170	6.53	6.14	6.78^a	5.97^a	6.51	6.10
Basketball	260	5.30	5.47	6.16^b	5.16^b	57.5	5.28
Bowling	82	4.60	4.12	3.73	4.34	3.39^a	4.44^a
Boxing	84	8.00	7.99	7.88	8.03	8.50	8.81
Field hockey	227	6.15	5.64	5.44	5.83	5.54	5.84
Figure skating	94	7.43	7.75	8.48	7.42	8.13	7.49
Football	327	6.90	7.03	6.72	7.13	6.67	7.14
Gymnastics	92	5.00	4.91	5.93^b	4.46^b	5.72^a	4.50^a
Ice hockey	129	6.12	5.95	5.72	6.07	5.95	6.00
Races	169	8.46	7.92	8.54^a	7.79^a	8.38	7.84
Racquet sports	299	5.76	6.11	4.65^b	6.01^b	5.63	6.22
Rifle, pistol, and archery	222	9.59	9.58	8.54^b	9.87^b	8.75^b	9.97^b
Soccer	123	7.21^a	6.38^a	6.48	6.72	6.92	6.49
Swimming	126	6.53	6.09	6.32	6.08	6.27	6.10
Volleyball	207	5.05	5.19	5.13	5.18	5.56	5.01

[a] Significant difference, $p < .05$.
[b] Significant difference, $p < .01$.

racquet sports (tennis, badminton, squash, and so forth) contain individuals of higher rated proficiency in the congruent hand-eye category. All explanations why a particular pattern of lateral preference favors a given set of coordinations must be speculative. However, we can suggest a number of possibilities.

The superiority of congruent hand-eye preference in racquet sports may arise from a visual control factor. If the preferred eye is on the same side of the body as the preferred hand, the individual has a larger useful visual field in the sector of the environment where most of the activity is occurring. If visual input is monitoring both the projectile to be hit and the racquet that will strike it, ipsi-lateral hand-eye positioning means that both the target and the racquet will enter the visual field of the preferred eye earlier than would be the case if moni-toring was done by a contralateral preferred eye. In this case the usable visual field would be truncated by the bridge of the nose. With the earlier appearance of the hand to the ipsilateral preferred eye, there is more time to make minor adjustments to the ongoing swing and hence to improve overall accuracy.

When dealing with the shooting sports, one might at first feel that the advant-age of congruency is somewhat artifactual. Most rifles are designed to be fired by right-handers, and since they are generally held against the right shoulder, it is more convenient for an individual to sight with the right eye. The experimental work reviewed earlier in this chapter indicated that there is some advantage conveyed by using the preferred hand and the preferred eye in shooting. Since the rifle itself favors ipsilateral individuals, one might argue that congruent hand-eye preference merely accommodates to the bias of the apparatus itself. However, a hand-held pistol does not have the same bias as a rifle. The pistol is not held against the shoulder and can be sighted easily with either eye. Nonetheless, even when we considered pistol shooters alone, those individuals who manifested congruent preference of hand and eye also showed higher proficiency scores. The exact reasons why congruent hand-eye (and foot-eye) lateral preference aids in the shooting sports must ultimately be solved by biomechanical and kinesiological study. Unfortunately, to date no direct experimentation on the relationship of lateral preference patterns to the dynamics of motion have been conducted. Nonetheless, the existing literature suggests some factors that might account for the observed pattern of results. Perhaps the most obvious factor involves shifts in the body's center of gravity (Broer & Zernicke, 1979). Most target shooters adopt a stance that orients their body at an angle to the target. The target weapons are heavy. When held, they tend to pull the body's center of gravity in their direction, applying a rotary torque in the general direction of the line of fire. The shooter adopts a specific posture at an angle to the target to compensate for this, usually spreading the legs to provide a firmer base and tilting the hip toward the rearmost leg. The hand on the trigger—the preferred hand—usually is held closer to the body. If the eye is on the same side as the preferred hand, the tilt of the head into alignment with the hand and weapon supports this action, and the resulting line of gravity will be quite stable, located somewhere near the middle of the body. However, if the contralateral eye is the sighting eye, the head and trunk of the body must be twisted to bring the eye into alignment with the sights. The resulting position is less stable (since the twist moves the center of gravity forward toward the weapon) and it requires more effort to maintain. The crossed-preferent shooter has a problem. Either a less stable and more fatiguing twisted stance must be adopted, which could reduce efficiency and accuracy, or the nonreferred eye must be used for sighting. As indicated in the previous section, use of the nonpreferred eye in a task having an aiming component results in poorer performance. Therefore, whatever strategy is employed by crossed-preferent shooters, their performance may not be at the level of shooters with congruent preference.

The remaining four significant hand-eye congruency findings all show higher proficiency ratings in the crossed, rather than the congruent, group. In three of these sports, gymnastics, running, and basketball, the performance advantage of preference may be related to postural considerations. For example, most activities involving reaching, pushing, lifting, or holding involve an initial shift of the center of gravity in the direction of the acting limb (Broer & Zernicke, 1979). If one assumes that most such manipulative activities will begin with the activity of the preferred hand or foot, this will mean a shift of the center of gravity in the direction of the preferred side. With countless repetitions during everyday activities, the lateral shift of weight probably becomes habitual and anticipates the limb extension through shifts of other bodily components (Page, 1968).

This is generally adaptive, since it brings the force of the body's weight into play and increases the power of the resulting movements. For sports, such as gymnastics, that favor bilateral movements (as in tumbling, vaulting, rings, and so forth) this shift will add a slight twisting torque to the activity, and such twisting is usually downgraded in the scoring during competition. An individual with crossed preference may have a center of gravity that is pulled slightly away from the preferred side (in other words, it is positioned more toward the body's midline). This could result in more balanced performance and better scoring during competition. The same aspects of bodily posture and center of gravity might be the cause of the greater proficiency of basketball players and runners who show patterns of crossed preference. As basketball players jump to shoot the ball, especially in one-handed shots, the slight torque on the body of the player with congruent preference requires more of a compensation than is required for the crossed-preferent player. This could affect throwing accuracy. For a runner, the location of the center of gravity in the midline reduces the likelihood of veering slightly from the chosen running ling. A tendency to veer would require one or two lateral or oblique steps to correct the error. These compensatory steps are, of course, relatively wasted activity, in that they move the individual laterally in the track or lane, and do not advance the running toward the finish line. A few such steps could make a large difference in short races, such as the hundred-meter dash, which are often won by centimeters. Compounded across a long race, such lateral components to forward strides could cost the runner a considerable distance. Crossed preference, by placing the center of gravity closer to the midline, reduces the necessity for such correction, and hence increases the forward speed of the runner.

The performance advantage of crossed preference in baseball may be due to the nature of the stance adopted by the baseball batter. A right-handed batter generally orients in a position parallel to the home plate. The baseball bat is held to the right side of the body, in preparation for a swing that will traverse in an arc from the right side of the body around toward the left. Since the player is standing with the right side oriented toward the catcher and the left side toward the pitcher, the eye facing the pitcher, which will monitor the trajectory of the ball, is the eye contralateral to the preferred hand (in this example, the left eye). If aiming coordinations with the preferred eye are more accurate, this stance favors the individual whose preferred eye is contralateral to the preferred hand.

These explanations of our results are only tentative suggestions. Many of these speculations assume a relationship between the sidedness of lateral preference and the location of the body's center of gravity. Also, many of the notions have assumed that lateral preference plays a role in body posturing and positioning. All of these assumptions need direct empirical tests before we can verify the notion that there is an interaction between the postural requirements of an activity and the pattern of lateral preference that results in the highest performance efficiency.

Earlier discussions suggested that the most important aspect of crossed versus congruent preference involved patterns between the hand and the eye. However, there are also some significant differences in terms of foot eye lateral preference. The hypothesis that crossed preference is of value for the maintenance of balance in gymnastics tends to be confirmed by the fact that individuals with crossed foot-eye preference show greater proficiency. Congruent foot-eye patterns seem to be of value in the shooting sports (rifle, pistol, and archery) and in bowling, another sport involving a ballistic aiming response. The only sport where hand-foot patterns seem to matter is soccer, where crossed-preferent individuals are more proficient. This result makes sense from a postural viewpoint, since the act of kicking requires a complex compensating shift of the body's center of gravity in order to maintain an upright stance. Normally, one does not fall toward the side of the lifted foot because one extends the contralateral arm. Perhaps the preferred arm can accomplish these adjustments more quickly and accurately. The most effective preference pattern, then, in a sport that involves kicking is for the foot preferred for kicking to be contralateral to the preferred hand.

Lateral preference seems to be related to some aspects of sensorimotor performance. In our laboratory study of a simple hand-eye coordination task, both the preferred hand and the preferred eye contributed independent advantages that acted to increase the speed of performance. The results of our large survey of lateral preference patterns in athletes indicated that sidedness itself may not be a variable that interacts with the skilled coordinations required in sport activities. However, the consistency of the displayed preference and the congruency patterns across the various indexes may affect the levels of ability that are achieved in some sports. Clearly, our results and suggestions concerning the findings from the athlete survey are only preliminary and suggestive. They do, however, demonstrate that any link between lateral preference and sensorimotor proficiency will be ability specific and not generalizable to all sensorimotor skills.

12

Sensory Preferences

Although we have discussed the two manifestations of sensory preference, eyedness and earedness, many times in the previous chapters, we have always done so in relation to limb preference or in the context of the general dimension of sidedness. As we noted in Chapter 3, there are significant but small correlations among the four preference indexes. The factor analytic analysis of Porac, Coren, Steiger, and Duncan (1980) discussed in Chapter 4 indicated that the preference dimensions underlying eyedness and earedness are separable from those of handedness and footedness, and are also independent of each other. This suggests that the functional significance of eyedness and earedness may be due to perceptual factors unique to each of these systems.

There are a number of problems in visual and auditory information processing that arise because human observers possess bilateral sense organs. The need to solve these problems could be enough to foster the use of a preferred eye or a preferred ear. We know much more about eyedness than we do about earedness, since ear preference has been comparatively ignored in the research literature. This means that the bulk of the discussion will deal with eye preference, and issues common to eye and ear preference will be presented first in the visual context before extending them to the auditory modality.

Eye Preference

The earliest reference to a *preferred* or *dominant* eye is a discussion by Giam Baptista del Porta (1593) in his book *De Refractione.* In order to appreciate Porta's (1593) treatment of the problem, one must know a few basic facts about normal human binocular (two-eyed) vision. When we look at, or *fixate,* a visual target, so that its image stimulates the fovea of each eye, the visual information is available to each retina separately and independently. We have two separate retinal images potentially contributing to the construction of our percept. These images are different in content because the two eyes view the world from slightly different directions as a result of the spatial separation caused by the nose. This image difference is called *binocular disparity*. An example of the type of disparity that can exist between the two eyes' views is shown in Figure 12-1. Binocular disparity has generated one of the most interesting, yet still unexplained, problems of human binocular vision, namely, how the two disparate monocular images combine into a stable single percept (see Dodwell & Engle, 1953; Gulick & Lawson, 1976; Helmholtz, 1909; Julesz, 1971; Nelson, 1975; Sperling, 1975). The issue is further complicated by the fact that under some conditions the visual system fails in its attempts to fuse the two monocular views. This occurs under conditions where one is dealing with targets at different distances from the observer. You can demonstrate this simply by fixating a distant target (e.g., a spot on the wall) and holding a pencil in the line of sight a few centimeters in front of the nose while continuing to fixate the distant target. These viewing conditions produce double images of the pencil, indicating a failure of fusion of the disparate binocular images.

There is a clearly defined region in visual space, called *Panum's area*, in which disparate images are fused. Its position in external visual space is determined by the viewing distance on which the eyes are converged, or in other words, by the

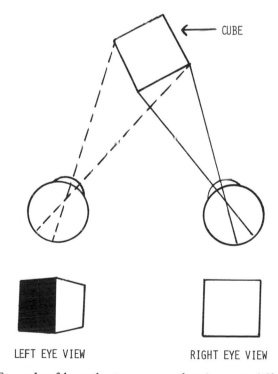

Figure 12-1. Example of how the two monocular views can differ during binocular viewing.

distance of the fixated target. All objects at about the same distance from the viewer as the fixated target are seen in single vision, while objects farther away from or closer to the observer than this distance are seen doubly. This is shown in Figure 12-2. The presence of diplopia (double images) in the visual field presents a perceptual problem. Suppose that while performing the demonstration with the pencil and the distant target, one had to locate the position of the pencil in space. It is impossible to do this, since there are two apparent pencils that occupy two different spatial directions relative to the observer. One way out of this dilemma is to close one eye, thus immediately restoring single vision.

In everyday coordinations, when pointing at or reaching for objects or viewing objects in the world, one is not aware of double images. Some investigators have suggested that this is because one psychologically closes one eye. To be more precise, these theories are based on the notion of the selection of input to one eye and the suppression of inputs to the other as a way of achieving single vision (Asher, 1961; Verhoeff, 1935). Perhaps the first example of a suppression theory of single vision appeared in 1593, when Porta discussed the difficulty in seeing with both eyes simultaneously with the following example:

> Nature has bestowed on us eyes in pairs, one at the right hand and one at the left, so that if we are to see anything at the right hand we make use of the right eye . . . whence we always see with one eye, although we think that both are open and that we see with both. . . . Between the two eyes let there

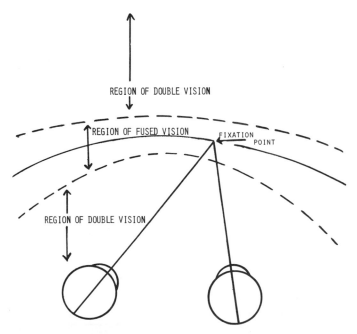

Figure 12-2. Notice that only a relatively narrow region of the visual field is seen in fused single vision. Objects nearer than or beyond the region of the fixated object are seen as double.

be placed a partition to divide the one from the other, and let us place a book
before the right eye and read. If anyone shows another book to the left eye
it will not only not be able to read, but it cannot even see the pages, unless
in a moment it withdraws the visual virtue from the right eye and changes it
to the left. (as quoted in Miles, 1929, p. 114)

In other words, the most efficient way of dealing with the inherent problems of
binocularity is to pay attention to only one eye (to prefer it over the other).
Porta (1593) also implies that it is impossible to maintain full attention to both
eyes even though both may be open and receiving visual stimulation. Thus, for
him, binocular vision always involves monocular preference of some type. A suppression theorist like Porta (1593) would contend that the lack of persistent
diplopia is the result of a habitual monocular preference of inputs to one eye
during binocular vision. We normally suppress one monocular input, and this
results in the conscious perception of a stable, unified, or single visual image. The
problem of the different monocular visual directions for a target is handled within this context by assuming that the visual direction of any single image, even
that resulting from actual binocular fusion, is determined by the preferred eye
alone. Eyedness may well reflect such unequal use of the input to the two eyes.

Varieties of Eye Preference

In Chapter 2 we discussed a number of different measures of eye preference.
These were presented in Tables 2-5 and 2-6. It might be useful to review some
aspects of the measurement of eyedness before continuing. Table 2-5 presented a
number of tests of eyedness based on the relative *proficiency* of the two eyes.
These measures could be subdivided easily into four subgroups on the basis of
the theoretical rationales used to derive each test. These subgroups can be called
physiological dominance, acuity dominance, motor dominance, and *perceptual
dominance,* and we will consider each group in turn.

Physiological dominance concerns specific physiological differences between
the two eyes that have been proposed as a way of accounting for eye preference.
There have been several attempts to tie eyedness to differences in pupil size
(postulating that the dominant eye has a larger pupil and thus receives more light
than the other eye) and to differences in photoreceptor innervation density,
with this being greater in the dominant or preferred eye (Kovac & Horkovic,
1970; Kovac & Ley, 1969). However, the two most common physiological asymmetries encountered in the literature at varying times are differences in muscular
control between the two eyes and differences in monocular refractive states.

Acuity dominance indicates the presence of a tested visual acuity difference
between the two eyes; in other words, the monocular refractive abilities differ,
resulting in asymmetries in the extent to which the two eyes can resolve the
properties of the visual input. This type of eye dominance is often referred to in
the optometric literature (Duke-Elder, 1952), and the dominant eye is defined as
the one that shows comparatively better performance on standard tests of visual
acuity, such as Landolt C's or Snellen letters.

Typically, differences in muscular strength, or the presence of *motor dominance,* has been tested by looking at the way in which the two eyes maintain fixation under conditions of relaxed and strained convergence (Ogle, 1964; Schoen & Scofield, 1935). It is assumed that the dominant eye is the eye that is less likely to shift its fixation as the conditions of muscular convergence change. Some investigators have tested muscular strength differences by looking at bilateral asymmetries in the ability to wink each eye (Danielson, 1930; Kovac & Horkovic, 1970). The dominant eye is supposedly the eye that is more difficult to wink or the eye that cannot be closed without some lowering of the lid of the other eye.

Perceptual dominance is an approach that maintains that the image of the preferred eye is perceptually more clear, intense, or stable than that of the non-preferred eye. This accounts for its perceptual dominance during binocular vision. One way this has been measured is by asking observers to rate the perceived saturation of colored stimuli presented alternately to the two eyes (Pascal, 1926). However, the most common method used to assess perceptual dominance is to place an observer in a *binocular rivalry* situation. Binocular rivalry is produced experimentally by presenting discrepant visual input to the two eyes. If the monocular stimuli are too dissimilar, a stable single percept will not emerge; rather, the two views will compete or rival each other in the combined view. For example, one could present a grid of vertical lines to one eye and a grid of horizontal lines to the other eye using a stereoscope or some other optical device that allows the presentation of visual information separately to each eye. The observer will typically perceive rivalry between the two views under these conditions, with the horizontal grid dominating the conscious view for brief periods and the vertical grid appearing at other times. The alternation between the two views continues because in this case the contours in the monocular images are too dissimilar to give rise to a single fused percept. If asymmetries are apparent during binocular rivalry, that is, if one eye is able to hold its view for longer periods of time during this visual competition, this could indicate the increased perceptual saliency of one monocular view. This is the rationale behind binocular rivalry tests for eye dominance. There is experimental evidence that asymmetrical dominance times exist for the two eyes; in other words, there is a *binocular rivalry dominance* (Cohen, 1952; Lack, 1973; Porac & Coren, 1975b, 1978b; Toch, 1960; Washburn, Faison, & Scott, 1934).

While the efficiency measures of eyedness seem to be quite heterogeneous, the *preference* measures, such as those described in Table 2-6, all have much in common, namely, the act of sighting. Thus all of these tests might be said to be measures of *sighting dominance.* The concept of sighting dominance is often associated with the notion that one eye dominates in the determination of visual direction (Walls, 1951). This theoretical substrate is detectable in a typical test used to determine the sighting eye. Suppose that an experimenter or tester stands facing an individual at a distance of about 3 meters. The observer is asked to keep both eyes open and to point quickly with an outstretched hand at the experimenter's nose, which is directly in front of him. An individual might be asked to perform this fingertip-nose alignment several times, alternating hands in order to control for any handedness bias. As the experimenter, you would notice that the individual aligns the outstretched fingertip with your nose by using only one eye's view; in other words, the fingertip is placed in front of one eye and the near-far alignment of fingertip and nose is effected. Figure 12-3 tries to duplicate the experimenter's view of such a situation. Both individuals are pointing with the right hand, but the male observer has positioned his fingertip in front of his left eye whereas the female observer has performed the same action by aligning her fingertip with her right eye. In both instances, full binocular vision is available, since both eyes are open, but one eye's view has been chosen to complete the task. Considering the two individuals pictured in Figure 12-3, we would call the male a left-sighter and the female a right-sighter. We have just described and seen the results of a common measure of sighting dominance, the *point test*.

What is happening in this situation? We have requested that the observers align a near and a far target, namely, their finger (near) and the experimenter's nose or the camera lens (far). To do this, each observer must choose a point on the body that will serve as a reference point and then align the near and the far target with it, so that the result is a straight line connecting the three points in external

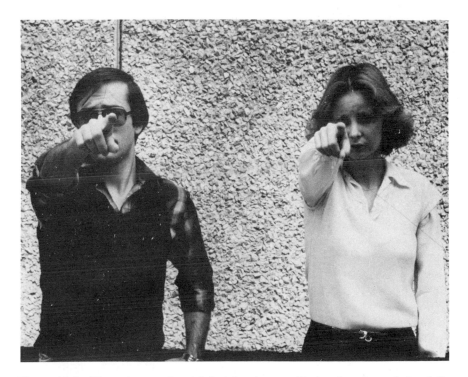

Figure 12-3. The point test for sighting dominance. Notice that the male is a left-sighter (hand aligned with left eye) while the female is a right-sighter (hand aligned with right eye).

space. The previous double vision demonstration showed that the positioning of visual targets at different distances from the observer is the type of situation that gives rise to visual diplopia. In order to complete the requested near-far alignment, the observer must solve a really difficult perceptual problem. Fixation of the near object (the fingertip) will bring about a diplopic view of the far object (the nose). Thus one must point to two apparent targets with one apparent finger. Fixation of the far target will cause a double image of the closer one, leaving you with two apparent fingers to point at one target. Either way, it is difficult to complete the task under these visual conditions, so as we suggested earlier, the problem is solved by using only one eye's view. Simultaneously, one eye is chosen as the bodily reference point and visual targets are positioned in a manner consistent with the visual direction of that eye. The competing or confusing view of the contralateral eye is suppressed, so the diplopia is not apparent. In effect, one sights or aligns with the dominant eye alone.

When sighting dominance, such as that shown in Figure 12-3, is displayed under conditions of full binocularity, it is called *unconscious sighting* because the observer seems unaware of the choice of one eye's view (Miles, 1929, 1930). Most observers are not aware of the monocularity of the behavior and think that they are performing the task by aligning the fingertip and the nose with a bodily reference point that lies between the two eyes. This would be the most reasonable location for the bodily referent if both eyes' views are used in this situation. However, one eye is consistently chosen as the point of origin of the near-far alignments. This fact indicates the close tie between visual directionalizing and one eye, the sighting eye. It is assumed that this eye's view is chosen because it, rather than its contralateral partner, more adequately maintains the stability of visual direction required by the task. Its image is chosen and one visual direction is perceived, while the view of the nonsighting eye is ignored or suppressed.

Sighting dominance is the form of eyedness that is most analogous to the other types of lateral preference. One eye is chosen in situations where the use of only one sense organ is the most efficient way to accomplish a task. This aspect of sighting dominance is especially apparent in *conscious sighting* tasks, such as those described in questionnaire items 1-5 of Table 2-8. In conscious sighting tasks, such as sighting through a telescope, a microscope, or a rifle, the observer is aware that only one eye can be used and acts accordingly. Our research has shown that conscious and unconscious sighting behaviors have an approximate agreement of 92% concerning the choice of right or left eye (Coren, Porac, & Duncan, 1979); thus one can talk comfortably about one type of sighting dominance that covers both covert and overt monocular (one-eyed) choice in certain viewing situations.

Sighting dominance is the form of eye preference encountered most often in the literature (see Porac & Coren, 1976). It has been reliably measured in infants, children, and adults (Coren, 1974; Porac, Coren, & Duncan 1980b) and cross-culturally (Porac & Coren, 1976). The eyedness data presented in this book are almost always based on sighting dominance measures. Sighting dominance has something else in common with all other forms of lateral preference, namely, the population tends to show a right-sided bias, with 65-70% of the population manifesting a preferred right eye. Finally, it is the most stable of the forms of lateral preference in that it shows very little evidence for a systematic shift with increasing chronological age, as we saw in Chapters 3 and 6.

Relationships among Eye Preference Behaviors

In the preceding section we noted that there are a variety of eyedness tests, each based on a different theoretical rationale. Thus, one can ask if there are one or several types of eye dominance or preference? If there is only one form of eye dominance, then we would expect that an individual who is a right-eyed sighter would be right eyed on tests of perceptual proficiency and motor performance, as well as on tests of visual acuity, for example. However, if there are several distinct types of eye dominance, then the eye preferred in one visual situation is not necessarily the one preferred in another. If this situation prevails, and there are a number of different types of eye dominance behaviors, can we identify the relationships among them? Is there a degree of overlap or commonality, or are they mutually exclusive, so that knowledge of displayed eye preference in one situation will not allow one to predict the results obtained under other testing conditions?

There have been several attempts to form taxonomics of eye preference or eye dominance behaviors based on the foregoing theoretical considerations. These attempts have generated estimates of eye dominance types that range from as few as two (Berner & Berner, 1953; Cohen, 1952; Schoen & Scofield, 1935; Walls, 1951) to as many as five (Lederer, 1961). A few studies have looked at the empirical relationship between two forms of eye dominance, usually the congruency of sighting and rivalry dominance (Porac & Coren, 1975b, 1978b; Washburn, Faison, & Scott, 1934) and of sighting and acuity dominance (Coons & Mathias, 1928; Crovitz, 1961; Cuff, 1931; Gahagan, 1933; Geldard & Crockett, 1930; Porac & Coren, 1975b; Porac, Whitford, & Coren, 1976; Snyder & Snyder, 1928; van Biervlet, 1901; Woo, 1928; Woo & Pearson, 1927). As is often the case when comparing studies that have used different procedures and testing instruments, the interpretation of the results of these studies is somewhat equivocal. Generally, there is greater support for an association between eye preference displayed in binocular rivalry and sighting situations than there is for an association between sighting dominance and asymmetries in visual acuity.

Two studies have addressed the taxonomic question directly, by measuring groups of observers on a number of eye dominance tests specifically chosen to cover the range of approaches described in the previous section (Coren & Kaplan, 1973; Gronwall & Sampson, 1971). This type of investigation is valuable, since it allows one to assess the congruency of a wide range of eye dominance behaviors within an individual; therefore, it is worthwhile to look more closely at the results of these two studies.

The study by Coren and Kaplan (1973) has already been discussed in Chapter 2. In that chapter we were interested in describing the intercorrelation among the measures, and these we have reproduced as Table 12-1A. Some of the

Table 12-1: Comparison of Correlations among Similar Measures of Eye Preference Obtained by Coren and Kaplan (1973) and Gronwall and Sampson (1971)

A. Matrix of correlations reported by Coren and Kaplan (1973)

					Eye preference measure					
	1	2	3	4	5	6	7	8	9	10
1. Point	—	$.64^b$	$.65^b$	$.64^b$	.06	-.11	$.53^b$	$.52^b$	.21	.16
2. Alignment		—	$.64^b$	$.64^b$	.07	-.21	$.30^b$	$.42^b$	$.28^a$	.22
3. Hole			—	$.84^b$	.12	-.01	$.35^b$	$.47^b$	.13	.08
4. Miles ABC				—	.06	-.14	$.28^a$	$.51^b$	.09	.06
5. Form rivalry					—	$.41^b$	.16	.17	.00	$.41^b$
6. Color rivalry						—	.08	.01	-.06	.16
7. Chromatic							—	.24	.06	.15
8. Convergence								—	.20	-.03
9. Wink									—	.14
10. Acuity										—

B. Matrix of correlations reported by Gronwall and Sampson (1971)

					Eye preference measure					
	1	2	3	4	5	6	7	8	9	10
1. Point (ring)	—	$.76^b$	$.83^b$	$.56^b$	$.33^b$	$.24^b$	-.08	$.38^b$	$.40^b$	$.29^b$
2. Alignment (box)		—	$.70^b$	$.51^b$	$.35^b$	$.36^b$	-.16	$.26^b$	$.38^b$	$.27^b$
3. Hole (card)			—	$.60^b$	$.34^b$	$.20^a$	-.06	$.28^b$	$.47^b$	$.33^b$
4. Miles ABC				—	$.35^b$	$.36^b$	-.03	$.37^b$	$.25^b$	.13
5. Form rivalry					—	$.47^b$	-.09	.12	.08	$.34^b$

6. Color rivalry	—	-.00	.06	.07	.16
7. Chromatic		—	.01	-.11	-.14
8. Convergence (Mills)			—	.19[a]	-.19[a]
9. Wink (eye closing)				—	.09
10. Acuity					—

Note. Tests are described in Tables 2-5 and 2-6.

[a] $p < .05$.
[b] $p < .01$.

measures are highly intercorrelated; for example, the five sighting measures (tests 1-5) have an average intercorrelation of .67. Others tend not to be related. For example, although the rivalry scores are correlated with each other, they do not appear to be related to the sighting measures or even to the other measures of perceptual dominance. In an attempt to reduce the correlation matrix to a smaller number of dimensions, the data were factor analyzed. Three separate factors emerged. The first factor, which accounted for the greatest proportion of the variance, correlated highly with the five sighting dominance tests as well as with the convergence and chromatic tests. The second factor contained high loadings with the rivalry tests, and the last factor (which accounted for the least amount of predictive variance) contained the acuity test and the dichoptic recognition test. Coren and Kaplan (1973) proposed that these represented different dimensions of eyedness and named them sighting, rivalry, and acuity dominance, respectively, to reflect the pattern of significant correlations found with each factor. This study was taken as empirical confirmation for the existence of several separate types of eye dominance.

However, to reach a final conclusion on this issue, we must consider a number of other aspects of the Coren and Kaplan (1973) study, both in isolation and in comparison with the highly similar investigation of Gronwall and Sampson (1971). First, we have mentioned previously that the sighting eye is the most commonly used indicator of eye dominance. It is quite common for investigators to use sighting dominance as the sole indicator of eye preference. Some support for this common experimental practice is found in the Coren and Kaplan (1973) study. Although the intercorrelation matrix could be reduced to three separable clusters or factors, sighting dominance measures form the most internally coherent and highly intercorrelated type of eye dominance. In addition, as Table 12-1 shows, the sighting behaviors are somewhat correlated with one measure of perceptual dominance (the chromatic test) and with one measure of motor efficiency (the convergence test). Gronwall and Sampson (1971) also looked at the intercorrelations within individuals of a large variety of measures for testing the dominant eye. Although the procedures in the two studies differ somewhat, we are able to extract 10 tests from each report that are virtually identical. Table 12-1 compares the two studies by showing the pattern of obtained measures. We have arranged the matrix so that the identical tests are vertically aligned in the table, and the tests are named as in Tables 2-5 and 2-6. The original Gronwall and Sampson (1971) labels are in parentheses.

A comparison of the intercorrelations among the 10 measures gives some interesting insights. For example, the Gronwall and Sampson (1971) study confirms that sighting measures tend to be highly intercorrelated; also, they are correlated with a measure of muscular superiority, thus replicating the results of Coren and Kaplan (1973). However, using slightly different methods of scoring form and color rivalry and slightly different stimuli, they have demonstrated a relationship between sighting and rivalry dominance. In addition, Gronwall and Sampson's (1971) results indicate that sighting preference might also be related to visual acuity asymmetries. In fact, they conclude that a single dimension might suffice to describe eyedness. Gronwall and Sampson (1971) used a dichotomous method of scoring their data, while Coren and Kaplan (1973) used a graded method of analysis that incorporated both the side and the strength of the displayed preference. Therefore, it is possible that the discrepancies in the various clusters of significant relationships are related to measurement differences between the two studies. The facts that Gronwall and Sampson (1971) provide empirical support for a more integrated and unidimensional approach to eye dominance and that sighting dominance is the largest single factor in the Coren and Kaplan study provide some justification for concentrating our attention on this aspect of eyedness.

We conducted a series of direct experimental tests to ascertain how well sighting dominance predicts the other dimensions of eyedness. We first explored the notion that the sighting eye is also the eye that would predominate (or show longer periods of perceptual dominance) during binocular rivalry. We conducted three studies using several different types of rivalrous stimuli. All of our observers had been tested for sighting dominance and had no measurable acuity differences between the two eyes. In addition, we used a more sensitive measure of scoring the dominance times for each eye, since we reasoned that differences in methodology might have caused the discrepancies between the results of the Coren and Kaplan (1973) and Gronwall and Sampson (1971) studies. The results of our investigations are shown in Table 12-2, where the entries indicate the mean number of seconds that each eye held its view during 60 seconds of binocular rivalry. All of the studies verify that the sighting eye is also the eye that predominates during binocular rivalry, although the time differences between the rivalry dominance of the sighting and the nonsighting eyes are not as large as some investigators have proposed (Washburn et al., 1934).

Coincident with our attempt to clarify the relationship between sighting and rivalry dominance, we endeavored to explore the connection between the sighting eye and monocular asymmetries in visual acuity. We knew from previous research that attempts to connect these two variables had produced equivocal

Table 12-2: Relation between Sighting and Rivalry Dominance as Indicated by Data from Three Studies

| | | Stimulus in view (Mean no. of seconds in 60-sec trial) | | |
	N	Sighting eye	Nonsighting eye	Difference
Porac and Coren (1975b)	48	32.5	27.5	5.0
Porac and Coren (1978b, Exp. 1)	40	32.0	28.0	4.0
Porac and Coren (1978b, Exp. 2)	8	34.3	25.7	8.6
Mean		32.9	27.7	5.8

results, with some studies finding that the sighting eye displays better performance on acuity tests (Crovitz, 1961; Gronwall & Sampson, 1971; Porac & Coren, 1975b; Porac, Whitford, & Coren, 1976; van Biervlet, 1901; Woo, 1928; Woo & Pearson, 1927), while others had not reported empirical confirmation for the association (Coons & Mathias, 1928; Coren & Kaplan, 1973; Cuff, 1931; Gahagan, 1933; Geldard & Crockett, 1930; Snyder & Snyder, 1928). Our own work on this issue had also produced mixed results, depending on the acuity test and the method of measurement that we used (Coren & Kaplan, 1973; Porac & Coren, 1975b; Porac, Whitford, & Coren, 1976). However, we knew that acuity asymmetries were not a necessary condition for the display of strong sighting behaviors. The observers, who were participants in most of our laboratory studies, were tested to ensure equal monocular acuity. Even given this constraint, subjects with strong consistent sighting preferences were not difficult to find. We reasoned that standard acuity tests may not provide a sensitive enough measuring device for the detection of small acuity asymmetries supporting sighting behaviors in observers with vision within the normal range. Therefore, we decided to approach the visual acuity-sighting dominance relationship in another way (Coren & Porac, 1977a).

We began with a sample of individuals with strong sighting dominance characteristics who, on a preliminary screening, had been judged to have approximately equal visual acuity between the two eyes. We then subjected them to the following experimental manipulation. By using a series of positive test lenses, which ranged in power from 0 to 10 diopters, we were able to degrade the vision in the sighting eye artificially (lenses of this type will tend to make the view of the eye wearing them increasingly more blurred as the strength increases). Ten right-sighters and 10 left-sighters were given repeated opportunities to perform the point test (described earlier in this chapter), while the sighting eye wore the lenses of varying strengths. Six repetitions of the point test were given to each observer under all conditions of blur, and the results of this study are shown in Figure 12-4. The ordinate is scaled using the laterality index of $(R-L)/N$ where R is right-eye preference, L is left-eye preference, and N is the number of test points at each degree of blur in the sighting eye. Thus a positive score represents right preference and a negative score represents left sighting. The abscissa is scaled in positive diopters of lens strength.

At 0 diopters (no distortion), both the left-sighters and the right-sighters show very strong left- and right-eye scores, respectively. As the vision to the sighting eye begins to degrade, however, the left-sighters shift toward the right eye and the right-sighters shift toward the left. In order to offset the initial sighting dominance, one needs to degrade the vision in the sighting eye with a lens more than 3 diopters in strength. This produces an amount of visual blurring that generally would be found only in eyes that were refractively poor, with acuity approaching 20/200. With lesser degrees of blurring, sighting behaviors become less consistent. However, subjects still use their habitual sighting dominant eye, even though its image is blurred while that of the nonsighting eye is clear. The results of this experiment indicate that established sighting dominance

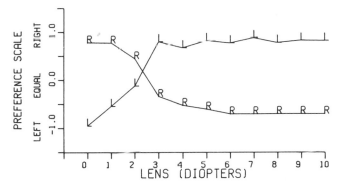

Figure 12-4. Shift in eye preference as blurring lenses are inserted in front of the naturally preferred sighting eye (R is the group of right-sighters, L the group of left-sighters). Degree of blur corresponds to lens diopters; the preference scale is based on performance in the point test.

in observers of normal visual acuity is relatively resistent to the normal range of monocular acuity differences. It takes rather large acuity asymmetries between the two eyes before the sighting behaviors shift. However, the results of this study tend to support the notion that eye dominance and visual acuity may be related in situations of ocular pathology. Given the nature of these results, we are confident that in studying sighting dominance in observers with normal visual acuity, we need not worry about minor acuity differences shifting or affecting the established sighting dominance behaviors.

If we consider the overall pattern revealed by the two large correlational studies (Coren & Kaplan, 1973; Gronwall & Sampson, 1971) and the pattern of data from the rivalry and acuity experiments that we have conducted, it seems clear that there may be separable dimensions of eyedness but they are not independent of one another. Sighting dominance provides the least ambiguous cluster of behaviors and does appear to be predictive of the other forms of eye preference, although the degree of association revealed seems to be sensitive to the specific methodologies employed.

Sighting Dominance: Its Maintenance and Function

Does the preferred eye, as measured by sighting tests, show either perceptual or motoric superiority when compared to its contralateral partner? It is important to answer this question before exploring the origin and function of eye dominance. We will deal with the motoric asymmetry question first, since it relates not only to the control of eye position, but also to the notion of subjective visual direction. It has been maintained that the dominant eye is motorically stronger, that it holds fixation more precisely, and in this way serves as the referent for visual direction (Ogle, 1964; Schoen & Scofield, 1935; Walls, 1951). For example, Ogle (1964) claimed that the sighting eye determines the direction of the viewed object while the nonsighting eye completes the act of binocular fixation by adjusting itself to the principal visual direction determined by the sighting eye. We previously discussed the notion that the determination of visual direction requires a bodily reference point to which the observer egocentrically refers the locus of all points in visual space. The straight line between the internal reference point (the sighting eye) and the target provides the basis for the perceived direction of the target.

The ability to locate visually the direction of targets requires not only a bodily or egocentric reference point, but also the maintenance of stable single vision. Meaningful perception of direction cannot be accomplished in the presence of double images, since by their very nature they have two visual directions. If one eye, the sighting eye in this case, determines the principal visual direction, then one would expect that a point in visual space that is perceived as lying subjectively straight ahead would be found to be biased toward the side of this eye; or one might expect that observers would indicate that they use the sighting eye as their reference point in determining the visual direction of targets. Some direct tests have been conducted on this issue and the experimental evidence supports the notion that knowledge of eyedness predicts some aspects of visual localization. Visual direction seems more likely to be referred to, or at least shifted toward, the side of the sighting eye (Barbeito, 1979; Charnwood, 1965; Foley & Held, 1972; Howard & Templeton, 1966; Ogle, 1964; Schneider, 1966).

As might be expected, this position also implies that the sighting eye would more efficiently extract visual spatial information, since visual direction is encoded with reference to its position. This has been demonstrated by Porac and Coren (1977), who used an illusion decrement procedure. This is basically a perceptual learning task in which an observer views a visual geometric illusion (e.g., the Mueller-Lyer illusion) with freely moving eyes. Eye movement errors tend to be made on the basis of the illusory distortion; thus the eye will tend to overshoot the ends of an apparently longer line and to undershoot the ends of an apparently shorter one (Festinger, White, & Allyn, 1968; Judd, 1905). On the basis of this erroneous eye movement information the observer encodes the fact that there is an illusion present and corrects for it, and gradually the magnitude of the distortion decreases (Coren & Girgus, 1974, 1978). In the absence of free eye movements, the error feedback is not available and no decrease occurs Coren & Hoenig, 1972; Day, 1962; Festinger, White, & Allyn, 1968). Porac and Coren (1977) used this procedure to test the relative efficiency of the two eyes in picking up information based on eye movements. They found that the sighting eye was more efficient at this task than the nonsighting eye. Furthermore, if one measures the amount of transfer between the two eyes (in other words, one eye is allowed to view the figure for the exploration interval but pre- and posttesting is done on the unexposed eye), one finds that the information in the sighting eye is more readily available to the nonsighting eye, while transfer of information from the nonsighting to the sighting eye is much less efficient.

The interaction between sighting dominance and other perceptual processes is much broader than merely motoric and directional. It seems to affect the perceived quality of the stimulus as well. These effects do not appear to reside in peripheral refractive differences between the two eyes (Coren & Porac, 1975; Porac, 1974) nor in asymmetries related to retinal functioning (Schoen & Wallace, 1936), but seem to be associated with the central processing of the information. We first noticed that there seem to be phenomenal differences between the two eyes when we found that targets in the sighting eye appeared to be larger than targets in the nonsighting eye (Coren & Porac, 1976). Recently we conducted a study that demonstrates some other aspects of the perceptual inequality between the views of the sighting and the nonsighting eyes (Coren & Porac, 1979a). We presented visual targets to observers under three exposure conditions: binocular, monocular to the sighting eye, or monocular to the non-sighting eye. The targets were presented in pairs, so that on some trials a target viewed with the sighting eye was paired with a binocular target, on other trials with a target viewed by the nonsighting eye, and so forth. All possible pairs were presented 96 times in random order. This type of presentation was accomplished by using a multichannel tachistoscope in which polaroid filters were used to separate the two eyes' views.

To permit assessment of perceptual quality, observers were asked to choose the target in each pair that appeared to be "more clear" to them. They were allowed to interpret this perceptual requirement in any way that seemed reasonable to them. They were also asked to rate the apparent saturation (intensity of the color) using a rating scale devised by Boynton and Gordon (1965). Saturation judgments were made on a 5-point scale, where a highly saturated target was said to contain five parts color whereas a very desaturated color was rated as containing only one part color. Ratings of 2, 3, and 4 represented degrees of perceived saturation between these endpoints. The data that resulted from these two types of perceptual judgments of binocular targets and those presented to the sighting and the nonsighting eyes are shown in Figures 12-5 and 12-6.

The binocular targets were most likely to be judged as clearer, regardless of the monocular view of comparison. However, on trials comparing views of the sighting and nonsighting eyes, the sighting eye was more likely to be judged as providing a clearer image, as can be seen in Figure 12-5. In like fashion, the binocular targets were judged to be the most deeply saturated, followed by the sighting eye and the nonsighting eye, respectively, as can be seen in Figure 12-6. This finding implies that on both the clarity and the saturation judgments, the rank order of binocular, sighting, and nonsighting represents the perceptual salience of the visual inputs. The sighting eye was generally judged to be higher on these perceptual dimensions than the nonsighting eye and observers could reliably detect these phenomenal differences in monocular exposure.

In another study, we were able to demonstrate that the image in the sighting eye is not only more salient, but also more stable and persistent (Porac & Coren, 1979d). In this study we looked at the disappearance of stabilized retinal image targets as a function of sighting dominance. A stabilized image is one that remains in the same retinal position regardless of how the eyes are moved. Such a situation is not like normal vision, in which retinal stimulation (or the visual

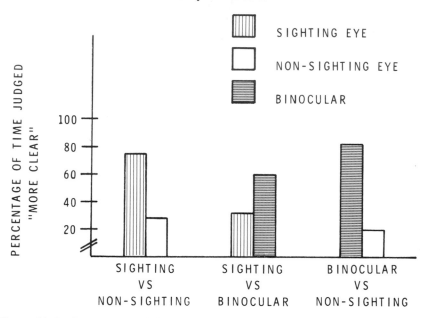

Figure 12-5. Comparison of the judged clarity of targets as a function of viewing condition.

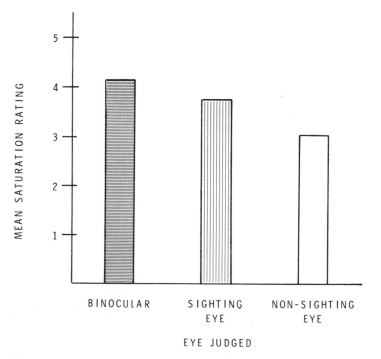

Figure 12-6. Judged saturation of colored targets as a function of viewing conditions (higher saturation ratings indicate more apparent color).

image) moves across the retinal surface when we move our eyes. The presence of continuous high frequency movements due to small amplitude, high freeye tremors and microsaccades also displaces the retinal image regardless of how steadily one attempts to fixate a target. Retinal receptors are responsive to change, and the continual displacement of the image over the retina is thought to be responsible for the ability to maintain target visability over long periods of time (see Heckenmueller, 1965). A stabilized retinal image disrupts this normal movement system, and usually such patterns fade from view in a few seconds. The study of the fading of stabilized retinal images has a long history, and the disappearance process has been attributed at various times to retinal, neural, and cortical fatigue, satiation, or disruption (Arend, 1973; Coren & Porac, 1974; Ditchburn & Ginsberg, 1952; Hecht, 1937; Krauskopf & Riggs, 1959; Riggs, Ratliff, Cornsweet, & Cornsweet, 1953). We explored the relative speed of the fading of such images in the sighting versus the nonsighting eye as a measure of the relative salience of their inputs.

Although there are many ways to achieve retinal image stabilization (see Heckenmueller, 1965), we chose to use an entopic phenomenon called *Haidinger's brush*. Under the appropriate blue polarized illumination, an observer can actually see the shadow of the retinal pigment cells as they converge into the center of the fovea (see Coren, 1971; Coren & Kaplan, 1972; Coren & Porac, 1974; for details of the apparatus used to achieve a visible Haidinger's brush). The resulting percept is of a tiny grey propeller-shaped target that is perfectly stabilized on the fovea of the eye. If one rotates the plane of polarization of the light that allows the brush to be perceived, the pattern rotates and is readily visible as a spinning propeller. When the rotation stops, completely stabilizing the pattern, it fades from view within 2-3 seconds.

We had observers with known sighting dominance characteristics observe the stabilized image while it rotated. We then halted the rotation so that the brush pattern stopped at various angles from horizontal through to vertical. As a measure of fading time, we asked the observers to tap a telegraph key when the image was no longer visible to them. The resulting time period between the halting of the rotation and the tapping of the telegraph key was a measure of the visual persistence of the stabilized target. We measured the fading times for the sighting and the nonsighting eyes separately, and the resulting data are shown in Figure 12-7. Regardless of the orientation (horizontal, oblique, or vertical), the image remains visible in the sighting eye for a longer period of time. Fading is faster in the nonsighting eye, leading one to conclude that perhaps its registered impression is less visually salient. This finding is consistent with the results of the image rating experiment described previously. The sighting eye tends to show perceptual asymmetries that indicate greater image saliency, or in this case, perhaps a lowered susceptibility to satiation or fatigue processes, when its input is compared to that of the nonsighting eye.

The results of the foregoing studies suggest that habitual sighting dominance behaviors are maintained by, or at least predictive of, detectable perceptual differences between the two eyes' views. In the first experiment that we described, input to the sighting eye was rated as being clearer and more saturated than that

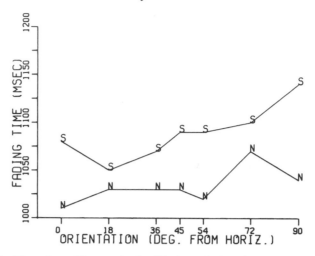

Figure 12-7. Time in milliseconds for Haidinger's brush pattern to completely disappear as a function of viewing condition (S is the sighting eye, N the non-sighting eye). Orientation refers to the angle at which the brush image was stopped in degrees from the horizontal.

to the nonsighting eye, while in the second experiment the sighting eye showed an ability to retain its view for longer time periods, even under conditions of image stabilization.

In the preceding sections we followed the line of reasoning proposed by Porac and Coren (1976), who maintained that under some conditions the use of the full input from the two eyes may be too much of a good thing. While full binocularity provides more accurate relative depth information, binocular vision also results in double images and concomitant directional confusions. Suppression of the input to the nondominant eye eliminates this problem. According to the experiments just described, we can suggest that the habitual use of the sighting eye in these circumstances may result from the fact that its input is better and perceptually more stable than that of its contralateral partner. Why this should be the right eye in the majority of the population, however, has yet to be ascertained.

One tradition that predicts performance asymmetries between the right and the left eyes, regardless of the sidedness of sighting behaviors, emanates from the optometric literature on eye movement control during reading. It is called the *binocular controlling eye hypothesis* and it proposes that one eye will take the lead during complex binocular coordinations, such as reading, where rapid movements and changes of fixation are necessary (Benton, 1968; Berner & Berner, 1953; Helveston, Billips, & Weber, 1970). Brod and Hamilton (1971) propose, in addition, that Indo-European reading patterns, involving left to right scans, dictate the development of a right controlling eye. In their theory, the controlling eye is favored during binocular viewing, and it need not be the sighting eye. There is some experimental support for the notion of a right eye-left eye asymmetry in visual information processing. For example, Porac & Coren (1979b) reported that recognition of a target presented immediately following initiation of an eye movement was better for the right eye than for the left eye, regardless of the individual's sighting dominance. The right eye-left eye asymmetry was enhanced under conditions of binocular viewing. Three additional studies have also found either faster reaction time to visual stimulation of the right eye or better target recognition in the right eye (Sampson & Spong, 1961, 1962; Sampson & Horrocks, 1966). Thus, it is possible that right eye-left eye asymmetries exist, perhaps fostered by habitual reading patterns, and that these operate irrespective of the side of eye preference or to enhance the occurrence of right-sided preference.

As discussed extensively in Chapter 4, there has been a tendency to explain all forms of lateral preference in terms of some aspects of cerebral hemispheric specialization. Attempts have also been made to explain eye preference in this fashion (Belmont & Birch, 1965; Berman, 1973; Delacato, 1967; Freidlander, 1971; Harris, 1957; Orton, 1937; Parsons, 1924). Unfortunately, the arguments for such an association are even weaker in the realm of sensory preferences than they are in limb preferences.

There are few neurological and physiological data to support the presence of any relationship between eye preference and cerebral specialization. Although it is true that motor innervations to the arms and legs are basically under the control of the contralateral cerebral hemisphere, such a simple relationship does not exist for the visual system. As any elementary sensory physiology or perception textbook will indicate, there is a semidecussation of the optic fibers at the optic chiasm before any information has reached even the lower cerebral centers. This results not in the information of one eye passing to a particular hemisphere, but rather in the information of one-half of each retina going to a particular hemisphere. Hence the neural messages from the right hemiretinas of both eyes travel to the right hemisphere, while those from the left hemiretinas of each eye travel to the left cerebral hemisphere. Stimulation of one eye results in inputs to both sides of the brain. Evidence from various types of brain lesions demonstrates how the fields of view of each eye are related to the bilateral nature of the optic projections. If one side of the brain is destroyed, the victim loses control of the contralateral hand and foot; however, the individual does not become blind in one eye, but exhibits hemianopsia or blindedness for half of the field of view in each eye. The neurological picture is further complicated by conflicting evidence concerning the bilateral versus unilateral nature of the representation of the foveal region of each eye (the region of maximal acuity). In cases of hemianopsia, one may find that foveal vision remains unimpaired and present in both sides of the brain, even in the presence of hemiretinal blindness (Halstead, Walker, & Bucy, 1940; Penfield & Rasmussen, 1950; Sanford & Bair, 1939). However, more recent evidence gathered with neurologically intact observers has not supported the notion of bilateral or dual foveal representation (Harvey, 1978). Since eye dominance is an exhibited preference for the input to one eye, these neurological facts militate against a simple relationship to a dominant cerebral hemisphere. It cannot be said that a right-eyed person is exhibiting preferential use of one hemisphere.

Because of the interest in hemispheric specialization, there are some data on how eye dominance (defined by sighting dominance) interacts with visual information processing in the right and left visual fields. Under conditions of binocular viewing, visual stimulation presented to the right of fixation (the right visual field) forms its image on the left hemiretina (the right-left reversal is due to the optics of the crystalline lens). With left hemiretinal stimulation, the information is first processed by the left cerebral hemisphere. Information presented to the left of fixation (the left visual field and right hemiretina) travels to the right cerebral hemisphere. These anatomical separations in the visual systems have fostered the experimental technique of stimulus presentation to the visual half fields as a means of studying hemispheric specialization for the processing of certain types of visual information. As a result, there is a vast literature using this technique. To simply and briefly summarize a complex and extensive body of data, these studies tend to report two findings. It seems that the processing of verbal information (e.g., words, letters, or nonsense syllables) is accomplished more efficiently when this material is presented to the right visual field and thus is first processed by the left hemisphere. Nonverbal visual information (e.g., faces or forms) is dealt with more expeditiously if the stimuli are presented to the left visual field, where the primary processing is by the right hemisphere (see Bryden, 1978; Hecaen & Albert, 1978; Krashen, 1976; White, 1969). The results of visual field stimulation studies, then, generally confirm expectations based on our current knowledge of cerebral localization of function. Verbal material is more efficiently processed when it is differentially channeled to the left hemisphere, which appears to be specialized for certain language functions. Alternatively, nonverbal information is better handled by the right hemisphere, which may be a specialized locus for certain nonlinguistic functions.

There is no reason to expect that eye preference behaviors should be related to visual field processing asymmetries or to mechanisms of hemispheric specialization for the anatomical reasons previously discussed. Thus, as the anatomy would lead one to expect, the majority of the reports have shown that there is little or no effect of eye dominance on performance of perceptual tasks where stimuli have been presented to the hemifields (Hayashi & Bryden, 1957; Keller, 1937; Jasper & Raney, 1937; Maddess, 1975a; Smith, 1938; White, 1969; Whelan, 1967). Studies that have reported positive eye dominance effects have shown either that they are specific to a certain type of visual task (Bryden, 1973) or that right- and left-eyed sighters are performing differently in *both* visual fields (Anderson & Crosland, 1933; Kershner & Jeng, 1972; Levy & Gur, 1980; Maddess, 1975b; McKinney, 1967; Porac & Coren, 1979b). The only data that suggest a link between eye preference and the cerebral hemispheres involve subjects who have undergone removal of an entire cerebral hemisphere. Following the complete ablation of one cerebral hemisphere in monkeys, it has been reported that they prefer to sight with the eye that is contralateral to the remaining hemisphere (Ettlinger & Dawson, 1969; Kruper, Boyle, & Patton, 1967; Kruper, Patton, & Koskoff, 1971; Lehman, 1970). Unfortunately, when similar studies have been carried out on humans who have brain lesions resulting in homonymous hemianopsia, the reports have been mixed in their findings. Williams and Gassel (1962) presented reports that agreed with the monkey studies, whereas Rothschild and Streifler (1952) reported the opposite finding. In the absence of a sound anatomical reason for these results, one can only say that they offer tentative support for some possible relationship between eye preference and hemispheric function. However, rather than indicating a hemispheric interaction, these results may merely reflect the relative processing dominance of the nasal, or crossed, fibers over the temporal, or uncrossed, fibers (Crovitz, 1964; Crovitz & Lipscomb, 1963; Doty, 1958; Hubel & Weisel, 1959, 1962; Polyak, 1957). Thus, this line of evidence, in the absence of any other supportive data, remains only suggestive. The overall negative flow of the other lines of evidence, combined with the lack of appropriate hemispheric separation of the inputs from each eye, suggests that any hemispheric link to eye preference is probably only secondary in nature, if it exists at all.

The eyedness data that we have reviewed may seem complex, but they can be summarized easily. The single most predictive manifestation of sidedness in eye use is sighting dominance. Generally, the sighting eye seems to process visual information more efficiently. There are, however, some other manifestations of sidedness. Right- and left-sighters do not always respond in the same manner, and the right eye, even of left-sighters, may be more efficient for some tasks in certain circumstances. Like limb preference, eyedness is a complex form of sidedness.

Ear Preference

The literature that addresses itself to the preferential use of one ear, it situations where only one can be used, is extremely sparse. As a consequence, knowledge about the mechanisms that maintain ear preference and about its function in auditory processing or in an overall system of side preferences is extremely limited. For this reason, any conclusions that we might draw must be extremely speculative. However, we can review the few explanations for earedness that have been offered and the data that suppport or contradict each point of view.

The sensory function of ear preference has never been clear. The auditory sytem does not suffer from the same problems encountered by the visual system in forming a single percept from discrepant images. The only naturally occurring discrepancies between the inputs to the two ears occur in the form of frequency content differences in the sound stimulus, intensity differences, or differences in the time of arrival of the stimulus to the ears. Consider the situation were one ear is closer to the stimulus than the other. Both ears will receive the stimulus input; however, the more distant ear will receive it a few milliseconds later because it is farther away from the sound source. Since the head is between the source and the more distant ear, the sound will be shadowed slightly and it will reach this ear at a somewhat lower intensity. This sound shadow effect will be most pronounced for the higher frequencies, slightly shifting the tonal composition of the sound. Such differences never result in the auditory analogue of diplopia (where a single sound source is heard as two); rather, the observer hears a single source and its apparent egocentric direction is given by the pattern of differences in the inputs (see Coren, Porac, & Ward, 1979, for a more complete explanation). One ear's input need not be suppressed to accomplish this fusion.

However, it seems reasonable to postulate that ear preference is related to some asymmetry of auditory processing. For this reason, several investigators have proposed, in a way that is analogous to some theories of eyedness, that the preferred ear is the one that is more sensitive. In other words, the preferred ear has a lower auditory threshold than the nonpreferred ear (Bilto & Peterson, 1944; Fridenberg, 1904; Koch, 1933). Both Koch (1933), and Bilto and Peterson (1944) present some data in support of this relationship. In the case of the Bilto and Peterson (1944) study, however, the preferred ear displayed a lower threshold only in observers who had large inequalities in threshold sensitivity between the two ears. We explored the connection between behavioral ear preference and auditory acuity in a study that we conducted with Dr. Frank Spellacy of the University of Victoria. We administered the lateral preference battery shown in Table 3-1 to a group of 227 university students. We also assessed the auditory acuity of each student. We determined the threshold for the detection of a pure tone at four sound frequencies—500, 1,000, 2,000, and 4,000 Hz—using the psychophysical method of limits. Two trials were administered at each frequency, one starting with a tone that was well above threshold and was gradually decreased in intensity until it was no longer detected, and one starting with a tone intensity that was clearly inaudible and was gradually increased until it was heard. The mean of these ascending and descending trials was computed for each frequency for every observer, and the resulting data are shown in Table 12-3.

The mean auditory threshold in decibels is shown for the right- and the left-eared groups, for the total sample, and for males and females separately. Since there was no interaction between the ear tested or the ear preferred and the test tone frequency, the data in Table 12-3 have been averaged across the four test frequencies. There are no significant differences as a function of ear preference. The only trend that appears in these data is the tendency for the right ear to have slightly lower thresholds (greater acuity) for all groups of observers. Thus, in a population where the threshold sensitivities of the two ears are approximately equal, there does not seem to be a relationship between ear preference and auditory acuity.

If the function of a dominant ear is not sensory in nature, perhaps it is motoric or postural. Since some of the behaviors used to measure ear preference also involve a hand action, such as the ear against which one places a telephone receiver, it has been proposed that the side of the preferred ear is determined by the side of the preferred hand (Clark, 1957; Fridenberg, 1904). Within this context, there seems to be a relationship between the two types of preference when

Table 12-3: Right and Left Ear Auditory Thresholds (Mean of Four Frequency Levels) for Right- and Left-Eared Subjects

	Auditory threshold (dB)		
	Right ear	Left ear	Mean
Females (N = 119)			
Right ear preferred	11.80	11.24	11.52
Left ear preferred	11.82	12.89	12.35
Mean	11.81	12.07	
Males (N = 108)			
Right ear preferred	11.99	12.81	12.40
Left ear preferred	11.75	13.04	12.40
Mean	11.86	12.94	
All subjects (N = 227)			
Right ear preferred	11.88	11.85	11.86
Left ear preferred	11.78	12.98	12.38
Mean	11.83	12.42	

the earedness measure involves some sort of preferred hand action (Clark, 1957). This is shown in our data presented in Table 4-3. Here, the highest correlations between a handedness and an earedness questionnaire item is found when the earedness question involves a hand action (earphone placement). The other ear preference items that involve no manual activity (listening to a heartbeat or a conversation behind a door) have lower correlations with the handedness items. However, this correlation is still small (.25) and accounts for only 5% of the variance. Other considerations also lead us to dismiss any causal relationship between handedness and earedness. For instance, the results of the factor analysis presented in Table 4-4 (Porac, Coren, Steiger, & Duncan, 1980) indicate that ear preference is separable from the other three forms of lateral preference. In addition, the data in Chapters 3 and 6 indicate an age trend toward the right for handedness, yet toward the left for ear preference. If these two behaviors share a common mechanism, they should show a common, rather than an opposite, age trend.

Another proposed explanation for ear preference is that it arises as a by-product of postural asymmetries. Humans, even from a very early age, exhibit asymmetries in the positioning of their heads and bodies. For example, Turkewitz (1977) reports that infants less than one week old lie with their heads turned out of the body midline, and that the turn is most often toward the right side. Some attempt has been made to use these early postural asymmetries as a predictor of later lateral preference (specifically, handedness) behaviors (Coryell & Michel, 1978). Since measures of ear preference often require postural asymmetry, for example, bending or tilting the head toward a sound source, it has been suggested that displayed earedness is really a manifestation of these habitual postural biases (Fridenberg, 1904). Unfortunately, there is no existing empirical evidence to either support or refute this contention. To provide some information on this issue, we decided to present subjects with a questionnaire item that asked them to designate whether they habitually tilted their heads to the right or to the left side. We can assess whether asymmetrical head carriage is associated with ear preference by comparing this set of responses to ear preference as determined by the earedness questions in Table 3-1. As can be seen in Table 12-4, based on a sample of 1,320 respondents, we find that the direction of habitual head tilt is related to the side of ear preference. A higher percentage of right-eared individuals report that they habitually tilt their head to the right side rather than to the left side, while the opposite result is found in the left-eared group. Of course, one cannot ascertain whether ear preference is *caused* by the head tilt, or if the head tilt is the *result* of the ear preference. However, such data do demonstrate a relationship between postural factors and ear preference.

Studies of hemispheric specialization have often used a technique of information input called dichotic listening. In a dichotic listening paradigm, discrepant auditory input is simultaneously presented to the right ear and to the left ear and observers are asked to respond to this input in some way. Most often, they are asked to report what is heard. This is an auditory analogue to the binocular rivalry task used in some eye dominance studies. Very early in the use of the dichotic listening paradigm, researchers demonstrated that the presentation of verbal material resulted in more information processing from the right ear than from the left (Broadbent, 1954). Later, this *right ear advantage* or *right ear preference* found in the dichotic presentation of verbal input was ascribed to left hemisphere dominance for speech processing and the preeminence of the contralateral auditory connections between the right ear and the left hemisphere (Kimura, 1961). Since that time there have been numerous reports of ear preference during dichotic listening, especially of right ear preference or advantage when verbal material, such as words or digits, is presented (see Berlin, 1977; Berlin & McNeil, 1976; Bryden, 1978; Krashen, 1976; Springer, 1977). The situation is, however, quite complex, and a number of alterations of stimulus parameters, presentation conditions, and subject instructions have been shown to affect the magnitude and even the existence of the dichotic right ear preference (see Berlin, 1977; Bryden, 1978).

Table 12-4: Percentage of Right and Left Habitual Head Tilt for Right- and Left-Eared Individuals ($N = 1,320$)

	Ear preference	
	Right	Left
Habitual head tilt (%)		
Right	54.0	44.4
Left	46.0	55.6

Note. Overall relationship significant with $p < .01$.

One can view asymmetries in dichotic listening performance as the selection of one ear's input in preference to the other. Thus it is not unusual to hear the ear that functions best in this task called the dominant or preferred ear. However, there is no existing experimental evidence that assesses whether dichotic listening is related empirically to the more behavioral manifestations of ear selection, which we are calling ear preference. We extended our study of auditory processing and ear preference to include a dichotic listening measure to provide these data. In addition to the completion of the lateral preference questionnaire (Table 3-1) and the testing of auditory acuity, each of the 227 observers also participated in a short dichotic listening experiment. We used a tape that presented dichotic verbal material. This tape had been prepared in the laboratories of Dr. Frank Spellacy at the University of Victoria and it had the following characteristics. Three discrepant word pairs were presented simultaneously to the right and to the left ears for a total of 22 trials (or 66 words in each ear). The word pairs were matched for their frequency of appearance in English language use and initial consonant, and they were either three, four, or five letters in length. Observers were asked to report all of the words that they could hear on each trial.

There are a number of ways to look at the data that resulted from this study. First, we dichotomized subjects into right- and left-eared groups, based both on the questionnaire responses and on their dichotic listening performance. This analysis is shown in Table 12-5. Overall, there is a preponderance of right-ear preference in both dichotic listening (166 subjects or 73%) and behavioral ear preference (123 subjects or 54%). In addition, 57% of the sample shows congruency between dichotic listening and behavioral ear preference. This value is statistically significant ($p < .05$). Of the right-ear preferent group (96 of 123), 78% shows a right-eared dichotic listening preference, while only 67% of the left-ear preferent group shows the same right-ear asymmetry. Thus, an individual classified as right eared on the questionnaire is 11% more likely than a person classified as left eared to be also classified as right eared in dichotic listening performance. The same type of asymmetry seems to hold for the left-eared group. Thirty-three percent (34 of 104) of the individuals displaying a left-ear preference show a left-eared dichotic listening superiority, while only 22% of the right-eared group is classified in this way. Thus, an individual displaying left-ear

Table 12-5: Number of Individuals Classified as Right and Left Eared Using Both an Ear Preference and a Dichotic Listening Performance Criterion (*N*=227)

	Ear preference		
	Left	Right	Total
Dichotic listening superiority			
Left	34	27	61
Right	70	96	166
Total	104	123	227

preference is 10% more likely than a right-eared individual to be classified as left eared in dichotic listening.

While this result shows an association between dichotic listening and ear preference, it is not robust. For instance, if we use a continuous measure to explore this relationship, namely, the number of words from each ear, the statistically significant association between ear preference and dichotic listening preference disappears, as shown in Table 12-6. When both strength and direction are encoded, the only significant difference is that more words are reported from the right than from the left ear, which is not surprising given the nature of the stimulus material. Both the right- and left-eared groups show this asymmetry, and they show it to the same extent. The absence of a statistically significant association between ear preference and dichotic listening when the mean values are used seems to arise from the fact that the left-ear preferent subjects are more variable in their performance than are the right-eared subjects. The standard deviation for the left-eared subjects is 12.76, while for the right-eared subjects it is 8.8 (this variability difference is statistically significant, $F = 1.45, 105/120, p < .05$). However, a sex-related trend emerges from this method of analysis. Males show a greater ear difference in dichotic listening performance than females. The ear asymmetry averages 12.7 words for males and 7.1 for females (this difference is also statistically significant, $t = 2.54, df = 225, p < .05$).

What is ear preference and what function does it serve? We have been able to show only that ear preference is related to asymmetries of head posture and is

Table 12-6: Mean Correct for Right and Left Ears during Dichotic Presentation of Word Pairs for Right- and Left-Eared Subjects

	Mean number of words correct		
	Right ear	Left ear	Mean
Females ($N = 119$)			
Right ear preferred	37.65	28.12	32.89
Left ear preferred	33.84	30.87	32.36
Mean	36.21	29.16	
Males ($N = 108$)			
Right ear preferred	38.30	25.68	31.99
Left ear preferred	39.36	26.66	33.01
Mean	38.90	26.23	
All subjects ($N = 227$)			
Right ear preferred	37.90	27.17	32.54
Left ear preferred	37.02	28.44	32.73
Mean	37.49[b]	27.77[b]	

[b] Significantly different with $p < .01$.

weakly related to dichotic listening behavior. The former suggests an interaction between bodily carriage and ear orientation, while the latter could suggest some hemispheric factor. Perhaps ear preference is not a true sensory lateral preference in the same way that eye preference seems to be, because it may not predict sensory information processing asymmetries in a manner analogous to eye preference. However, behavioral ear preference has been a relatively neglected phenomenon in terms of research, and we do not yet possess the data needed to evaluate these questions. Perhaps this brief discussion will encourage some research into this potentially interesting but relatively ignored form of lateral preference.

13

Reformulation

Since the first chapter, it has been clear that human behavior is predictably asymmetrical. Human beings consistently use one limb or sense organ rather than the other in many of their behavioral coordinations. Furthermore, human populations are predominantly right sided in that the majority of them tend to show a preference for the right hand, right foot, right eye, and right ear. At the outset of our enquiry these lateral preferences seemed to be a simple set of behaviors, presumably with easily specified functions, causes, and correlates. Unfortunately this presumption was an oversimplification, and the implications of these simple asymmetries are much broader than we expected initially. Our investigation of lateral preferences has forced us to consider a broad spectrum of variables, including neurological and physiological factors, genetics, pathological conditions, cognitive and language skills, sensorimotor coordination, individual differences, and developmental processes. We have surveyed nearly 1,000 published reports, and we have gathered new data from some 20,000 subjects. All of this effort has resulted from an attempt to answer supposedly simple questions about simple behaviors.

Has the totality of this exploration brought us closer to answering the questions that initiated this study? We must give both an affirmative and a negative response to this question. Our search for the causes and functions of laterally biased behaviors has not produced the definite answers we sought; however, we now possess enough of the appropriate data to state that some of the previous approaches to the problem need revision. In fact, some of the questions that we have asked need reformulation. We think that we now have some hints as to how to reformulate these questions in order to indicate possible new directions for future research. In the remainder of this last chapter, rather than repeat detailed arguments and reintroduce data that we have discussed earlier, we will simply refer to specific sections of the book through parenthetical references. When needed, one can glance back to the indicated places in the text to refresh the memory or to review the material in light of the ongoing discussion. We will begin by considering some of the approaches, beliefs, and theories that we have encountered during our study of lateral preferences, and we will briefly note the data that support or contradict them. Each approach can be summarized in the form of a simple statement, which we will then examine.

Right-sidedness is a universal human characteristic. The normative data in Chapter 3 showed that human populations are predominantly right handed, right footed, right eyed, and right eared. When faced with a unilateral task, the majority of the population prefers the limb or the sense organ on the right side of the body. While it is true that the majority of human beings are predominantly right sided, the degree of displayed dextrality differs among the various indexes of lateral preference. The dextral bias is most strongly apparent in handedness, where approximately 9 out of 10 individuals show a right-sided preference. The other indexes of preference are not as markedly dextral; 8 out of 10 individuals show right-footedness, 7 out of 10 show right-eyedness, and 6 out of 10 show right-earedness (Table 3-3). Thus, the degree of right-sided bias in the population depends on the specific index of lateral preference. As a group, humans range from being very right sided (handedness) to only moderately right sided (earedness).

The degree of manifest right-sidedness also depends on the gender, age, psychological status, neurological integrity, and cultural milieu of the sample under consideration. For example, both males and females prefer the right side over the left in all four preference indexes; however, in handedness, footedness, and earedness females are more strongly right-sided, while males are more strongly right sided in eye preference (Chapters 3 and 6). Age is a variable in that older individuals are proportionately more right handed and right footed but less right eared. Cultural factors and family membership also affect manifest dextrality, as shown in Chapters 5 and 6.

These considerations make it clear that the statement that humans are, as a population, right sided in their lateral preference behaviors has to be qualified with some restrictions. Although the general assertion of dextrality is true, right-sidedness is not a fixed or immutable characteristic of the species.

An individual can be described adequately as right or left sided on an index of lateral preference. Perhaps one of the oldest methodological assertions about lateral preference behaviors is that one can adequately describe a person as right or left handed, footed, and so forth in a dichotomous manner. To say that Queen Victoria of England was left handed is thus taken as a complete description of her asymmetrical hand use. One virtually never hears the question, "How left handed was she?" When conceptualizing a problem, it is often convenient and perhaps comforting to view behaviors as dichotomous entities. However, in many instances, such a simple separation of individuals into theoretical bins labeled "right" and "left" does not suffice (Chapter 2). Individuals differ in the strength of their lateral preference, defined by the consistency with which a particular limb or sense organ is selected in various unilateral tasks, as well as on the basis of the chosen side. These differences do not simply represent measurement artifacts, or random variability, but they can be used to define subgroups within the population. For example, females demonstrate stronger lateral preferences than do males, and older individuals demonstrate stronger lateral preferences than do those who are younger (Chapter 3, Table 3-4, and Chapter 6).

As a variable, the strength of the lateral preference also acts somewhat independently of the side of the preference. For instance, although family members may not resemble each other in terms of side of preference, they do in terms of the strength of preference (Chapter 5). Thus while left-handedness might not be common to members of the same family, ambi-handedness might. Clinically defined groups also show patterns of lateral preference that differ in both side and strength from typical populations. Retardates (Chapter 8) have been found to be not only less right sided, but also more mixed or weakly preferent than control groups. Conversely, weaker patterns of lateral preference are found to correlate with improved performance on some classes of cognitive and sensorimotor skills among clinically unaffected subjects (Chapters 10 and 11).

This evidence demonstrates that an individual's lateral preference behavior is *not* adequately described as simply right or left sided on an index. The additional dimension denoting consistent (strong) versus mixed (weak) preference should be part of the description, since this dimension is often independently predictive of other behavioral and subject variables. Perhaps it is best to view lateral preference behaviors as a continuous vector, with side as the direction and strength as the magnitude.

Lateral preference is unidimensional and one-sidedness is the norm. We have considered the various indexes of lateral preference as if they are independent of one another. Actually, most of the theories that we have encountered do not make such an assumption. A right-handed individual has been presumed to be right footed, right eyed, and right eared, as opposed to a left-handed individual, who is supposed to be completely left sided for foot, eye, and ear preference. Thus, congruent sidedness has been the assumed norm. Within this context, it has been presumed that there is a single mechanism producing a generalized dimension of lateral preference. Given this postulated unidimensionality, it is presumed that if one isolates the factors determining any one aspect of lateral preference, one has isolated the factors that determine all of the others. The hypothesized general mechanism has varied among different researchers, and has included genetic, physiological, pathological, and environmental mechanisms.

The issue here is not whether any of these variables contributes to the formation of a type of lateral preference, but rather whether all forms of lateral preference reflect the same single underlying sidedness factor. Unfortunately, many of the studies that have implicitly or explicitly postulated a generalized dimension of lateral preference have not incorporated appropriate measures to test this issue. Unidimensionality is simply assumed and variables are assessed that bear directly on the presumed general mechanism. Most investigators do not even question this unicausal postulate; typically, they measure only one form of lateral preference (usually handedness) and then assume that the other manifestations of sidedness respond in a similar fashion. However, while this may be a methodological simplification, measuring only one preference index does not allow the unidimensional hypothesis to be tested empirically. Furthermore, when several preference indexes are tested simultaneously in the same individuals, one quickly finds reasons to doubt the sufficiency of any unidimensional theory of lateral preference. For instance, only one out of three individuals is congruently sided, preferring the hand, foot, eye, and ear on the same side of the body (Chapter 3). This low rate of congruency is difficult to explain given the notion of a single dimension of lateral preference. Furthermore, the correlations among preference indexes are low and average only .3 (Chapter 3, Table 3-10, and Chapter 4).

Patterns of congruency across indexes often act as if they are a separate, or at least a separable, aspect of lateral preference in much the same way that side and strength seem to be. Subgroups can be distinguished on the basis of the degree of observed congruency, and these patterns can be related to individual difference factors. For instance, females show more congruency than males (Chapters 3 and 6), young children are less congruent than adults (Chapter 6), and very low congruency rates are found in some clinical groups (Chapters 8 and 9). Even considering each index separately provides evidence for several, rather than one, dimensions of lateral preference. For example, although the normative sample is predominantly right sided, the degree of right-sidedness significantly differs among the indexes (Chapter 3). There are also different age trends for the four forms of lateral preference (Chapter 3, Figure 3-2, and Chapter 6). Most important, when we conducted multivariate analyses of lateral preference behaviors, we found three independent factors of lateral preference, a general limb factor representing hand and foot, and two separate dimensions for eye and ear preference, respectively (Chapter 4).

Other data also support the notion that lateral preferences are multidimensional and multiply caused. For example, we presented evidence that suggests a possible genetic component for the strength of handedness and footedness; however, the case for ear preference is ambiguous and for eye preference it is clearly negative (Chapter 5). In addition, variables that alter the distribution of lateral preference work selectively. For instance, pathological factors, such as those surrounding the birth process, have an effect on hand and foot preference but do not affect sense organ preference in a similar fashion (Chapter 7). Generally, handedness and footedness patterns predict variations in cognitive skills (Chapters 9 and 10). However, eye and ear preference do not predict variations in any of these behaviors. Thus, we have not obtained convincing evidence to support the notion that all manifestations of lateral preference behaviors are derived from a single process and act in the same manner. Rather our data indicate that there are several (rather than one) dimensions of sidedness.

Humans are right sided because they are left brained. One of the most prevalent explanations for lateral preference behaviors is based on the notion of hemispheric specialization of function. Since there is contralateral organization of neural control of motor behavior, the centers for the motor control of the right limbs reside in the left hemisphere of the brain. The left hemisphere is also the hemisphere that is thought to be specialized for speech production and language processing in most individuals. It is often also assumed that because of this function the left hemisphere is the "dominant" hemisphere. This notion of left cerebral dominance has been used as an explanation for the predominance of right-sidedness, especially right-handedness, in human populations. In other words, we are right sided because we are left brained. An extension of this reasoning leads to the conclusion that left-handers should exhibit right hemisphere dominance.

This argument persists in the literature, even though much data indicate that it is untenable. Simple neurological considerations suggest that although cerebral functional specialization could contribute to the formation of a preferred limb, it cannot account for sensory preferences. The neural control systems connecting the brain and limbs are primarily contralateral but the sense organs project equally to both cerebral hemispheres. Hence, we do not have the right hemisphere controlling the left eye, and so forth (Chapter 12).

Unfortunately, the available data do not support a cerebral dominance notion for limb preference either. In Chapter 4 we reviewed a number of studies that obtained direct physiological measurements of the brains of individuals with known handedness. This review of 13 different measures of cerebral asymmetry (Table 4-1) showed that an average of 29% of the right-handed subjects actually showed right-hemispheric superiority. A sizable proportion of both groups also showed no clearly defined hemispheric asymmetry. Since the cerebral dominance notion stresses the contralateral nature of the dominant hemisphere-preferred hand connection, it must deal with the problem of explaining why one out of three subjects manifests a cerebral asymmetry in the direction opposite to that theoretically predicted, and a nearly equal proportion shows no clearly defined asymmetry. Simply put, knowledge of an individual's cerebral structural asymmetries does not allow accurate prediction of lateral preference patterns, even if one considers only the limbs. Consideration of localization of speech function alone does not improve the situation. Most individuals exhibit left hemisphere localization of speech function. This is the case for most left-handers as well as most right-handers (Chapter 4). There are right-handers with right hemisphere speech function and a somewhat greater proportion of left-handers with right-hemispheric speech function. Again, however, simple knowledge of the hemispheric location of the primary speech centers does not allow us to predict lateral preferences.

There are other conflicts between this theory and the available data. For instance, females are thought to be physiologically less laterally specialized than males (Chapters 4 and 6). If the cerebral dominance-limb preference dependency exists, females should show weaker preference patterns than those seen in males, since their cerebral functional asymmetries are not as pronounced as those of males. However, females actually show more consistent and more dextral patterns of lateral preference than do males (Chapters 3 and 6).

We are not suggesting that lateral asymmetries in the structural or functional characteristics of the human brain do not exist, nor are we stating that there are no relationships between cerebral asymmetries and lateral preferences. However, to treat lateral preferences as though they are a direct consequence of any specific pattern of cerebral organization certainly appears to be an overstatement of the contribution of this mechanism and an oversimplification of the etiology of lateral preference. While cerebral localization of function may contribute to the manifest pattern of lateral preference in some way, the degree of association is ill specified, and a convincing case for hemispheric involvement cannot be made on the basis of the available evidence.

Lateral preference patterns are genetically determined. The historical record indicates that humans have always been right handed (Chapter 1) and there has never been a predominantly left-handed culture (Chapter 6). This has been used as evidence that the dextral bias of the population may be genetic in its origin. However, the nature of such genetic transmission is far from clear. It does not follow simple Mendelian transmission models, and knowledge of parental patterns of lateral preference is not sufficient to allow reliable prediction of offspring preferences. Although family members do not resemble each other in the side of preference, there are familial similarities in the consistency of lateral preferences (Chapter 5). Offspring of parents with consistent lateral preference (regardless of side) are more apt to show strong preferences than are offspring of parents with inconsistent patterns, at least for handedness, footedness, and earedness. There seems to be some factor in the physiological heritage of our species that predisposes human populations toward dextrality; however, individual deviations from this norm do not seem to be genetically determined. The only genetic factor seems to be associated with the display of consistent versus mixed patterns of preference.

Lateral preference patterns are determined by social and environmental pressures. Environmental determination of lateral preferences, either through biases in the world or social pressure and learning, has been an explanation held in opposition to genetic determination. Some of the same evidence used to support genetic hypotheses directly contradicts environmental ones. Thus, environmental and learning theorists are embarrassed to note the absence of a predominantly left-handed culture or the lack of any historical trends in the population norms. However, evidence suggests that the degree of manifest dextrality, at least for hand preference, can be affected by societal membership and various social pressures. Left-handedness can be altered by training, and individuals can be induced to show more consistently dextral behaviors through the operation of covert environmental pressures in the form of right-handed tools, machines, and so forth. Such pressures may account for the age trends in lateral preference that we have observed (Chapters 3 and 6). However, despite such pressures, a substantial minority of left-handers persists in all cultures. It is also difficult to determine the nature of any social, cultural, and environmental pressure that might cause individuals to be predominantly right footed, right eyed, or right eared, or the existence of any consistent cultural attitudes about these indexes. The evidence suggests, at best, that environmental pressures sustain and perhaps strengthen some of the dextral tendencies in individuals; however, it does not seem to be the primary cause for lateral preferences (Chapter 6).

Left-sidedness is a sign of abnormality or pathology. This assertion arises from observations as well as assumptions. The major assumption is that individuals are normally right sided. The major observation is that there is a higher incidence of left-sidedness in some clinically affected groups (Chapters 7 and 8). We have found that left-sidedness and mixed sidedness patterns are characteristic of atypical groups of individuals, such as retardates. However, to leap from the observation that sinistrality is more prevalent in clinical samples to the assumption that all manifestations of sinistrality are signs of some form of overt or covert abnormality is not justifiable. First, the normative data in Chapter 3 indicates that there are large numbers of left-sided, mixed-sided, and crossed-preferent individuals in the general population. Second, among typical samples that we have studied, we find that left-sided individuals, except for their lateral preference patterns, are indistinguishable from their dextral peers both physiologically (Chapter 4) and, for the most part, behaviorally (Chapters 9 and 10).

One can summarize the relationship between pathology and lateral preferences as indicating that atypical individuals are more likely to show, as a population, preference patterns that differ from those of normal control populations. Since the norm is dextrality, especially for handedness and footedness, these differences will take the form of decreases in right-sidedness (increases in left-sidedness). However, while left-sidedness and mixed sidedness may be elevated in groups with manifest or implied pathology, the relationship between these two phenomena is not bidirectional, since it cannot be said that these patterns of lateral preference *imply* abnormality. Left-sidedness is found in sizable proportions in normal and even superior samples, and the majority of retardates and other atypical or clinically affected populations still show a predominance of manifest dextrality.

Reformulation

This summary and evaluation of the more frequently encountered statements about lateral preference behaviors was done in light of the literature that we have reviewed and the data that we have presented. Although it seems clear that no single mechanism provides a coherent explanation for the range of lateral preference behaviors, the resultant picture is far from bleak. If one is willing to adopt the less parsimonious, but apparently more defensible, multicausal approach, we have uncovered enough information to allow us to construct a tentative theoretical framework. In outlining this approach, we will concentrate on handedness as the typical expression of lateral preference and then see if the same reasoning can be extended to the other indexes.

At the behavioral level, there is more to hand preference than simply choosing to perform an activity with a given hand. One can view the development of lateral preference as primarily an evolutionary step toward specialization of function. The hand that we designate as preferred is generally the hand used in skilled activities requiring fine motor coordination. To unscrew the lid of a jar, one uses the preferred hand to turn the lid. Yet without the use of the nonpreferred hand to support, hold, and steady the jar, the task is impossible to perform without mechanical aids. One could say, then, that the nonpreferred hand is skilled in these more passive, supportive functions. It grasps, holds, steadies, and is in fact the preferred hand for this class of activities. This notion implies not a loss of skill in one limb relative to the other, but rather that the two limbs are specialized, or differentiated, according to distinct sets of functional activities. It is probably more accurate to refer to the preferred hand as the skilled-active hand and the nonpreferred as the skilled-passive hand than to refer to one hand as the dominant one. While the skilled-active (preferred) hand interacts with the world and causes environmental changes, the nonpreferred (skilled-passive) hand serves a support function and facilitates the action of its partner by steadying the body and keeping the material needed for task completion within its reach. This same pattern of specialization of the two limbs, one for manipulation and the other for support, is also found in infrahuman species. For example, although nonhuman primates do not show the population bias toward dextrality found in humans, each monkey demonstrates hand preference in a variety of active functions. Each monkey has one limb specialized for most active, manipulative behaviors, while the more passive, supportive behaviors are the function of the other limb (Beck & Barton, 1972; Cole, 1957; Ettlinger & Moffett, 1964; Finch, 1941; Gautrin & Ettlinger, 1970; Hall & Mayer, 1966; Kamai, 1967; Rothe, 1973; Warren, Abplanalp, & Warren, 1967). The skilled-active/skilled-passive specialization is still clearly evident.

Once one recognizes that separate functions are often performed by the two hands, one can ask about the adaptive significance of having one hand specialized for a class of functions. Why is it less adaptive to have both hands performing either active or passive functions at different times? Suppose that an individual begins early in life to perform some active, manipulative tasks with one hand, using the other for supportive functions. Repetition of these activities will soon give this limb facility in this set of activities. Skill learning is generally specific to the practiced limb. Although some of the newly learned activity patterns may be available to the unpracticed limb, it will not be as proficient at these activities (Adams, 1969; Cook, 1933, 1935; Kimble, 1952), and evidence indicates that practice effects may even be limited to the specific effectors used (Walker, DeSoto, & Shelly, 1957). This could start the process whereby the muscle groups involved in the active behaviors of one hand or the supportive behaviors of the other became selectively skilled or specialized. In effect, a biasing factor has been created. The active hand is already trained in movement patterns that are common to other active behaviors. Thus it is easier for this hand to learn new activities, since many elements have already been learned and are common to the old and the new activity (Ellis, 1969; Postman, 1971). It is simply easier for the previously active limb to learn new active behaviors. Once an individual has selected a preferred limb for one set of skilled movements, it is more likely that

that same limb will be used on successive occasions. It will develop proficiency in an entire constellation of skilled motoric coordinations. Regardless of the side of the body selected, individuals should become more consistent in their limb use for particular coordinations, since that limb is better at such tasks, and the consistency will increase over time through simple repetition and reinforcement. Such a pattern of increasing consistency of preference is what one finds when one looks at changes in lateral preferences over the life span (Chapters 3 and 6). Not only does *practice make perfect,* but *practice* also *makes preference.* Each member of the paired limbs become specialized and preferred for a specific set of activity patterns.

We have shown how an initial set of spontaneously emitted unilateral responses coupled with simple learning mechanisms can produce laterally asymmetrical behaviors. However, how does this hypothesized development of lateral preferences relate to neurological asymmetries or genetic predispositions? In this context, Reynolds (1975) has proposed an interesting theoretical position to explain hand preference in both primates and humans. He suggested that the specialization of manual function (or at least the tendency toward such specialization) may have evolved prior to the lateral differentiation of neural control in primates. According to our extension of this hypothesis, the development of handedness in humans, accompanied by some lateralization of neurological functioning, represents an evolutionary advance whereby the organization of the nervous system evolved to support the adaptive active-passive differentiation of the paired limbs. If such bilateral specialization conveyed an adaptive advantage to the organism through increased skill, selective pressure on the species would lead to higher survival rates of individuals with strong manifest lateral preferences. The side of preference is not important, since either the right or the left side serves equally well in the active or passive function. It is only important for each side to develop a primary specialized set of functions. This reasoning leads to the expectation that the aspect of lateral preference that is transmitted genetically is the propensity toward consistent versus weak lateral preference response patterns, which is, of course, the pattern of genetic involvement observed in Chapter 5.

Selective pressure favoring individuals with lateral preferences, who have laterally specialized neural organizations to support such behaviors, implies the existence of neurophysiological correlates to lateral preference. However, this does not imply a perfect correlation between neural asymmetries and these behaviors. A specific form of neurological organization may support the specialization of the two sides, but such specialization could have occurred in the absence of neural biases. This last statement is supported by the relatively symmetrical brain organization in primates, who nonetheless still show lateral preferences (Chapters 4 and 5). It may be easier for one side to develop a particular function, given a particular pattern of cerebral asymmetries; however, this effect may be a statistical bias in the population, rather than a direct cause. The weak relationship between handedness and cerebral asymmetries observed in Chapter 4 are quite compatible with this line of reasoning.

Why is the right side the preferred side in the majority of humans? This may be a completely spurious aspect of an evolutionary process that originally emerged to support some form of lateral specialization but did not specify a particular side. In the first stages of lateral preference development, as we outlined it previously, the specialization of function in the hands becomes a behavioral fact with the continued practice of various active or passive activities. In the absence of lateral biasing pressures, causing one side to be preferentially chosen for a particular class of activities, each hand would be exercised randomly during the early learning stage. Chance would dictate the hand used a few more times for active behaviors, which would then assume the lead in the acquisition of these patterns of skill. If the development of lateral preference conveys an adaptive advantage, the earlier the development of lateral preferences, the more practice time the individual has, and thus the faster the development of facility in these specialized activities. This process only requires that the majority of early movements favor one side. If one could build into the developing child or the developmental sequence some process or set of processes that cause one set of specialized behaviors (skilled active) to be systematically biased to one side, the patterns of practice would thus focus more consistently on an individual limb and the development of lateral specialization would be speeded. If all individuals shared a similar bias to one side, a biased population would be the result. What types of biasing predispositions are sufficient? Any number of minor ones, acting singly or in concert, would serve this purpose. For example, postural asymmetries have been noted in neonates older than 12 hours in which infants preferentially turn their heads toward the right side (Liederman & Kinsbourne, 1980; Turkewitz, Gordon, & Birch, 1965; Turkewitz & Creighton, 1974). Such a simple behavior could increase the likelihood that visible targets are on the right side, hence reached for with the near (i.e., right) hand (Coryell & Michel, 1978). Furthermore, active movements of the right hand would be frequently in the infant's field of view. These events could result in a biasing of early active sensorimotor behaviors toward the right. Similarly, if neurological development begins earlier on the left side (Corballis & Morgan, 1978; Morgan & Corballis, 1978), then the contralateral control pattern for limb function could bias some of the early postural or balance reflexes toward the right side. A prime candidate for a possible mechanism is the palmer reflex, whereby objects placed against the palm are grasped firmly. If the faster maturation of the left hemisphere causes the right hand to grasp a few moments longer, then individuals have become biased toward a preferred hand for grasping and manipulating.

This line of reasoning also predicts greater left-sidedness or mixed lateral preference in clinically affected populations. Neuropathy results in alterations, disruptions, or delays of the usual course of motoric development. These may produce postural changes or suppress some of the typical reflex patterns in infants (such as the palmer reflex). These disruptions could delay the development of lateral specialization, since the normal motoric and reflex supports toward the right are absent. More ambilaterality and left-sidedness result as first one side is practiced and then the other in a mixed fashion, retarding the development of clear specialization. The occurrence of more left-sidedness and ambilaterality in clinically retarded and other groups of low performers (Chapters 7-10) is explainable also given that there is a learning component in this conception of the genesis of lateral preferences. Such groups, because of their cognitive deficiencies, may simply be slower at learning the specialization. If they need more repetitions of a coordination for acquisition, less consistency may develop along with more ambilaterality. Furthermore, most of the infant reflexes, which might bias an individual toward the right, tend to disappear within the first year of development. Hence, if skill learning is slow, it may develop late, and this slight pressure toward dextrality will have gone, resulting in higher incidences of left-sidedness. A typical nonpathological left-handed minority is not a problem within this thesis, since the biases toward the right are minor and serve only to raise the probability that the initial active responses will be dextral. If, as a result of chance, environmental factors, or some aspect of early prenatal or neurological intervention, the first few active responses have a leftward bias, the gradual skill acquisition process will strengthen this tendency, producing a left-handed individual.

This theoretical framework is speculative, but it incorporates some of the trends that have emerged from the literature and from our data. Lateral preferences represent lateral specialization of skills, and as such are susceptible to learning effects (Chapters 6 and 11). There is evidence for genetic involvement in the strength or consistency of preferences (Chapter 5); there are some weak neurological correlates (Chapter 4); there are developmental trends (Chapters 3 and 6) and alterations in the normative pattern of preference in clinical samples (Chapters 7-9). There are gaps in the theory because of missing empirical evidence; however, such a multicausal, multiple-mechanism approach seems closer to accounting for the phenomena than any unicausal theory.

Although we have concentrated on handedness in this theoretical sketch, we can extend this argument easily to foot preference. There is also lateral specialization of foot use. While one foot kicks an object, the other supports the weight of the body. Once again, there is differentiation of movement pattern according to the active and manipulative functions versus the passive and supportive functions. Foot use is also subject to many of the same influences as hand use. Foot preference is affected by learning processes (Chapters 6 and 11), shows some genetic component for strength (Chapter 5), has a neural motor control system that is contralateral (Chapter 4), and shows shifts toward mixed preference and left-sidedness in clinical groups (Chapters 7-9). It also shows developmental trends and individual difference patterns similar to those of handedness (Chapters 3 and 6). Finally, hand and foot represent a common dimension of lateral preference (Chapter 4); hence, it is possible that they share a common mechanism.

Extension of this explanation to the sense organ preferences is more difficult. There are no direct data about whether or not the preferred and nonpreferred sense organ partners are specialized for a different set of functions. The two eyes act asymmetrically at times, but the nature of these differences is not clear.

As we noted in Chapter 12, there are some visual functions, such as the maintenance of single vision, which require that the input to the two eyes be separated
and used differentially. The central nervous system must be able to identify the
right and the left eye input for organized recombination of the inputs in the
stereoscopic view. However, this process requires identifiability, or an eye signature, not a difference in function. The data on sense organ preference are different from those on the limbs. Eye preference shows only a slight age changes,
and ear preference loses its dextral bias in older individuals (Chapter 6). Eyedness shows no familial similarities, while there may be genetic involvement in
determining both the side and the strength of ear preference (Chapter 5). Sensory preferences are different from limb preferences, and eyedness and earedness
themselves may serve different purposes. At present, however, we know too
little to speculate further.

We have shown that lateral preferences are an easily and reliably measured
aspect of human behavior. They show a general asymmetry in human behavioral
coordinations for both the limbs and the sense organs. Human populations are
biased predominantly toward the right side, but the degree of biasing is not
immutable. Lateral preference patterns are subject to influence by individual
difference factors such as age, gender, and familial and societal membership,
and are perhaps influenced by physiological and environmental histories. But
lateral preferences are not unitary phenomena, and those of limb and sense
organ seem to be quite different. They probably represent different functions
and seem to be supported by different causal structures. Furthermore, one
causal mechanism cannot account for the total array of lateral preferences.
Lateral preferences vary in side and in strength, and individuals may differ in the
consistency of these behaviors as well as in the overall sidedness congruency
across indexes of preference. There are also neurological, cognitive, and coordination correlates of lateral preference behaviors that can be measured. Based on
this information, we have tried to present a theoretical framework that demonstrates how genetics, learning, physiological considerations, life history, pathological interventions, and even chance may interact to produce some forms of
lateral preference. Yet there is much that we do not as yet understand. We feel
that we have made a first step toward a full exploration of these interesting
asymmetries in human behavior. Yet sometimes we find ourselves mentally
returning to the issues which we still do not fully understand and to those
aspects of the problem that remain on the hypothetical level. At such times, we
are reminded of a passage in a children's book:

> Pooh looked at his two paws. He knew that one of them was the right, and
> he knew that when you had decided which one of them was the right, then
> the other one was the left, but he never could remember how to begin.
> "Well," he said slowly. . . . (A. A. Milne, 1926, *House at Pooh Corner*, p. 118)

References

Achenbach, T. M. Comparison of Stanford-Binet performance of non-retarded and retarded persons matched for MA and sex. American Journal of Mental Deficiency, 1970, **74**, 488-494.

Achenbach, T. M. Developmental Psychopathology. New York: Ronald Press, 1974.

Adams, G. L. Effect of eye dominance on baseball batting. The Research Quarterly, 1965, **36**, 3-9.

Adams, J. A. Acquisition of motor responses. In M. H. Marx (Ed.), Learning Processes. London: Macmillan, 1969, pp. 481-494.

Allen, M., & Wellman, M. M. Hand position during writing, cerebral laterality and reading: age and sex differences. Neuropsychologia, 1980, **18**, 33-40.

Allison, R. B. The relationship between handedness in elementary school children and reading skills, school achievement, and perceptual-motor development. Dissertation Abstracts, 1966, **27**, 5-A, 1256.

Anderson, I., & Crosland, H. R. The effects of eye-dominance on "range of attention" scores. Studies in Psychology, Bulletin 4. Eugene, Oregon: University of Oregon, 1933.

Annett, J., & Sheridan, M. R. Effects of S-R and R-R compatibility on bimanual movement time. Quarterly Journal of Experimental Psychology, 1973, **25**, 247-252.

Annett, M. A model of the inheritance of handedness and cerebral dominance. Nature, 1964, **204**, 59-60.

Annett, M. The binomial distribution of right, mixed and left handedness. Quarterly Journal of Experimental Psychology, 1967, **19**, 327-333.

Annett, M. A classification of hand preference by association analysis. British Journal of Psychology, 1970, **61**, 303-321. (a)

Annett, M. The growth of manual preference and speed. British Journal of Psychology, 1970, **61**, 545-558. (b)

Annett, M. The distribution of manual asymmetry. British Journal of Psychology, 1972, **3**, 343-358.

Annett, M. Handedness in families. Annals of Human Genetics, 1973, 37, 93-105.

Annett, M. Handedness in the children of two left-handed parents. British Journal of Psychology, 1974, 65, 129-131.

Annett, M. Genetic and nongenetic influences on handedness. Behavior Genetics, 1978, 8, 227-249. (a)

Annett, M. A single gene explanation of right and left handedness and brainedness. Coventry, England: Lanchester Polytechnic, 1978. (b)

Annett, M., & Turner, A. Laterality and the growth of intellectual abilities. British Journal of Educational Psychology, 1974, 44, 37-46.

Arend, L. E. Spatial differential and integral operations in human vision: implications of stabilized retinal image. Psychological Review, 1973, 80, 374-395.

Asher, H. Experiments in Seeing. New York: Basic Books, 1961.

Bakan, P. The eyes have it. Psychology Today, 1971, 96, 64-67. (a)

Bakan, P. Handedness and birth order. Nature, 1971, 229, 195. (b)

Bakan, P. Left-handedness and alcoholism. Perceptual and Motor Skills, 1973, 36, 514.

Bakan, P. The right brain is a dreamer. Psychology Today, 1976, 10, 66-68.

Bakan, P. Left handedness and birth order revisited. Neuropsychologia, 1977, 15, 817-839.

Bakan, P. Why left handedness? Behavioral and Brain Sciences, 1978, 2, 279-280.

Bakan, P., Dibb, G., & Reed, P. Handedness and birth stress. Neuropsychologia, 1973, 11, 363-366.

Baldwin, J. M. Origin of right or left handedness. Science, 1890, 16, 247-248.

Baldwin, J. M. Dextrality. Baldwin's Dictionary of Philosophy and Psychology. New York: Macmillan, 1911.

Balow, I., & Balow, B. Lateral dominance and reading achievement in the second grade. American Educational Research Journal, 1964, 1, 139-143.

Banister, H. A study of eye dominance. British Journal of Psychology, 1935, 26, 34-42.

Bannatyne, A. Language, Reading and Learning Disabilities. Springfield, Ill.: Charles C Thomas, 1971.

Barbeito, R. Ocular dominance: an explanation based on sighting behavior. Unpublished doctoral dissertation, York University, 1979.

Barsley, M. Left-handed People. North Hollywood: Wilshire Book Co., 1976.

Barnsley, R. H., & Rabinovitch, M. S. Handedness: Proficiency versus stated preference. Perceptual and Motor Skills, 1970, 30, 343-362.

Bastian, H. C. On the specific gravity of different parts of the human brain. Journal of Mental Science, 1869, 14, 454-460.

Bateman, F. On aphasia or loss of speech in cerebral disease. Journal of Mental Science, 1869, 15, 367-392; 489-502.

Beck, C. H. M., & Barton, R. L. Deviation and laterality of hand preference in monkeys. Cortex, 1972, 8, 339-363.

Beck, E. C., & Dustman, R. E. Changes in evoked responses during maturation and aging in man and macaque. In N. Burch, and H. I. Altshuler (Eds.), Behavior and Brain Electrical Activity. New York: Plenum, 1975, pp. 431-472.

Beckman, L., & Elston, R. Data on bilateral variation in man: handedness, hand clasping and hand folding in Swedes. Human Biology, 1962, **34**, 99-103.

Bell, C. The Hand: It's Mechanism and Vital Endowments as Evincing Design. London: Pickering, 1833.

Bell, J. Our president, the south-paw. San Francisco Examiner and Chronicle, October 20, 1974.

Belmont, L., & Birch, H. G. Lateral dominance, lateral awareness, and reading disability. Child Development, 1965, **36**, 57-71.

Bender, L. Neuropsychiatric disturbances. In A. H. Keeney and V. T. Keeney (Eds.), Dyslexia: Diagnosis and Treatment of Reading Disorders. St. Louis: Mosby, 1968, pp. 42-48.

Benton, A. L., Meyers, R., & Pobler, G. J. Some aspects of handedness. Psychiatric Neurology, 1962, **144**, 321-337.

Benton, C. D. Management of dyslexia associated with binocular control abnormalities. In A. H. Keeney and V. T. Keeney (Eds.), Dyslexia: Diagnosis and Treatment of Reading Disorders. St. Louis: Mosby, 1968.

Berlin, C. I. Hemispheric asymmetry in auditory tasks. In S. Harnad, R. W. Doty, L. Goldstein, J. Jaynes, and G. Krauthamer (Eds.), Lateralization in the Nervous System. New York: Academic Press, 1977, pp. 303-324.

Berlin, C. I., & McNeil, M. R. Dichotic listening. In N. J. Lass (Ed.), Contemporary Issues in Experimental Phonetics. New York: Academic Press, 1976.

Berman, A. Reliability of perceptual-motor laterality tasks. Perceptual and Motor Skills, 1973, **36**, 599-605.

Berner, G. E., & Berner, D. E. Relation of ocular dominance, handedness and the controlling eye in binocular vision. A. M. A. Archives of Ophthalmology, 1953, **50**, 603-608.

Bethe, A. von. Zur statistik der links und rechtshaendigkeit und der vorherrschaft einer hemisphaere. Deutsche Medizinische Wochenschrift, 1925, **17**, 681-683.

Bever, T. G., & Chiarello, R. J. Cerebral dominance in musicians and nonmusicians. Science, 1974, **184**, 537-539.

Biervlet, J. J. van. L'asymétrie sensorielle. Bulletin de l'Académie Royale de Belgique, 1897, **34**, 326-366.

Biervlet, J. J. van. Nouvelle contribution à l'étude de l'asymétrie sensorielle. Bulletins de l'Académie Royale des Sciences de Belgique, 1901, 3, 679-694.

Bilto, E. W., & Peterson, G. E. The relation between ear preference and hearing acuity. Journal of Speech Disorders, 1944, **9**, 123-125.

Bingley, T. Mental symptoms in temporal lobe epilepsy and temporal lobe gliomas. Acta Psychiatrica Neurologica Scandinavia, 1958, **120**, 151.

Blau, A. The Master Hand. New York: American Orthopsychiatric Association, 1946.

Boklage, C. E. The sinistral blastocyst: An embryologic perspective on the development of brain function asymmetries. In J. Herron (Ed.), Neuropsychology of Left-Handedness. New York: Academic Press, 1980, pp. 115-138.

Bolin, B. J. Left-handedness and stuttering as signs diagnostic of epileptics. Journal of Mental Science, 1953, **99**, 483-488.

Boyd, R. Tables of the weights of the human body and internal organs of the sane and insane of both sexes of various ages arranged from 2,114 postmortum examinations. Philosophical Transactions of the Royal Society, London, 1861, **151**, 241-262.

Boynton, R. M., & Gordon, J. Bezold-Brucke hue shift measured by color naming technique. Journal of the Optical Society of America, 1965, **55**, 78-86.

Brain, R. Speech Disorders (2nd ed.). London: Butterworth, 1965.

Braitenberg, V., & Kemali, N. Exceptions to bilateral symmetry in the epithalamus of lower vertebrates. Journal of Comparative Neurology, 1971, **138**, 137-146.

Brewster, E. T. The ways of the left hand. McClure's Magazine, 1913, pp. 168-183.

Briggs, G., Nebes, R. P., & Kinsbourne, M. Intellectual differences in relation to personal and family handedness. Quarterly Journal of Experimental Psychology, 1976, **28**, 591-601.

Brister, B. Master eyes and misses. Field and Stream, 1975, August, pp. 66-70.

Broadbent, D. E. The role of auditory localization in attenuation and memory span. Journal of Experimental Psychology, 1954, **47**, 191-196.

Broca, P. Recherches sur la circulation cérébrale. Bulletin de l'Académie de Médecine, 1877, **6**, 508-539 (2ème série).

Brod, N., & Hamilton, D. Monocular-binocular coordination vs. hand-eye dominance as a factor in reading performance. American Journal of Optometry and Archives of the American Academy of Optometry, 1971, **48**, 123-129.

Broer, N. R., & Zernicke, R. F. Efficiency of Human Movement. Philadelphia: Saunders, 1979.

Broman, S. H., Nichols, P. L., & Kennedy, W. A. Pre-school IQ: Prenatal and Early Developmental Correlates. Hillsdale, N.J.: Lawrence Erlbaum Associates, 1975.

Brookshire, K. H., & Warren, J. M. The generality and consistency of handedness in monkeys. Animal Behavior, 1962, **10**, 222-227.

Brown, J. S., Knauft, E. B., & Rosenbaum, G. The accuracy of positioning movements as a function of their direction and extent. American Journal of Psychology, 1948, **61**, 167-182.

Browne, T. *Pseudoxia epidemica, or, Enquiries into vary many received tennents and commonly presumed truths.* London: printed by T. H. for Edward Dod, 1646.

Bryant, D. N., & Patterson, P. Reading disability: part of a syndrome of neurologic dysfunctioning. Paper presented at the meetings of the International Reading Association, 1962.

Bryden, M. P. Perceptual asymmetry in vision: relation to handedness, eyedness, and speech lateralization. Cortex, 1973, **11**, 418-432.

Bryden, M. P. Measuring handedness with questionnaires. Neuropsychologia, 1977, **15**, 617-624.

Bryden, M. P. Strategy effects in the assessment of hemispheric asymmetry. In G. Underwood (Ed.), Strategies of Information Processing. London: Academic Press, 1978, pp. 117-149.

Bryden, M. P. Possible genetic mechanisms of handedness and laterality. Paper presented at the meeting of the Canadian Psychological Association, Quebec City, Quebec, June, 1979.

Buchanan, A. Mechanical theory of the predominance of the right hand over the left. Philosophical Society of Glasgow, Proceedings, 1862, 5, 142-167.

Burt, C. The Backward Child. London: University of London Press, 1937.

Buxton, C. E. A comparison of preferred and motor-learning measures of handedness. Journal of Experimental Psychology, 1937, 24, 464-469.

Calnan, M., & Richardson, K. Developmenal correlates of handedness in a national sample of 11-year-olds. Annals of Human Biology, 1976, 3, 329-342.

Carey, S., & Diamond, R. From piecemeal to configurational representation of faces. Science, 1977, 195, 312-314.

Carlyle, T. Diary for June 15, 1871. In J. A. Froide, Thomas Carlyle (Vol. 2). London: Longmans, Green, 1884, p. 407.

Carmon, A. P., & Gombos, G. M. A physiological vascular correlate of hand preference: possible implications with respect to hemispheric cerebral dominance. Neuropsychologia, 1970, 8, 119-128.

Carmon, A. P., Harishanu, Y., Lowinger, E., & Lavy, S. Asymmetries in hemispheric blood volume and cerebral dominance. Behavioral Biology, 1972, 7, 853-859.

Carter-Saltzman, L. Biological and socio-cultural effects on handedness: comparison between biological and adoptive families. Science, 1980, 209, 163-165.

Carter-Saltzman, L., Scarr-Salapatek, S., Barker, W. B., & Katz, S. Left handedness in twins: incidence and patterns of performance in an adolescent sample. Behavior Genetics, 1976, 6, 189-294.

Cattell, R. B. Abilities: Their Structure, Growth and Action. Boston: Houghton-Mifflin, 1971.

Cavalli-Sforza, L. L., & Bodmer, W. F. The Genetics of Human Populations. San Francisco: W. H. Freeman, 1971.

Cernacek, J., & Podivinsky, F. Ontogenesis of handedness and somatosensory cortical response. Neuropsychologia, 1971, 9, 219-232.

Chamberlain, H. D. The inheritance of left handedness. Journal of Heredity, 1928, 19, 557-559.

Chan, K. S. F., Hsu, F. K., Chan, S. T., & Chan, Y. B. Scrotal asymmetry and handedness. Journal of Anatomy, 1960, 94, 543-548.

Chandler, C. M. Hand, eye and foot preference of two hundred psychotic patients and two hundred college students. Psychological Bulletin, 1934, 31, 593-594.

Charman, D. K. Note on a failure to find hemispheric asymmetries for a small sample of strongly left- and right-handed males and females using verbal and visuo-spatial recall. Perceptual and Motor Skills, 1980, 51, 139-145.

Charnwood, L. An Essay on Binocular Vision. New York: Hafner, 1965.

Chayatte, C., Abern, S. B., Reddy, A. M., & Bottichelli, R. M. Left handed people. Irish Medical Journal, 1979, 72, 511.

Chayatte, C., Chayatte, C., & Althoff, D. Left-handedness and vegetarianism. South African Medical Journal, 1979, 56, 505-506.

Chorazyne, H. Shifts in laterality in a baby chimpanzee. Neuropsychologia, 1976, **14**, 381-384.

Churchill, J. A., Inga, E., & Senf, R. The association of position at birth and handedness. Pediatrics, 1962, **29**, 307-309.

Clark, M. M. Left Handedness: Laterality Characteristics and Their Education Implications. London: University of London Press, 1957.

Clark, M. M. Reading Difficulties in Schools. Harmondsworth: Penguin Books, 1970.

Clarke, J. C., & Whitehurst, G. I. Asymmetrical stimulus control and the mirror-image problem. Journal of Experimental Child Psychology, 1974, **17**, 147-166.

Clements, S. D., & Peters, J. E. Minimal brain dysfunction in the school-age child. Archives of General Psychiatry, 1962, **6**, 185-197.

Cohen, J. Eye dominance. American Journal of Psychology, 1952, **65**, 634-636.

Cole, J. Paw preference in cats related to hand preference in animals and man. Journal of Comparative and Physiological Psychology, 1955, **48**, 137-140.

Cole, J. Laterality in the use of the hand, foot and eye in monkeys. Journal of Comparative and Physiological Psychology, 1957, **50**, 296-299.

Coleman, R. I., & Deutsch, C. P. Lateral dominance and right-left discrimination: a comparison of normal and retarded readers. Perceptual and Motor Skills, 1964, **19**, 43-50.

Collins, R. L. On the inheritance of handedness, I: Laterality in inbred mice. Journal of Heredity, 1968, **59**, 9-12.

Collins, R. L. On the inheritance of handedness, II: Selection for sinistrality in mice. Journal of Heredity, 1969, **60**, 117-119.

Collins, R. L. The sound of one paw clapping: an inquiry into the origin of left-handedness. In F. Lindzey & D. D. Thiessen (Eds.), Contributions to Behavior-Genetic Analysis: The Mouse as a Prototype. New York: Appleton, 1970, pp. 115-136.

Collins, R. L. When left handed mice live in right handed worlds. Science, 1975, **187**, 181-184.

Collins, R. L. Toward an admissible genetic model for the inheritance of the degree and direction of asymmetry. In S. Harnard, R. W. Doty, J. Jaynes, L. Goldstein, & G. Krauthamer (Eds.), Lateralization in the Nervous System. New York: Academic Press, 1977, pp. 137-150.

Collins, R. L. In the beginning was the asymmetry gradient even when it was null: A propositional framework for a general theory of the inheritance of asymmetry. The Behavioral and Brain Sciences, 1978, **2**, 290-291.

Cook, T. W. Studies in cross education, I: Mirror tracing and the star shaped maze. Journal of Experimental Psychology, 1933, **16**, 144-210.

Cook, T. W. Studies in cross education, IV: Permanence of transfer. Journal of Experimental Psychology, 1935, **18**, 255-266.

Coons, J. C., & Mathias, R. S. Eye and hand preference tendencies. Journal of Genetic Psychology, 1928, **35**, 629-632.

Corballis, M. C. Is left-handedness genetically determined? In J. Herron (Ed.), Neuropsychology of Left-Handedness, New York: Academic Press, 1980, 159-176. (a)

Corballis, M. C. Laterality and myth. American Psychologist, 1980, 35, 284-295. (b)

Corballis, M. C., & Beale, I. L. The Psychology of Left and Right. Hillsdale, N.J.: Lawrence Erlbaum Associates, 1976.

Corballis, M. C., & Morgan, M. J. On the biological basis of human laterality, I: Evidence for a maturational left-right gradient. The Behavioral and Brain Sciences, 1978, 2, 261-336.

Coren, S. The use of Haidinger's brushes in the study of stabilized retinal images. Behaviour Research Methods and Instrumentation, 1971, 3, 295-297.

Coren, S. The development of ocular dominance. Developmental Psychology, 1974, 10, 304.

Coren, S., & Girgus, J. S. Transfer of illusion decrement as a function of perceived similarity. Journal of Experimental Psychology, 1974, 102, 881-887.

Coren, S., & Girgus, J. S. Seeing is Deceiving: The Psychology of Visual Illusions. Hillsdale, N.J.: Lawrence Erlbaum Associates, 1978.

Coren, S., & Hoenig, P. Eye movements and decrement in the Oppel-Kundt illusion. Perception and Psychophysics, 1972, 12, 224-225.

Coren, S., & Kaplan, C. P. Clarity of Haidinger's brushes as a function of luminance. Behaviour Research Methods and Instrumentation, 1972, 4, 314-324.

Coren, S., & Kaplan, C. P. Patterns of ocular dominance. American Journal of Optometry and Archives of the American Academy of Optometry, 1973, 50, 283-292.

Coren, S., & Porac, C. The fading of stabilized images: eye movement and information processing. Perception and Psychophysics, 1974, 16, 529-534.

Coren, S., & Porac, C. Ocular dominance: an annotated bibliography. JSAS Catalogue of Selected Documents in Psychology, 1975, 4, 229-230.

Coren, S., & Porac, C. Size accentuation in the dominant eye. Nature, 1976, 260, 527-528.

Coren, S., & Porac, C. Effects of simulated refractive asymmetries on eye dominance. Bulletin of the Psychonomic Society, 1977, 9, 269-271. (a)

Coren, S., & Porac, C. Fifty centuries of right-handedness: the historical record. Science, 1977, 198, 631-632. (b)

Coren, S., & Porac, C. The validity and reliability of self-report items for the measurement of lateral preference. British Journal of Psychology, 1978, 69, 207-211.

Coren, S., & Porac, C. Eye signature: phenomenal differences as a function of sighting dominance. Paper presented at the meetings of the Psychonomic Society, Phoenix, Arizona, November 1979. (a)

Coren, S., & Porac, C. Normative data on hand position during writing. Cortex, 1979, 15, 679-682. (b)

Coren, S., & Porac, C. Birth factors in laterality: effects of birth order, parental age, and birth stress on four indices of lateral preference. Behavior Genetics, 1980, 10, 123-138. (a)

Coren, S., & Porac, C. Family patterns in four dimensions of lateral preference. Behavior Genetics, 1980, 10, 333-348. (b)

Coren, S., Porac, C., & Duncan, P. A behaviorally validated self-report inventory to assess four types of lateral preference. Journal of Clinical Neuropsychology, 1979, 1, 55-64.

Coren, S., Porac, C., & Duncan, P. Lateral preference in pre-school children and young adults. Child Development, 1981.

Coren, S., Porac, C., & Ward, L. M. Sensation and Perception. New York: Academic Press, 1979.

Coryell, J. F., & Michel, G. F. How supine postural preferences of infants can contribute toward the development of handedness. Infant Behavior and Development, 1978, 1, 245-257.

Court-Brown, W. M., Jacobs, P. A., Buckton, K. E., Tough, I. M., Kuenssberg, E. V., & Knox, J. A. F. Chromosome Studies on Adults. New York and London: Cambridge University Press (Eugenics Laboratory Memoirs No. 42), 1966.

Court-Brown, W. M., Jacobs, P. A., & Tough, I. M. Some types of information obtainable from chromosome studies on defined population groups. In Human Radiation Cytogenics: Proceedings of an International Symposium (Edinburgh, October 12-15, 1966). New York: Wiley, 1967, pp. 115-121.

Crider, B. The relationship of eye muscle balance to the sighting eye. Journal of Experimental Psychology, 1935, 18, 152-154.

Crider, B. The importance of the dominant eye. Journal of Psychology, 1943, 16, 145-151.

Crider, B. A battery of tests for the dominant eye. Journal of General Psychology, 1944, 31, 179-190.

Critchley, M. The Dyslexic Child. London: Heinemann, 1970.

Crovitz, H. F. Differential acuity of the two eyes and the problem of ocular dominances. Science, 1961, 134, 614.

Crovitz, H. F. Retinal locus in tachistoscopic binocular color rivalry. Perceptual and Motor Skills, 1964, 19, 808-819.

Crovitz, H., & Lipscomb, D. Dominances of the temporal visual fields at short duration of stimulation. American Journal of Psychology, 1963, 76, 631-637.

Crovitz, H. F., & Zener, K. A group-test for assessing hand and eye dominances. American Journal of Psychology, 1962, 75, 271-276.

Cuff, N. B. Eyedness and handedness-report of paper. American Journal of Psychology, 1930, 42, 459-460. (a)

Cuff, N. B. The relationship of eyedness and handedness to psychopathic tendencies. Journal of Genetic Psychology, 1930, 37, 530-536. (b)

Cuff, N. B. A study of eyedness and handedness. Journal of Experimental Psychology, 1931, 14, 164-175.

Cunningham, D. J. Contribution to the Surface Anatomy of the Cerebral Hemispheres, with a Chapter upon Cranio-cerebral Topography by Victor Horsley. Dublin: Royal Irish Academy (Cunningham Memoirs), 1892.

Cunningham, D. J. Right-handedness and left-brainedness (The Huxley Lecture for 1902). Journal of the Royal Anthropological Institute of Great Britain and Ireland, 1902, 32, 273-296.

Dahlberg, G. Twin Births and Twins from a Heredity Point of View. Stockholm: Tidens, 1926.

Daniels, F. S. Do the eyes have it? American Rifleman, March 1981, **129**, 38-39; 79.

Danielson, R. W. A study of unilateral voluntary winking: some modifying factors and associated phenomena. University of Colorado Studies, 1930, **18**, No. 2.

Darwin, C. A biographical sketch of an infant. Mind, 1877, **2**, 199-265.

Davidson, W. P. A study of confusing letters b, d, p, q. Journal of Genetic Psychology, 1935, **47**, 458-468.

Dawson, J. L. M. Temne-arunta hand-eye dominance and cognitive style. International Journal of Psychology, 1972, **7**, 219-233.

Dawson, J. L. M. B. Anthropological perspective on the evolution and lateralization of the brain. In S. J. Dimond & D. A. Blizard (Eds.), Evolution and lateralization of the brain. Annals of the New York Academy of Sciences, 1977, **299**, 424-447.

Day, R. H. The effects of repeated trials and prolonged fixation on errors in the Mueller-Lyer figure. Psychological Monographs, 1962, **76**, No. 14 (Whole No. 53).

Dearborn, W. F. Ocular and manual dominance in dyslexia. Psychological Bulletin, 1931, **28**, 704.

de Fleury, A. Sur la pathogenie du langage articlé. Letter to l'Académie des Sciences, Belles Lettres et Arts de Bordeaux, 9 February, 1865.

De Hirsch, K., Jansky, J. J., & Langford, W. S. Predicting Reading Failure: A Preliminary Study. New York: Harper & Row, 1966.

Delacato, C. H. The Treatment and Prevention of Reading Problems (The Neuropsychological Approach). Springfield, Ill.: Charles C Thomas, 1963.

Dennis, M., & Whitaker, H. A. Hemispheric equipotentiality and language acquisition. In S. J. Segalowitz & F. A. Gruber (Eds.), Language Development and Neurological Theory. New York: Academic Press, 1977, pp. 93-107.

Dennis, W. Early graphic evidence of dextrality in man. Perceptual and Motor Skills, 1958, **8**, 147-149.

Denny-Brown, D., Mayer, J. S., & Horenstein, S. The significance of perceptual rivalry resulting from parietal lesions. Brain, 1952, **75**, 433-471.

DeRenzi, E., & Faglioni, P. The relationship between visuospatial impairment and constructional apraxia. Cortex, 1967, **3**, 327-342.

Diagnostic Reading Test. Mountain Home, N.C.: The Committee on Diagnostic Reading Tests, Inc., 1966.

Di Chiaro, G. Angiographic patterns of cerebral convexity veins and superficial dural sinuses. American Journal of Roentgenology Radium Therapy and Nuclear Medicine, 1962, **87**, 308-321.

Dimond, S. J., & Beaumont, J. G. Hemispheric Function in the Human Brain. London: Elek Science, 1974.

Ditchburn, R. W., & Ginsberg, B. L. Vision with a stabilized retinal image. Nature, 1952, **170**, 36-38.

Dodwell, P. C., & Engel, G. R. A theory of binocular vision. Nature, 1953, **198**, 73-74.

Doll, E. A. Psychological significance of cerebral birth lesions. American Journal of Psychology, 1933, **45**, 444-452.

Dolman, P. The relation of the sighting eye to the measurement of heterophoria: a preliminary report. American Journal of Opthalmology, 1920, **3**, 258-261.

Doty, R. W. Potentials evoked in cat cerebral cortex by diffuse and punctate photic stimulation. Journal of Neurophysiology, 1958, **21**, 437-464.

Downey, J. Types of dextrality and their implications. American Journal of Psychology, 1927, **38**, 317-367.

Downey, J. E. Back-slanted writing and sinistral tendencies. Journal of Educational Psychology, 1932, **23**, 277-286.

Doyne, R. W. Eye in sport shooting. Ophthalmoscope, 1915, **13**, 119.

Duke-Elder, W. S. Textbook of Ophthalmology (Vol. 4). London: Henry Kimpton, 1952.

Dunn, L. M. Studies of reading and arithmetic in mentally retarded boys, I: A comparison of the reading processes of mentally retarded and normal boys of the same mental age. Monographs of Social Research and Child Development, 1954, **19**, 7-99.

Durost, W. N. The development of a battery of objective groups tests of manual laterality, with the results of their application to 1300 children. Genetic Psychology Monographs, 1934, **16**, 229-235.

Dwight, T. Right and left-handedness. Journal of Psychological Medicine, 1870, **4**, 535-542.

Eberstaller, O. Zur oberflachen-anatomie der Grosshirn-hemispharen. Weiener Medizinische Blaetter, 1884, **7**, 479-482; 542-582; 644-646.

Eeg-Olofsson, O. The development of the EEG in normal children from the age of 1 to 15 years: 14- and 6- persecond positive spike phenomena. Neuropadiatrie, 1971, **4**, 405-427. (a)

Eeg-Olofsson, O. The development of the EEG in normal young persons from the age of 16 to 21 years. Neuropadiatrie, 1971, **3**, 11-45. (b)

Ellis, H. C. Transfer: empirical findings and theoretical interpretations. In M. H. Marx (Ed.), Learning Processes. London: Macmillan, 1969, pp. 400-423.

Elworthy, F. T. The Evil Eye. London: John Murray, 1895, p. 429.

Enstrom, E. A. The extent of the use of the left hand in handwriting. Journal of Educational Research, 1962, **55**, 234-235.

Etaugh, C., & Brausam, M. Sensitivity to laterality as a function of handedness. Perceptual and Motor Skills, 1978, **46**, 420-422.

Ettlinger, G., & Dawson, R. F. Hand preferences in the monkey: the effect of unilateral cortical removals. Neuropsychologia, 1969, **7**, 161-166.

Ettlinger, G., Jackson, C. V., & Zangwill, O. L. Cerebral dominance in sinistrals. Brain, 1956, **79**, 569-588.

Ettlinger, G., & Moffett, A. Lateral preference in the monkey. Nature, 1964, 204-206.

Fagan-Dubin, L. Lateral dominance and development of cerebral specialization. Cortex, 1974, **10**, 69-74.

Falek, A. Handedness: a family study. American Journal of Human Genetics, 1959, **11**, 52-62.

Festinger, L., White, C. W., & Allyn, M. R. Eye movements and decrement in the Mueller-Lyer illusion. Perception and Psychophysics, 1968, 3, 376-382.

Finch, G. Chimpanzee handedness. Science, 1941, 94, 117-118.

Fincher, J. Sinister people. New York: Putnam, 1977.

Fink, W. H. The dominant eye: its clinical significance. Archives of Ophthalmology, 1938, 4, 555-582.

Flechsig, P. Anatomie des menschlichen gehirns und ruckenmarks auf myelognetischer grundlage. Leipzig: Georg Thiem, 1920.

Fleishman, E. A. On the relation between abilities, learning, and human performance. American Psychologist, 1972, 27, 1017-1032.

Fleishman, E. A., & Ellison, G. D. A factor analysis of five manipulative tests. Journal of Applied Psychology, 1962, 46, 96-105.

Fleishman, E. A., & Hempel, W. E., Jr. A factor analysis of dexterity tests. Personnel Psychology, 1954, 7, 15-32.

Fleminger, J. J., Dalton, R., & Standage, K. F. Age as a factor in the handedness of adults. Neuropsychologia, 1977, 15, 471-473.

Flick, G. Sinistrality revisited: a perceptual-motor approach. Child Development, 1966, 37, 613-622.

Flor-Henry, P. Psychosis and temporal lobe epilepsy. Epilepsia, 1969, 10, 363-395.

Flor-Henry, P. Lateralized temporal-limbic disfunction and psychopathology. Annals of the New York Academy of Science, 1976, 280, 777-797.

Flowers, K. Handedness and controlled movement. British Journal of Psychology, 1975, 66, 39-52.

Foley, J. E., & Held, R. Visually directed pointing as a function of target distance, direction and available cues. Perception and Psychophysics, 1972, 12, 263-268.

Forness, S. R., & Weil, M. C. Laterality in retarded readers with brain dysfunction. Exceptional Children, 1970, 36, 684-695.

Freeman, G. L., & Chapman, J. S. Minor studies from the psychological laboratory of Northwestern University. American Journal of Psychology, 1935, 47, 146-151.

Fridenberg, P. Binocular single vision and hypothesis of the dominant eye. Ophthalmology, 1904, 1, 196-212.

Friedlander, W. J. Some aspects of eyedness. Cortex, 1971, 7, 357-371.

Fritsch, B. Left and Right in Science and Life. London: Barrie and Rockliff, 1968.

Fromkin, V. A., Krashen, S., Curtiss, S., Rigler, D., & Rigler, M. The development of language in Genie: a case of language acquisition beyond the critical period. Brain and Language, 1974, 1, 81-108.

Gahagan, L. Visual dominance-acuity relationships. Journal of General Psychology, 1933, 9, 455-459.

Gainotti, G. Emotional behavior and hemispheric side of the lesion. Cortex, 1972, 8, 41-55.

Galaburda, A. M., LeMay, M., Kemper, T. L., & Geschwind, N. Right-left asymmetries in the brain. Science, 1978, 199, 852-856.

Galin, D. Implications for psychiatry of left and right cerebral specialization: a neurophysiological context for unconscious processes. Archives of General Psychiatry, 1974, 31, 572-583.

Gardner, M. The Ambidextrous Universe. London: Allen Lane, Penguin Press, 1964.

Gasparrine, M. A., Satz, P., & Heilman, K. N. Hemispheric asymmetries of affective processing as determined by the MMPI. Journal of Neurological and Neurosurgical Psychiatry, 1978, 41, 470-473.

Gautrin, D., & Ettlinger, G. Lateral preferences in the monkey. Cortex, 1970, 6, 287-292.

Geldard, F. A., & Crockett, W. B. The binocular-acuity relation as a function of age. Journal of Genetic Psychology, 1930, 37, 139-145.

Geschwind, N. The anatomical basis of hemispheric differentiation. In S. J. Dimond & J. G. Beaumont (Eds.), Hemisphere Function in the Human Brain. London: Elek Science, 1974.

Geschwind, N., & Levitsky, W. Human brain: left-right asymmetries in temporal speech region. Science, 1968, 161, 186-187.

Gesell, A., & Ames, L. B. The development of handedness, Journal of Genetic Psychology, 1947, 70, 155-175.

Giannitrapani, D. Laterality preference, electrophysiology and the brain. Electromyography and Clinical Neurophysiology, 1979, 19, 105-123.

Giesecke, M. The genesis of hand preference. Monographs of the Society for Research in Child Development, 1936, 1, No. 5.

Gilbert, C. Strength of left-handedness and facial recognition ability. Cortex, 1973, 9, 145-151.

Gilkey, B. G., & Parr, F. W. Analysis of the reversal tendency of fifty selected elementary school pupils. Journal of Educational Psychology, 1944, 35, 284-292.

Gloning, I., Gloning, K., Haub, G., & Quatember, R. Comparison of verbal behavior in right-handed and non-right-handed patients with anatomically verified lesion of one hemisphere. Cortex, 1969, 5, 43-52.

Goldstein, K. The Organism: A Holistic Approach to Biology, Derived from Pathological Data in Man. New York: American Book, 1939.

Gooddy, W., & Reinhold, M. Congenital dyslexia and asymmetry of cerebral function. Brain, 1961, 84, 231-242.

Goodglass, H., & Quadfasal, F. A. Language laterality in left-handed aphasics. Brain, 1954, 77, 521-548.

Gordon, H. Left handedness and mirror writing, especially among defective children. Brain, 1921, 43, 313-368.

Gould, G. M. Right Handedness and Left Handedness with Chapters Treating of the Writing Posture. The Rule of the Road, etc. Philadelphia and London: J. P. Lippincott, 1908.

Granet, M. Right and left in china. In R. Needham (Ed.), Right and Left. Chicago: University of Chicago Press, 1973.

Granjon-Galifret, N., & de Ajuriaguerra, J. Troubles de l'apprentissage de la lecture et dominance latérale. Encéphale, 1951, 40, 385-398.

Gronwall, D. M., & Sampson, H. Ocular dominance: a test of two hypotheses. British Journal of Psychology, 1971, 62, 175-185.

Gross, C. G., & Bornstein, M. H. Left and right in science and art. Leonardo, 1977, 11, 29-38.

Groves, C. P., & Humphrey, N. K. Asymmetry in gorilla skulls: evidence of lateralized brain function? Nature, 1973, 244, 53-54.

Gruen, G. E., & Vore, D. A. Development of conservation in normal and retarded children. Developmental Psychology, 1972, 6, 146-157.

Guilford, J. P. Psychometric Methods. New York: McGraw-Hill, 1954.

Gulick, W. L., & Lawson, R. B. Human Stereopsis: a Psychophysical Approach. New York and London: Oxford University Press, 1976.

Hakstian, A. R., & Cattell, R. B. The checking of primary ability structure on a broader basis of performance. British Journal of Educational Psychology, 1974, 44, 140-154.

Hakstian, A. R., & Cattell, R. B. Manual for the Comprehensive Ability Battery (CAB). Champaign, Ill.: Institute for Personality and Ability Testing, 1976.

Halgren, B. Specific dyslexia ("congenital word blindness"): a clinical and genetic study. Acta Psychiatrica et Neurologica (Suppl. 65). Copenhagan: Munsgaard, 1950.

Hall, G. S. Notes on the study of infants. Pedagogical Seminary, 1891, 1, 127-138.

Hall, K. R. L., & Mayer, B. Hand preferences of captive patas monkeys. Folia Primatologica, 1966, 4, 169-185.

Halstead, W. C., Walker, A. E., & Bucy, P. C. Sparing and nonsparing of "macular vision" associated with lobectomy in man. Archives of Ophthalmology, 1940, 24, 948.

Hamburger, F. A. Monocular dominance in binocular vision. Monatsblatter für Augenheilkunde, 1943, 109, 1.

Hardyck, C., Goldman, R., & Petrinovich, L. Handedness and sex, race, and age. Human Biology, 1975, 47, 369-375.

Hardyck, C., Petrinovich, L., & Goldman, R. Left-handedness and cognitive deficit. Cortex, 1976, 12, 266-279.

Hare, R. D. Psychopathy and laterality of cerebral function. Journal of Abnormal Psychology, 1979, 88, 605-610.

Hare, R. D. A research scale for the assessment of psychopathy in criminal populations. Personality and Individual Differences, 1980, 1, 111-119.

Harman, D. W., & Ray, W. J. Hemispheric activity during affective verbal stimuli: an EEG study. Neuropsychologia, 1977, 15, 457-460.

Harris, A. J. Lateral dominance, directional confusion, and reading disability. Journal of Psychology, 1957, 44, 283-294.

Harris, L. J. Sex and handedness differences in well educated adults' self-descriptions of left-right confusability. Archives of Neurology, 1978, 35, 773.

Harris, L. J. Left handedness: early theories, facts, and fancies. In J. Herron (Ed.), Neuropsychology of Left-Handedness. New York: Academic Press, 1980, pp. 3-78.

Harris, L. J., & Gitterman, S. R. University professors self-description of left-right confusability: sex and handedness differences. Perceptual and Motor Skills, 1978, 47, 819-823.

Harshman, R. A., & Remington, R. Sex, language and the brain, Part one: a review of the literature on adult sex differences in lateralization. Unpublished manuscript, 1975.

Harvey, L. O. Single representation of the visual midline in humans. Neuropsychologia, 1978, 16, 601-610.

Hatta, T., & Nakatsuka, Z. Note on hand preference in Japanese people. Perceptual and Motor Skills, 1975, 42, 530.

Hayashi, T., & Bryden, M. P. Ocular dominance and perceptual asymmetry. Perceptual and Motor Skills, 1957, 25, 605-612.

Hecaen, H., & Albert, M. L. Human Neuropsychology. New York: Wiley, 1978.

Hecaen, H., & de Ajuriaguerra, J. Left Handedness: Manual Superiority and Cerebral Dominance. New York: Grune & Stratton, 1964.

Hecaen, H., & Piercy, M. Paroxysmal dysphasia and the problems of cerebral dominance. Journal of Neurology, Neurosurgery and Psychiatry, 1956, 19, 194-201.

Hecaen, H., & Sauget, J. Cerebral dominance in left-handed subjects. Cortex, 1971, 7, 19-48.

Hecht, S. Rods, cones and the chemical basis of vision. Psychological Review, 1937, 17, 239-290.

Heckenmueller, E. G. Stabilization of the retinal image: a review of method, effects and theory. In R. N. Haber (Ed.), Contemporary Theory and Research in Visual Perception. New York: Holt, Rinehart and Winston, 1965, pp. 280-294.

Heim, A. W., & Watts, K. P. Handedness and cognitive bias. Quarterly Journal of Experimental Psychology, 1976, 28, 355-360.

Heinlein, J. H. A study of dexterity in children. Journal of Genetic Psychology, 1929, 36, 91-117.

Hellebrandt, F. A., & Houtz, S. J. Ergographic study of hand dominance. American Journal of Physical Anthropology, 1950, 8, 225-236.

Helmholtz, H. E. S. von. Handbuch der Physiologischen Optik. Dritte Auflage. Hamborg: Leopold Voss, 1909, 1910, 1911. English translation, J. P. C. Southall (Ed.). The Optical Society of America, 1924; reissued by Dover, New York, 1962.

Helveston, E. M., Billips, W. C., & Weber, J. C. Controlling eye-dominant hemisphere relationship as a factor in reading ability. American Journal of Ophthalmology, 1970, 70, 96-100.

Herrmann, D. J., & Van Dyke, K. A. Handedness and the mental rotation of perceived patterns. Cortex, 1978, 14, 521-529.

Herron, J. Two hands, two brains, two sexes. In J. Herron (Ed.), Neuropsychology of Left-Handedness. New York: Academic Press, 1980, pp. 233-262.

Hertz, R. A study in religious polarity. In R. Needham (Ed.), Right and Left. Chicago: University of Chicago Press, 1973, pp. 3-31.

Hicks, R. A., & Beveridge, R. Handedness and intelligence. Cortex, 1978, 14, 304-307.

Hicks, R. A., Evans, E. A., & Pellegrini, R. J. Correlation between handedness and birth order: compilation of five studies. Perceptual and Motor Skills, 1978, 46, 53-54.

Hicks, R. A., Pellegrini, R. J., & Evans, E. Handedness and birth risk. Neuropsychologia, 1978, 16, 243-245.

Hicks, R. A., Pellegrini, R. J., Evans, E. A., & Moore, J. D. Birth risk and left handedness reconsidered. Archives of Neurology, 1979, 36, 119-120.

Hicks, R. E., & Barton, K. A note on left-handedness and severity of mental retardation: replications and refinements. Journal of Genetic Psychology, 1975, 127, 323-324.

Hicks, R. E., & Kinsbourne, M. Human handedness: a partial cross-fostering study. Science, 1976, 192, 908-910.

Hildreth, G. The development and training of hand dominance, I-II. Journal of Genetic Psychology, 1949, 75, 197-275.

Hildreth, G. Development and training of hand dominance, IV-V. Journal of Genetic Psychology, 1950, 75, 39-144.

Hillerich, R. L. Eye-hand dominance and reading achievement. American Educational Research Journal, 1964, 1, 121-126.

Hochberg, F. H., & Le May, M. Arteriographic correlates of handedness. Neurology, 1975, 25, 218-222.

Horn, J. L. Human abilities: a review of research and theory in the early 1970's. In M. R. Rosenzwieg & L. W. Porter (Eds.), Annual Review of Psychology (Vol. 2). Palo Alto, Calif.: Annual Reviews, Inc., 1976.

Howard, I. P., & Templeton, W. B. Human Spatial Orientation. New York: Wiley, 1966.

Hubbard, J. I. Handedness not a function of birth order. Nature, 1971, 232, 276-277.

Hubel, D. H., & Wiesel, T. N. Receptive fields of single neurons in the cat's striate cortex. Journal of Physiology, 1959, 148, 574-591.

Hubel, D. H., & Wiesel, T. N. Receptive fields, binocular interaction and functional architecture in the cat's visual cortex. Journal of Physiology, 1962, 160, 106-154.

Huber, J. B. Why are we right handed? Scientific American, 1910, 102, 260-261; 268-269.

Hudson, P. T. W. The genetics of handedness—a reply to Levy and Nagylaki. Neuropsychologia, 1975, 13, 331-339.

Hughes, H. An investigation into ocular dominancy. British Journal of Physiological Optics, 1953, 3, 119-143.

Huheey, J. E. Concerning the origin of handedness in humans. Behavior Genetics, 1977, 7, 29-32.

Hull, C. J. A study of laterality test items. Journal of Experimental Education, 1936, 4, 287-290.

Humphrey, M. E. Consistency of hand usage. British Journal of Educational Psychology, 1951, 21, 214-225.

Hyrdl, J. Handbuch der topographischen Anatomie (4th ed.). Vienna: Brau-mueller, 1860.

Imus, H. A., Rothney, J. W. M., & Bear, R. M. An Evaluation of Visual Factors in Reading. Hanover, N.H.: Dartmouth College, 1938.

Ingram, D. Motor asymmetries in young children. Neuropsychologia, 1975, **13**, 95-102.

Ingram, T. T. S., & Reid, J. F. Developmental aphasia observed in a department of child psychiatry. Archives of Disabled Children, 1956, **31**, 161-172.

Jackson, J. Ambidexterity or Two-handedness and Two-brainedness. London: Kegan Paul, Trench, Trubner and Co., 1905.

James, W. E., Mefferd, R. B., & Wieland, B. A. Repetitive psychometric measures: handedness and performance. Perceptual and Motor Skills, 1967, **25**, 209-212.

Jasper, H. H., & Raney, E. T. The phi test of lateral dominance. American Journal of Psychology, 1937, **49**, 450-457.

Johnstone, J., Galin, D., & Herron, J. Choice of handedness measures in studies of hemispheric specialization. International Journal of Neuroscience, 1979, **9**, 71-80.

Jones, H. F. Dextrality as a function of age. Journal of Experimental Psychology, 1931, **14**, 125-144.

Jones, W. F. The problem of handedness in education. Journal of Proceedings and Addresses of the National Educational Association, 1915, **53**, 959-963.

Jordan, H. E. The inheritance of left-handedness. American Breeder's Magazine, 1911, **2**, 19-28; 113-124.

Jordan, H. E. Hereditary left handedness with a note on twinning. Journal of Genetics, 1914, **4**, 67-81.

Jordan, H. E. The crime against left-handedness. Good Health, 1922, **57**, 378-383.

Jowett, B. (trans.) The Dialogues of Plato (4th ed., Vol. 4). New York and London: Oxford University Press, 1953.

Judd, C. H. The Mueller-Lyer illusion. Psychological Review Monograph Supplement, 1905, No. 29, 55-82.

Julesz, B. Foundations of Cyclopean Perception. Chicago, Ill.: University of Chicago Press, 1971.

Kaes, T. Die grossnirnrinde des menschen. Ein gehir Anatomischer Atlas. Jena Verlag von Gustov Fischer, 1907.

Kamai, M. Catching behavior observed in the Koshima troop—a case of newly acquired behavior. Primates, 1967, **8**, 181-188.

Keller, J. F., Croake, J. W., & Riesenman, E. Relationships among handedness intelligence, sex, and reading achievement of school age children. Perceptual and Motor Skills, 1973, **37**, 159-162.

Keller, M. Ocular dominance and the range of visual apprehension. Journal of Experimental Psychology, 1937, **21**, 545-553.

Kephart, N. C., & Revesman, S. Measuring differences in speed performance. Optometric Weekly, 1953, **44**, 1965-1967.

Kershner, J. R., & Jeng, A. G. Dual functional hemispheric asymmetry in visual perception: effects of ocular dominance and postexposural processes. Neuropsychologia, 1972, **10**, 437-445.

Kertesz, A., & Geschwind, N. Patterns of pyramidal decussation and the relationship to handedness. Archives of Neurology, 1971, **24**, 326-332.

Kidd, D. Savage Childhood. London, 1906, p. 296.

Kimble, G. A. Transfer of work inhibition in motor learning. Journal of Experimental Psychology, 1952, **43**, 391-392.

Kimura, D. Cerebral dominance and perception of visual stimuli. Canadian Journal of Psychology, 1961, **15**, 166-171.

Kimura, D. The neural basis of language qua gesture. In W. Haiganoosh & H. A. Whitaker (Eds.), Studies in Neurolinguistics (Vol. 2). New York: Academic Press, 1976, pp. 145-156.

Kobyliansky, E., Micle, S., & Arensburg, B. Handedness, hand-clasping and arm-folding in Israeli maks. Annals of Human Biology, 1978, **5**, 247-251.

Koch, H. L. A study of the nature, measurement, and determination of hand preference. Genetic Psychology Monographs, 1933, **13**, 117-221.

Komai, T., & Fukuoka, G. A study on the frequency of left-handedness and left-footedness among Japanese school children. Human Biology, 1934, **6**, 33-41.

Koos, E. M. Manifestations of cerebral dominance and reading retardation in primary grade children. Journal of Genetic Psychology, 1964, **104**, 155-166.

Kovac, D., & Horkovic, G. How to measure lateral preference, I. Studia Psychologica, 1970, **12**, 5-11.

Kovac, D., & Ley, I. Visual differentiation and lateral preference. Studia Psychologica, 1969, **11**, 237-239.

Krashen, S. D. Cerebral asymmetry. In W. Haiganoosh & H. A. Whitaker (Eds.), Studies in Neurolinguistics (Vol. 2). New York: Academic Press, 1976, pp. 157-191.

Krauskopf, J., & Riggs, L. A. Interocular transfer in the disappearance of stabilized images. American Journal of Psychology, 1959, **72**, 248-252.

Kruper, D. C., Boyle, B., & Patton, R. A. Eye preference in hemicerebectomized monkeys. Psychonomic Science, 1967, **7**, 105-106.

Kruper, D. C., Patton, R. A., & Koskoff, Y. D. Hand and eye preference in unilaterally brain ablated monkeys. Physiology and Behavior, 1971, **7**, 184-185.

Kucera, O., Matejcek, Z., & Langmier, J. Some observations on dyslexia in children in Czechoslovakia. American Journal of Orthopsychiatry, 1963, **33**, 448-456.

Lack, L. C. Amplitude of visual suppression during the control of binocular rivalry. Perception and Psychophysics, 1973, **13**, 374-378.

LaGrone, C. W., & Holland, B. F. Accuracy of perception in peripheral vision in relation to dextrality, intelligence and reading ability. American Journal of Psychology, 1943, **56**, 592-598.

Lake, D. A., & Bryden, M. P. Handedness and sex differences in hemispheric asymmetries. Brain and Language, 1976, **3**, 266-282.

250 References

Landers, D. M. Moving competitive shooting into the scientist's lab. American Rifleman, April, 1980, **128**, 36-38.

Lansdell, H. The effect of neurosurgery on a test of proverbs. American Psychologist, 1961, **16**, 448.

Landsdell, H. A sex difference in effect of temporal-lobe neurosurgery on design preference. Nature, 1962, **194**, 852-854.

Lansdell, H. The use of factor scores from the Wechsler-Bellevue Scale of Intelligence in assessing patients with temporal lobe removals. Cortex, 1968, **4**, 257-268.

Lansdell, H. Effect of neurosurgery on the ability to identify popular word associations. Journal of Abnormal Psychology, 1973, **81**, 255-258.

Lansdell, H., & Davie, J. C. Mass intermedia: possible relation to intelligence. Neuropsychologia, 1972, **10**, 207-210.

Lattes, L. Destrismo e mancinismo in relazione colle asimmetrie funzionali del cervello. Archivo di Psichiatria, Neuropatalogia, Antropologia criminale e medicina legale, 1907, **28**, 281-303.

Lauterbach, C. E. Studies in twin resemblance. Genetics, 1925, **10**, 525-568.

Lavery, F. S. Ocular dominance. Transactions of the Ophthalmological Society of the United Kingdom, 1943, **63**, 409-435.

Lebensohn, J. E. Ocular dominance and marksmanship. U.S. Navy Medical Bulletin, 1942, **40**, 590-594.

Lederer, J. Ocular dominance. Australian Journal of Optometry, 1961, **44**, 531-574.

Lehman, R. A. Hand preference and cerebral dominance in 24 rhesus monkeys. Journal of Neurological Science, 1970, **10**, 185-192.

Le May, M. Asymmetries of the skull and handedness. Journal of the Neurological Sciences, 1977, **32**, 243-253.

Le May, M., & Culebras, A. Human brain morphologic differences in the hemispheres demonstrable by carotid arteriography. New England Journal of Medicine, 1972, **287**, 168-170.

Le May, M., & Geschwind, N. Hemispheric differences in the brains of great apes. Brain Behavior and Evolution, 1975, **11**, 48-52.

Leonard, A. G. The Lower Niger and Its Tribes. New York: Macmillan, 1906.

Lepori, N. G. Sur le genèse des structures asymétriques chez l'embryon des oiseaux. Monitore Zoologico Italiano, 1969, **3**, 33-53.

Le Roux, A. Sex differences and the incidence of left-handedness. Journal of Psychology, 1979, **102**, 261-262.

Lesinski, J. High risk pregnancy: unresolved problems of screening, management and prognosis. Obstetrics and Gynecology, 1975, **46**, 599-603.

Leviton, A., & Kilty, T. Birth order and left-handedness. Archives of Neurology, 1976, **33**, 664.

Leviton, A., & Kilty, T. Seasonal variation in the births of left-handed schoolgirls. Archives of Neurology, 1979, **36**, 115-116.

Leviton, M., & Montagu, A. Textbook of Human Genetics. New York and London: Oxford University Press, 1971.

Levy, J. Possible basis for the evolution of lateral specialization of the human brain. Nature, 1969, 224, 614-615.

Levy, J. Lateral specialization of the human brain. Behavioral manifestation and possible evolutionary bias. In J. Kiger (Ed.), The Biology of Behavior. Corvallis: Oregon State University Press, 1973.

Levy, J. Psychobiological implications of bilateral asymmetry. In S. J. Dimond & J. Beaumont (Eds.), Hemispheric Function in the Human Brain. London: Elek Science, 1974, pp. 212-283.

Levy, J. A review of evidence for a genetic component in the determination of handedness. Behavior Genetics, 1976, 6, 429-453.

Levy, J. A reply to Hudson regarding the Levy-Nagylaki model for the genetics of handedness. Neuropsychologia, 1977, 15, 187-190.

Levy, J., & Gur, R. C. Individual differences in psychoneurological organization. In J. Herron (Ed.), Neuropsychology of Left-Handedness. New York: Academic Press, 1980, pp. 199-210.

Levy, J., & Levy, J. M. Human lateralization from head to foot: sex-related factors. Science, 1978, 200, 1291-1292.

Levy, J., & Nagylaki, T. A model for the genetics of handedness. Genetics, 1972, 72, 117-128.

Levy, J., & Reid, M. Variations in writing posture and cerebral organization. Science, 1976, 194, 337-339.

Levy, J., & Reid, M. Variations in cerebral organization as a function of handedness, hand posture in writing, and sex. Journal of Experimental Psychology: General, 1978, 107, 119-144.

Liederman, J., & Kinsbourne, M. Rightward motor bias in newborns depends upon parental right-handedness. Neuropsychologia, 1980, 18, 579-584.

Lindsley, D. B. A longitudinal study of the occipital alpha rhythm in normal children: frequency and amplitude standards. Journal of Genetic Psychology, 1939, 55, 197-213.

Lipman, R. S. Children's manifest anxiety in retardates and approximately equal M.A. normals. American Journal of Mental Deficiency, 1960, 64, 1027-1028.

Lombroso, C. The Man of Genius. London: Walter Scott Co., 1891.

Lombroso, C. Left-sidedness. North American Review, 1903, 170, 440-444.

Lueddeckens, R. Rechts und Linkshandigkett. Leipzig, 1900.

Lund, F. H. Physical asymmetries and disorientation. American Journal of Psychology, 1930, 42, 51-62.

Lund, F. The dependence of eye-hand coordinations upon eye-dominance. American Journal of Psychology, 1932, 44, 756-762.

Luria, S. M. Swimming, accuracy and consistency of scuba divers under conditions of low visibility. Aviation, Space and Environmental Medicine, 1979, 233-238.

Macmeeken, A. M. Ocular dominance in relation to developmental aphasia. London: University of London Press, 1939.

Maddess, R. J. Bilateral tachistoscopic presentation of letters and line orientation in bisected visual fields at three visual angles. Unpublished doctoral dissertation, University of Victoria, 1975. (a)

Maddess, R. J. Reaction time to hemiretinal stimulation. Neuropsychologia, 1975, **13**, 213-218. (b)

Marcel, T., Katz, L., & Smith, M. Laterality in reading proficiency. Neuropsychologia, 1974, **12**, 131-139.

Margoshes, A., & Collins, G. Right-handedness as a function of maternal heartbeat. Perceptual and Motor Skills, 1965, **20**, 443-444.

Marlowe, W. B. Hemisphere laterality effects for trigram reproduction and face recognition in dextrals and two groups of sinistrals. Unpublished doctoral dissertation, University of Victoria, 1977.

Matsunaga, E. Effect of changing parental age patterns on the chromosomal aberrations and mutations. Social Biology, 1973, **20**, 82-88.

McClearn, G. E., & DeFries, J. C. Introduction to Behavioral Genetics. San Francisco: W. H. Freeman and Company, 1973.

McCullough, C. The Thornbirds. New York: Harper & Row, 1977.

McGee, M. G. Laterality, hand preference, and human spatial ability. Perceptual and Motor Skills, 1976, **42**, 781-782.

McGee, M. G. Handedness and mental rotation. Perceptual and Motor Skills, 1978, **47**, 641.

McGee, M. G. Human spatial abilities: Psychometric studies and environmental, genetic, hormonal and neurological influences. Psychological Bulletin, 1979, **86**, 889-918.

McGee, M. G., & Cozad, T. Population genetic analysis of human hand preference: evidence for generation differences, familial resemblance, and maternal effects. Behavior Genetics, 1980, **10**, 263-276.

McGlone, J., & Kertesz, A. Sex differences in cerebral processing of visuospatial tasks. Cortex, 1973, **9**, 313-320.

McKeever, W. F. Handwriting posture in left-handers: sex, familial sinistrality and language laterality correlates. Neuropsychologia, 1979, **17**, 429-444.

McKeever, W. F., & Hoff, A. L. Evidence of a possible isolation of left hemisphere visual and motor areas in sinistrals employing an inverted handwriting posture. Neuropsychologia, 1979, **17**, 445-455.

McKeever, W. F., & Van Deventer, A. D. Familial sinistrality and degree of left-handedness. British Journal of Psychology, 1977, **68**, 469-471.

McKeever, W. F., & Van Deventer, A. D. Inverted handwriting position, language laterality, and the Levy-Nagylaki genetic model of handedness and cerebral organization. Neuropsychologia, 1980, **18**, 99-102.

McKinney, J. P. Handedness, eyedness and perceptual stability of the left and right visual field. Neuropsychologia, 1967, **5**, 339-344.

McManus, I. C. Scrotal asymmetry in man and in ancient sculpture. Nature, 1976, **259**, 426.

McManus, I. C. Handedness in twins: A critical review. Neuropsychologia, 1980, **18**, 347-355.

McMeekan, E. R. L., & Lishman, W. A. Re-test reliabilities and interrelationship of the Annett Hand Preference Questionnaire. British Journal of Psychology, 1975, **66**, 53-59.

McRae, D. L., Branch, C. L., & Milner, B. The occipital horns and cerebral dominance. Neurology, 1968, 18, 95-98.

Merrell, D. J. Dominance of eye and hand. Human Biology, 1957, 29, 314-328.

Miles, W. R. Ocular dominance demonstrated by unconscious sighting. Journal of Experimental Psychology, 1929, 12, 113-126.

Miles, W. R. Ocular dominance in human adults. Journal of General Psychology, 1930, 3, 412-420.

Miller, E. Handedness and the pattern of human ability. British Journal of Psychology, 1971, 62, 111-112.

Miller, M. B. A group visual exploratory technique. Perceptual and Motor Skills, 1971, 33, 51-54.

Mills, L. Eyedness and handedness. American Journal of Ophthalmology, 1925, 8, 933-941.

Mills, L. Unilateral sighting. California and West Medicine, 1928, 28, 189-195.

Milne, A. A. The House at Pooh Corner. Toronto: McClelland & Stewart, 1926.

Milner, B. Hemispheric specialization: scope and limits. In F. O. Schmitt and F. G. Worden (Eds.), The Neurosciences: Third Study Program. Cambridge, Mass.: MIT Press, 1974, pp. 75-89.

Milner, B., Branch, C., & Rasmussen, T. Observations on cerebral dominance. In A. V. S. Dee Rueck & M. O'Conner (Eds.), Ciba Foundation Symposium on Disorders of Language. London: Churchill, 1964.

Milstein, V., Small, I. F., Malloy, F. W., & Small, J. G. Influence of sex and handedness on hemispheric functioning. Cortex, 1979, 15, 439-449.

Mintz, A. Lateral preferences of a group of mentally subnormal boys. Journal of Genetic Psychology, 1947, 71, 75-84.

Mittwoch, U. Lateral asymmetry and function of the mammalian Y chromosome. In K. Jones and P. E. Brandham (Eds.), Current Chromosomes Research. Amsterdam: North-Holland, 1976.

Monroe, M. Children Who Cannot Read. Chicago: University of Chicago Press, 1932.

Montagu, A. Prenatal Influences. Springfield, Ill.: Charles C Thomas, 1962.

Moore, K. L. The Developing Human. Philadelphia: Saunders, 1973.

Moorhead, T. G. The relative weights of the right and left sides of the body in the foetus. Journal of Anatomy and Physiology, 1902, 36, 400-404.

Morgan, M. Embryology and the inheritance of asymmetry. In S. Harnad, R. W. Doty, L. Goldstein, J. Jaynes, & G. Krauthamer (Eds.), Lateralization in the Nervous System. New York: Academic Press, 1977, pp. 173-194.

Morgan, M. J., & Corballis, M. C. Scrotal asymmetry and Rodin's dyslexia. Nature, 1976, 264, 295-296.

Morgan, M. J., & Corballis, M. C. On the biological basis of human laterality, II: The mechanisms of inheritance. The Behavioral and Brain Sciences, 1978, 2, 270-277.

Moscovitch, M. The development of lateralization of language functions and its relation to cognitive and linguistic development: A review and some theoretical speculations. In S. J. Segalowitz & F. A. Gruber (Eds.), Language Development and Neurological Theory. New York: Academic Press, 1977, pp. 194-212.

Nagamata, H. Study on ocular dominance, Pt. 3. Acta Society of Ophthalmology Japan, 1951, **55**, 314-318.

Nagylaki, T., & Levy, J. "The sound of one paw clapping" isn't sound. Behavior Genetics, 1973, **3**, 379-392.

Naidoo, S. An investigation into some aspects of ambiguous handedness. Unpublished master's thesis, University of London, 1961.

Nakamura, R., & Saito, H. Preferred hand and reaction time in different movement patterns. Perceptual and Motor Skills, 1974, **39**, 1275-1286.

Nakamura, R., Taniguchi, R., & Oshima, Y. Synchronization error in bilateral simultaneous flexion of elbows. Perceptual and Motor Skills, 1975, **42**, 527-532.

Nebes, R. D. Handedness and the perception of part-whole relationship. Cortex, 1971, **7**, 350-356. (a)

Nebes, R. D. Superiority of the minor hemisphere in commissurotomized man for the perception of part-whole relations. Cortex, 1971, **7**, 333-349. (b)

Nebes, R. D., & Briggs, G. C. Handedness and the retention of visual material. Cortex, 1974, **10**, 209-214.

Needham, R. The left hand of the Mugwe: an analytical note on the structure of Meru symbolism. In R. Needham (Ed.), Right and Left. Chicago, Ill.: University of Chicago Press, 1973, pp. 109-127.

Nelson, J. I. Globality and stereoscopic fusion in binocular vision. Journal of Theoretical Biology, 1975, **49**, 1-88.

Newcombe, F., & Ratcliff, G. Handedness, speech lateralization and ability. Neuropsychologia, 1971, **9**, 97-113.

Newland, J. Children's knowledge of left and right. Unpublished master's thesis, University of Auckland, 1972.

Newman, H. H. Asymmetry reversal or mirror imaging in identical twins. Biological Bulletin, 1928, **55**, 298-315.

Newman, H. H., Freeman, F. N., & Holzinger, K. J. Twins: A Study of Heredity and Environment. Chicago, Ill.: University of Chicago Press, 1937.

Nottebohm, F. Neurolateralization of vocal control in a passerine bird, I: Song. Journal of Experimental Zoology, 1971, **177**, 229-262.

Nottebohm, F. Neurolateralization of vocal control in a passerine bird, II: Subsong, calls and a theory of vocal learning. Journal of Experimental Zoology, 1972, **179**, 25-50.

Oddy, H. C., & Lobstein, T. J. Hand and eye dominance in schizophrenia, British Journal of Psychiatry, 1972, **120**, 331-332.

Ogle, K. N. Researches in Binocular Vision. New York: Hafner, 1964.

Ogle, S. W. On dextral pre-eminence. Transactions of the Royal Medical and Chirurgical Society, 1871, **35**, 279-301.

Ojemann, R. H. Technic for testing unimanual handedness. Journal of Educational Psychology, 1930, **21**, 597-611.

Oldfield, R. C. The assessment and analysis of handedness: the Edinburgh inventory. Neuropsychologia, 1971, **9**, 97-113.

Ondercin, P., Perry, N. W., & Childers, D. G. Distribution of ocular dominance and effect of image clarity. Perception and Psychophysics, 1973, **13**, 5-8.

Ong, J., & Rodman, T. Sex and eye-hand preferential difference in star-tracing performance. American Journal of Optometry and Archives of the American Academy of Optometry, 1972, **49**, 436-438.

Orme, J. E. Left-handedness, ability and emotional instability. British Journal of Social and Clinical Psychology, 1970, **9**, 87-88.

Orton, S. T. "Word-blindness" in school children. Archives of Neurology and Psychiatry, 1925, **14**, 581-615.

Orton, S. T. Specific reading disability-strephosymbolia. Journal of the American Medical Association, 1928, **90**, 1095-1099.

Orton, S. T. A physiological theory of reading disability and stuttering in children. New England Journal of Medicine, 1929, **199**, 1046-1052.

Orton, S. T. Reading, Writing and Speech Problems in Children. New York: Norton, 1937.

Page, M. M. Modification of figure-ground perception as a function of awareness of demand characteristics. Journal of Personality and Social Psychology, 1968, **9**, 59.

Palmer, M. F. Studies in clinical techniques. Journal of Speech Disorders, 1947, **12**, 415-418.

Parsons, B. S. Left-handedness. New York: Macmillan, 1924.

Pascal, J. I. The chromatic test for the dominant eye. American Journal of Ophthalmology, 1926, **9**, 357-358.

Pasteur, L. Proceedings of the Academie des Sciences, 1874.

Payne, B. B., Elberger, A. J., Berman, N., & Murphy, E. H. Binocularity in the cat visual cortex is reduced by sectioning the corpus collosum. Science, 1980, **207**, 1097-1099.

Pelecanos, M. Some Greek data on handedness, hand clasping and arm folding. Human Biology, 1969, **41**, 275-278.

Penfield, W., & Rasmussen, T. The Cerebral Cortex of Man: A Clinical Study. New York: Macmillan, 1950.

Penfield, W., & Roberts, L. Speech and Brain Mechanisms. Princeton: Princeton University Press, 1959.

Perry, N. W., & Childers, D. Monocular contribution to binocular vision in normals and amblyopes. In G. B. Arden (Ed.), The Visual System: Neurophysiology, Biophysics and Their Clinical Applications. New York: Plenum, 1972.

Peters, M., & Durding, B. M. Footedness of left- and right-handers. American Journal of Psychology, 1979, **92**, 133-142. (a)

Peters, M., & Durding, B. Left-handers and right-handers compared on a motor test. Journal of Motor Behavior, 1979, **11**, 103-111. (b)

Peters, M., & Pedersen, K. Incidence of left-handers with inverted writing position in a population of 5910 elementary school children. Neuropsychologia, 1978, **16**, 743-746.

Petersen, I., & Eeg-Olofsson, D. The development of the EEG in normal children from the age of 1 through 15 years: non-paroxysmal activity. Neuropadiatria, 1971, **3**, 277-304.

Peterson, J. M., & Lansky, L. M. Left-handedness among architects: some facts and speculation. Perceptual and Motor Skills, 1974, **38**, 547-550.

Peterson, J. M., & Lansky, L. M. Left-handedness among architects: partial replication and some new data. Perceptual and Motor Skills, 1977, **45**, 1216-1218.

Plomin, R., DeFries, J. C., & McClearn, G. E. Behavioral Genetics. San Francisco: W. H. Freeman, 1980.

Polednak, A. P. Paternal age in relation to selected birth defects. Human Biology, 1976, **48**, 727-739.

Polyak, S. The Vertebrate Visual System. Chicago, Ill.: University of Chicago Press, 1957.

Porac, C. Ocular dominance and suppressive processes in binocular vision (Doctoral dissertation, Graduate Faculty of the New School for Social Research, 1974). Dissertation Abstracts International, 1975, 35, 4229b. (University Microfilms No. 75-2323)

Porac, C., & Coren, S. Is eye dominance a part of generalized laterality? Perceptual and Motor Skills, 1975, **40**, 763-769. (a)

Porac, C., & Coren, S. Suppressive processes in binocular vision: ocular dominance and amblyopia. American Journal of Optometry and Physiological Optics, 1975, **52**, 651-657. (b)

Porac, C., & Coren, S. The dominant eye. Psychological Bulletin, 1976, **83**, 880-897.

Porac, C., & Coren, S. The assessment of motor control in sighting dominance using an illusion decrement procedure. Perception and Psychophysics, 1977, **21**, 341-346.

Porac, C., & Coren, S. Relationship between lateral preference behaviors in humans. The Behavioral and Brain Sciences, 1978, **2**, 311-312. (a)

Porac, C., & Coren, S. Sighting dominance and binocular rivalry. American Journal of Optometry and Physiological Optics, 1978, **55**, 208-213. (b)

Porac, C., & Coren, S. Individual and familial patterns in four dimensions of lateral preference. Neuropsychologia, 1979, **17**, 543-548. (a)

Porac, C., & Coren, S. Monocular asymmetries in recognition after an eye movement: sighting dominance and dextrality. Perception and Psychophysics, 1979, **25**, 55-59. (b)

Porac, C., & Coren, S. A test of the validity of offsprings' report of parental handedness. Perceptual and Motor Skills, 1979, **49**, 227-231. (c)

Porac, C., & Coren, S. Sighting dominance and the disappearance of stabilized retinal images. Paper presented at the meetings of the Canadian Psychological Association, Quebec City, Quebec, June 1979. (d)

Porac, C., Coren, S., & Duncan, P. Lateral preference in retardates: Relationships between hand, eye, foot and ear preference. Journal of Clinical Neuropsychology, 1980, **2**, 173-187. (a)

Porac, C., Coren, S., & Duncan, P. Life-span age trends in laterality. Journal of Gerontology, 1980, **35**, 715-721. (b)

Porac, C., Coren, S., Steiger, J. S., & Duncan, P. Human laterality: a multidimensional approach. Canadian Journal of Psychology, 1980, **34**, 91-96.

Porac, C., Whitford, F. W., & Coren, S. The relationship between eye dominance and monocular acuity: an additional consideration. American Journal of Optometry and Physiological Optics, 1976, 53, 803-806.

Porta, G. B. del. *De refractione.* Optics Parte: Libri Novem. Ex Officina Horatij Salvania. Naples: Apud Io Iacobum Carlinum and Anotinium Pacem, 1593.

Postman, L. Transfer interference and forgetting. In J. W. Kling & L. A. Riggs (Eds.), Experimental Psychology. New York: Holt, Rinehart, and Winston, 1971, pp. 1019-1132.

Pratt, R. T. C., & Warrington, E. K. The assessment of cerebral dominance with unilateral ECT. British Journal of Psychiatry, 1972, 121, 327-328.

Pringle, K. M. L., Butler, N. R., & Davie, R. 11,000 Seven-Year-Olds. London: Longmans, Green, 1966.

Provins, K. A. Handedness and motor skill. Medical Journal of Australia, 1967, 53, 468-470. (a)

Provins, K. A. Motor skills, handedness and behavior. Australian Journal of Psychology, 1967, 19, 137-150. (b)

Provins, K. A., & Cunliffe, P. Motor performance tests of handedness and motivation. Perceptual and Motor Skills, 1972, 35, 143-150.

Pyre-Smith, P. H. Left-handedness. Guy's Hospital Reports (3rd series), 1871, 16, 141-146.

Quinan, C. Sinistrality in relation to high blood pressure and defects of speech. Archives of Internal Medicine, 1921, 27, 255-261.

Raczkowski, D., Kalat, J. W., & Nebes, R. Reliability and validity of some handedness questionnaire items. Neuropsychologia, 1974, 12, 43-47.

Ramaley, F. Inheritance of left-handedness. American Naturalist, 1913, 47, 730-738.

Ramsay, D. S. Manual preferences for tapping in infants. Developmental Psychology, 1979, 15, 437-442.

Ramsay, D. S., Campos, J. J., & Fenson, L. Onset of bimanual handedness of infants. Infant Behavior and Development, 1979, 2, 69-76.

Rasmussen, T., & Milner, B. Clinical and surgical studies of the cerebral speech areas in man. In K. J. Zuelch, O. Creutzfeldt, & G. Galbraith (Eds.), Otfrid Foerster Symposium on Cerebral Localization. Heidelberg: Springer, 1976.

Reed, G. F., & Smith, A. C. Laterality and directional preferences in a simple perceptual-motor task. Quarterly Journal of Experimental Psychology, 1961, 13, 122-124.

Rengstorff, R. H. The types of incidence of hand-eye preference and its relationship with certain reading abilities. American Journal of Optometry and Archives of the American Academy of Optometry, 1967, 44, 233-235.

Reynolds, P. Handedness and the evolution of the primate forelimb. Neuropsychologia, 1975, 13, 499-500.

Rhoades, J. G., & Damon, A. Some genetic traits in Solomon Island populations, II: Hand clasping, arm folding and handedness. American Journal of Physical Anthropology, 1973, 39, 179-184.

Richardson, J. A factor analysis of self-reported handedness. Neuropsychologia, 1978, 16, 747-748.

Rife, D. C. Handedness of twins. Science, 1939, **89**, 178-179.

Rife, D. C. Handedness with special reference to twins. Genetics, 1940, **25**, 178-186.

Rife, D. C. An application of gene frequency analysis to the interpretation of data from twins. Human Biology, 1950, **22**, 736-745.

Riggs, L. A., Ratliff, F., Cornsweet, J. C., & Cornsweet, T. N. The disappearance of steadily fixated visual test objects. Journal of the Optical Society of America, 1953, **43**, 495-501.

Roberts, J., & Engle, A. Family Background, Early Development, and Intelligence of Children 6-11 Years (National Center for Health Statistics; data from the National Health Survey, Series 11, No. 142). DHEW Publication No. (HRA) 75-1624. Washington, D.C.: U.S. Government Printing Office, 1974.

Roberts, L. Handedness and cerebral dominance. Transactions of the American Neurological Association, 1955, **80**, 143-148.

Roberts, L. Aphasia, apraxia and agnosia in abnormal states of cerebral dominance. In P. J. Vinken and G. W. Bruyn (Eds.), Handbook of Clinical Neuropsychology (Vol. 4). Amsterdam: North-Holland, 1969.

Rock, I. Orientation and Form. New York: Academic Press, 1974.

Romer, A. S. The Vertebrate Body. Philadelphia: Saunders, 1962.

Roos, M. M. Variations with age in frequency distributions of degrees of handedness. Child Development, 1935, **6**, 259-268.

Roscoe, J. The Bakitara. London: Macmillan, 1923.

Rossi, G. F., & Rosadini, G. Experimental analysis of cerebral dominance in man. In C. H. Millikan and F. L. Darley (Eds.), Brain Mechanisms Underlying Speech and Language. New York: Grune & Stratton, 1967.

Rothe, H. Handedness in the common marmoset (Callithrix jacchus). American Journal of Physical Anthropology, 1973, **38**, 561-565.

Rothschild, F. S., & Streifler, M. On eyedness in homonymous hemianopia. Journal of Nervous and Mental Disease, 1952, **116**, 59-64.

Rudel, R. G., & Teuber, H. L. Discrimination of direction of line in children. Journal of Comparative and Physiological Psychology, 1963, **56**, 892-898.

Russell, R. W., & Espir, M. L. E. Traumatic Aphasia. New York and London: Oxford (Clarendon Press), 1961.

Sabatino, D., & Becker, J. Relationship between lateral preference and selected behavioral variables for children failing academically. Child Development, 1971, **42**, 2055-2060.

Sachs, B., & Peterson, F. A study of cerebral palsies of early life based upon an analysis of 140 cases. Journal of Neural and Mental Diseases, 1890, **17**, 395-433.

Salk, L. Mother's heartbeat as an imprinting stimulus. Transactions of the New York Academy of Sciences, 1962, **24**, 753-763.

Salk, L. The role of the heartbeat in the relations between mother and infant. Scientific American, 1973, **228**, 24-29.

Saltzman, L. C., Scarr-Salapatek, S., Barker, W. B., & Katz, S. Left-handedness in twins: incidence and patterns of performance in an adolescent sample. Behavior Genetics, 1976, **2**, 189-203.

Sampson, H., & Horrocks, J. B. Binocular rivalry and immediate memory. Quarterly Journal of Experimental Psychology, 1966, **18-19**, 224-231.

Sampson, H., & Spong, P. Binocular fixation and immediate memory. British Journal of Psychology, 1961, **52**, 239-248.

Sampson, H., & Spong, P. Handedness, eye-dominance, and immediate memory. Quarterly Journal of Experimental Psychology, 1962, **13**, 173-180.

Sanford, M. C., & Bair, H. L. Visual disturbance associated with tumors of the temporal lobe. Archives of Neurology and Psychiatry, 1939, **42**, 21.

Satz, P. Pathological left-handedness: an explanatory model. Cortex, 1972, **8**, 121-135.

Satz, P. Left-handedness and early brain insult: an explanation. Neuropsychologia, 1973, **11**, 115-117.

Satz, P. Cerebral dominance and reading disability: an old problem revisited. In R. M. Knights & D. J. Bakker, (Eds.), The Neuropsychology of Learning Disorders: Theoretical Approaches. Baltimore: University Park Press, 1976, pp. 273-296.

Satz, P. Incidence of aphasia in left-handers: a test of some hypothetical models of cerebral speech organization. In J. Herron (Ed.), Neuropsychology of Left-Handedness. New York: Academic Press, 1980, pp. 189-198.

Satz, P., Achenbach, K., & Fennel, E. Correlations between assessed manual laterality and predicted speech laterality in a normal population. Neuropsychologia, 1967, **5**, 295-310.

Satz, P., & Friel, J. Some predictive antecedents of specific reading disability: a preliminary two-year follow-up. Journal of Learning Disabilities, 1974, **7**, 437-444.

Schneider, C. W. Monocular and binocular perception of verticality and the relationship of ocular dominance. American Journal of Psychology, 1966, **79**, 632-636.

Schoen, Z. J., & Scofield, C. F. A study of the relative neuromuscular efficiency of the dominant and non-dominant eye in binocular vision. Journal of General Psychology, 1935, **11**, 156-181.

Schoen, Z. J., & Wallace, S. R. Ocular dominance: its independence of retinal events. Archives of Ophthalmology, 1936, **15**, 890-897.

Schonblum, J. E. On the problem of pathological right-handedness. Cortex, 1977, **13**, 213-214.

Schulter-Ellis, F. P. Evidence of handedness on documented skeletons. Journal of Forensic Science, 1980, **25**, 624-630.

Schwartz, M. Left-handedness and high risk pregnancy. Neuropsychologia, 1977, **15**, 341-344.

Searleman, A., Tweedy, J., & Springer, S. Interrelationships among subject variables believed to predict cerebral organization. Brain and Language, 1979, **7**, 267-276.

Selvin, S., & Garfinkel, J. The relationship between paternal age and birth order with the percentage of low weight infants. Human Biology, 1972, **44**, 501-510.

Selzer, C. A. Lateral Dominance and Visual Fusion. Cambridge, Mass.: Harvard University Press, 1933.

Semmes, J. Hemispheric speculation: a possible clue to mechanisms. Neuropsychologia, 1968, **6**, 11-26.

Serpell, R. Discrimination of orientation by Zambian children. Journal of Comparative Physiology, 1971, **75**, 312.

Seth, G. Eye/hand coordination and "handedness": a developmental study of visuo-motor behavior in infancy. British Journal of Psychology, 1973, **64**, 25-49.

Shankweiler, D. P. A study of developmental dyslexia. Neuropsychologia, 1963, **1**, 267-286.

Shanon, B. Writing positions in Americans and Israelis. Neuropsychologia, 1978, **16**, 587-591.

Shaw, S. Right-handedness and left-brainedness. Lancet, 1902, **2**, 1486.

Shepherd, G. Selected factors in the reading ability of educable mentally retarded boys. American Journal of Mental Deficiency, 1967, **71**, 563-570.

Sheridan, M. R. Effects of S-R compatibility and task difficulty on unimanual time. Journal of Motor Behavior, 1973, **5**, 199-205.

Sherman, J. A. Field articulation, sex, spatial visualization, dependency, practice, laterality of the brain and birth order. Perceptual and Motor Skills, 1974, **38**, 1223-1235.

Shick, J. Relationship between depth perception and hand-eye dominance and free-throw shooting in college women. Perceptual and Motor Skills, 1971, **33**, 539-542.

Shick, J. Relationship between hand-eye dominance and lateral errors in free-throwing shooting. Perceptual and Motor Skills, 1974, **39**, 325-326.

Shimrat, N. The impact of laterality and cultural background on the development of writing skills. Neuropsychologia, 1973, **11**, 239-242.

Sidman, M., & Kirk, B. Letter reversals in naming, writing, and matching to sample. Child Development, 1974, **45**, 616-625.

Siemens, H. W. Die Bedeutung der Zwillingspathologie fur die Actiologische Forschung erlautert an Beispiel der Linkshandigkelt. 1924.

Simpson, R. G., & Sommer, R. C. Certain visual functions as related to rifle marksmanship. School and Society, 1942, **55**, 677-679.

Sinclair, C. Ear dominance in pre-shcool children. Perceptual and Motor Skills, 1968, **26**, 510.

Sinclair, C. B., & Smith, I. M. Laterality in swimming and its relationship to dominance of hand, eye, and foot. Research Quarterly, 1957, **28**, 395-402.

Smart, J. C., Jeffery, C., & Richards, B. A retrospective study of the relationship between birth history and handedness at six years. Early Human Development, 1980, **4**, 79-88.

Smith, F. O. An experimental study of the reaction time of the cerebral hemispheres in relation to handedness and eyedness. Journal of Experimental Psychology, 1938, **22**, 75-83.

Smith, L. G. A brief survey of right- and left-handedness. Pedagogical Seminary, 1917, **24**, 19-35.

Snyder, A. M., & Snyder, M. A. Eye preference tendencies. Journal of Educational Psychology, 1928, **19**, 431-435.

Sparrow, S., & Satz, P. Dyslexia, laterality and neuropsychological development. In D. J. Bakker and P. Satz (Eds.), Specific Reading Disability: Advances in Theory and Method. Rotterdam: Rotterdam University Press, 1970, pp. 41-60.

Spemann, H., & Falkenberg, H. Uber asymmetrische Entwicklung und situs inversus bei Zzwillingen und Doppelbildungen. Wilhelm roux Archiv fur Entwicklungsemechanik, 1919, 45, 341-422.

Sperling, G. Binocular vision: a physical and a neural theory. American Journal of Psychology, 1970, 83, 461-534.

Sperry, R. W. Lateral specialization in the surgically separated hemispheres. In F. O. Schmidt and F. G. Worden (Eds.), The Neurosciences Third Study Program. Cambridge, Mass.: MIT Press, 1974, pp. 5-19.

Spong, G. Recognition and Recall of Retarded Readers: A Developmental Study (Winifred Gimble Report). Auckland, New Zealand: University of Auckland, 1962.

Springer, S. P. Tachistoscopic and dichotic listening investigations of laterality in normal, human subjects. In S. Harnad, R. W. Doty, L. Goldstein, J. Jaynes, & G. Krauthamer (Eds.), Lateralization in the Nervous System. New York: Academic Press, 1977, pp. 325-338.

Springer, S. P., & Deutsch, G. Left Brain, Right Brain. San Francisco: W. H. Freeman, 1981.

Springer, S. P., & Searleman, A. Left-handedness in twins: implications for the mechanisms underlying cerebral asymmetry of function. In J. Herron (Ed.), Neuropsychology of Left-Handedness. New York: Academic Press, 1980, pp. 139-158.

Steffen, H. Cerebral dominance: the development of handedness and speech. Acta Paedopsychiatrica, 1975, 41, 223-235.

Steingrueber, H. J. Handedness as a function of test complexity. Perceptual and Motor Skills, 1975, 40, 263-266.

Stellingwerf, Y. M. Laterality in families with reading disability. Unpublished doctoral dissertation, University of Colorado, 1975.

Stephens, W. E., Cunningham, E. S., & Stigler, B. J. Reading readiness and eye-hand preference patterns in first grade children. Exceptional Children, 1967, 33, 481-488.

Stevenson, L., & Robinson, H. Eye-hand preferences, reversals, and reading progress. In H. M. Robinson (Ed.), Clinical Studies in Reading (Vol. 2). Chicago, Ill.: University Press, 1953.

Stocks, P. A biometrical investigation of twins and their brothers and sisters. Annals of Eugenics, 1933, 5, 1-55.

Struthers, J. On the relative weight of the viscera on the two sides of the body; and on the consequent position of the center of gravity to the right side. Edinburgh Medical Journal, 1863, 8, 1086-1104.

Subirana, A. The prognosis in aphasia in relation to the factor of cerebral dominance and handedness. Brain, 1958, 81, 415-425.

Subirana, A. Handedness and cerebral dominance. In P. S. Vinken and G. W. Bruyen (Eds.), Handbook of Clinical Neurology (Vol. 4). Amsterdam: North-Holland, 1969, pp. 248-273.

Suchman, R. G. Visual testing of pre-verbal and non-verbal young children. American Journal of Optometry and Archives of the American Academy of Optometry, 1968, **45**, 642-647.

Sutton, P. R. N. Handedness and facial asymmetry: lateral position of the nose in two racial groups. Nature, 1963, **221**, 909.

Teegarden, L. Clinical identification of the prospective non-reader. Child Development, 1932, **3**, 346-358.

Teng, E. L., Lee, P., Yang, K., & Chang, P. C. Handedness in a Chinese population: biological, social, and pathological factors. Science, 1976, **193**, 1148-1150.

Teng, E. L., Lee, P., Yang, K., & Chang, P. C. Lateral preferences for hand, foot and eye and their lack of association with scholastic achievement. Neuropsychologia, 1979, **17**, 41-48.

Thompson, A. L., & Marsh, J. F. Probability sampling of manual asymmetry. Neuropsychologia, 1976, **14**, 217-223.

Thompson, M. Laterality and reading attainment. British Journal of Educational Psychology, 1975, **45**, 317-321.

Tinker, K. J. The role of laterality in reading disability. In Reading and Inquiry, Proceedings of the International Reading Association Annual Convention, Detroit, 1964.

Toch, H. H. Can eye dominance be trained? Perceptual and Motor Skills, 1960, **11**, 31-34.

Todor, J. I., & Doane, T. Handedness classification: Preference versus proficiency. Perceptual and Motor Skills, 1977, **45**, 1041-1042.

Todor, J. I., & Kyprie, P. M. Hand differences in the rate and variability of rapid tapping. Journal of Motor Behavior, 1980, **12**, 57-62.

Trankell, A. Aspects of genetics in psychology. American Journal of Human Genetics, 1955, **7**, 264-276.

Travis, L. E., & Lindsley, D. B. An action current study of handedness in relation to stuttering. Journal of Experimental Psychology, 1933, **16**, 258-270.

Tucker, D. M., Stenslie, C. E., Roth, R. S., & Shearer, S. L. Right frontal lobe activation and right hemisphere performance decrement during a depressed mood. Archives of General Psychiatry, 1979, **20**.

Turkewitz, G. The development of lateral differences in the human infant. In S. Harnad, R. W. Doty, L. Goldstein, J. Jaynes, & G. Krauthamer (Eds.), Lateralization in the Nervous System. New York: Academic Press, 1977, pp. 251-260.

Turkewitz, G., & Creighton, S. Changes in lateral differentiation of head posture in the human neonate. Developmental Psychology, 1974, **8**, 85-89.

Turkewitz, G., Gordon, E. W., & Birch, H. W. Head turning in the human neonate: spontaneous patterns. Journal of Genetic Psychology, 1965, **107**, 143-158.

Turner, E. Eye, hand and foot preferences of emotionally unstable adolescents compared with stable adolescents. Journal of Juvenile Research, 1938, 22, 122-124.

Tuttle, W. W., & Travis, L. E. The relation of precedence of movement in homologous structures to handedness. Research Quarterly, 1935, 6, 2-15.

Updegraff, R. Ocular dominance in young children. Journal of Experimental Psychology, 1932, 15, 758-766.

Vanderwolf, K. W. Problem solving and language. Archives of General Psychiatry, 1970, 23, 337.

Verhaegen, P., & Ntumba, A. Note on the frequency of left-handedness in African children. Journal of Educational Psychology, 1964, 55, 89-90.

Verhoeff, F. A new theory of binocular vision. Archives of Ophthalmology, 1935, 13, 151-175.

Vernon, M. D. Backwardness in Reading: A Study of Its Nature and Origin. New York and London: Cambridge University Press, 1957.

Verschuer, O. von. Der Vererbungsbiologische Zwillingsforchung. Ergebnisse der inneren Medizin und Kinderheilkunde, 1927, 31.

Wada, J. A. Morphological asymmetry of human cerebral hemispheres: temporal and frontal speech zones in 100 adult and 100 infant brains. Neurology, 1974, 24, 39.

Wada, J., & Rasmussen, T. Intracarotid injection of sodium amytal for the lateralization of cerebral speech dominance: experimental and clinical observations. Journal of Neurosurgery, 1960, 17, 266-282.

Wada, J. A., Clarke, R., & Hamm, A. Cerebral hemispheric asymmetry in humans. Archives of Neurology, 1975, 32, 239-246.

Walker, L. C., DeSoto, C. B., & Shelly, M. W. Rest and warm-up in bilateral transfer on a pursuit rotor task. Journal of Experimental Psychology, 1957, 53, 394-398.

Wall, W. D. Reading backward among men in the army, I. British Journal of Educational Psychology, 1945, 15, 28-40.

Wall, W. D. Reading backward among men in the army, II. British Journal of Educational Psychology, 1946, 16, 133-148.

Walls, G. L. A theory of ocular dominance. A. M. A. Archives of Ophthalmology, 1951, 45, 387-412.

Warren, J. M. The development of paw preference in cats and monkeys. Journal of Genetic Psychology, 1958, 93, 229-236.

Warren, J. M., Aplanalp, S. M., & Warren, H. B. The development of handedness in cats and rhesus monkeys. In H. Stevenson, E. Hess, & H. L. Rheingold (Eds.), Early Behavior: Comparative and Developmental Approaches. New York: Wiley, 1967, pp. 73-101.

Warrington, E. K., & Pratt, R. T. C. Language laterality in left-handers assessed by unilateral E.T.C. Neuropsychologia, 1973, 11, 423-428.

Washburn, M. F., Faison, C., & Scott, R. A comparison between the Miles ABC method and retinal rivalry as tests of ocular dominance. American Journal of Psychology, 1934, 46, 633-636.

Watson, J. B. Psychology from the Standpoint of a Behaviorist. Philadelphia: Lippincott, 1919.

Watson, J. B. What the nursery has to say about instincts. Journal of Genetic Psychology, 1925, **32**, 293-327.

Weitz, W. Studien an eineiigen Zwillingen. Zeitschrift fur Klinische Medizin, 1924, **101**.

Weiland, H. Heartbeat rhythm and maternal behavior. American Academy of Child Psychiatry Journal, 1964, **3**, 161-164.

Weiland, I. H., & Sperber, Z. Patterns of mother-infant contact: the significance of lateral preference. Journal of General Psychology, 1970, **117**, 157-165.

Westermarck, E. A. Ritual and Belief in Morocco (Vol. 2). London: Macmillan, 1926.

Weybrew, B. B., & Noddin, E. M. Hand preference and the MPI profiles of nuclear submariners. Psychological Reports, 1979, **45**, 107-110.

Weyl, H. Symmetry. Princeton: Princeton University Press, 1952.

Whelan, E. Visual perception and cerebral dominance. Unpublished doctoral dissertation, University of Sheffield, 1967.

Whipple, G. M. Manual of Mental and Physical Tests, Pt. 1. Baltimore: Warwick and York Inc., 1914.

White, K., & Ashton, R. Handedness assessment inventory. Neuropsychologia, 1976, **14**, 261-264.

White, M. J. Laterality differences in perception. Psychological Bulletin, 1969, **72**, 387-405.

Wiggins, J. S. Personality and Prediction: Principles of Personality Assessment. Reading, Mass.: Addison-Wesley, 1973.

Wile, I. S. Handedness: Right and Left. Boston: Lothrop, Lee, & Sheppard, 1934.

Williams, D., & Gassel, M. M. Visual functions in patients with homonymous hemianopia. Brain, 1962, **85**, 175-250.

Wilson, D. Paloeolithic dexterity. Transactions of the Royal Society of Canada, 1885, **3**, 119-133. (a)

Wilson, D. Primaeval dexterity. Royal Canadian Institute Proceedings, 1885, **3**, 125-143. (b)

Wilson, E. B. Notes on the reversal of asymmetry in the regeneration of chelae in Alpheus heterochelis. Biological Bulletin (of the Marine Biological Laboratory, Woods Hole, Mass.), 1903, **4**, 197-210.

Wilson, J. R., & Sanders, B. Evidence on handedness from the Hawaii Family Study. Behavior Genetics, 1978, **8**, 574-575.

Wilson, M. O., & Dolan, J. B. Handedness and ability. American Journal of Psychology, 1931, **43**, 261-266.

Wilson, P. T., & Jones, H. E. Left-handedness in twins. Genetics, 1932, **17**, 560-571.

Witelson, S. F. Abnormal right hemisphere specialization in developmental dyslexia. In R. M. Knights & D. J. Bakker (Eds.), The Neuropsychology of Learning Disorders: Theoretical Approaches. Baltimore: University Park Press, 1976, pp. 233-256.

Witelson, S. F. Anatomical asymmetry in the temporal lobes: its documentation, phylogenesis and relationship to functional asymmetry. Annals of the New York Academy of Sciences, 1977, **299**, 328-356. (a)

Witelson, S. F. Developmental dyslexia: two right hemispheres and none left. Science, 1977, **195**, 309-311. (b)

Witelson, S. F. Neuroanatomical asymmetry in left-handers: a review and implications for functional asymmetry. In J. Herron (Ed.), Neuropsychology of Left-Handedness. New York: Academic Press, 1980, pp. 79-114.

Wittenborn, J. R. Correlates of handedness among college freshmen. Journal of Educational Psychology, 1946, **37**, 161-170.

Witty, P. A., & Kopel, D. Sinistral and mixed manual ocular behavior in reading disability. Journal of Educational Psychology, 1936, **27**, 119-134.

Wold, R. Visual and perceptual aspects for the achieving and underachieving child. Washington, D.C.: Special Child Publication, 1969.

Wolf, C. W. An experimental investigation of specific language disability (dyslexia). Bulletin of the Orton Society, 1967, **17**.

Woo, T. L. Dextrality and sinistrality of hand and eye: second memoir. Biometrika, 1928, **20**, 79-158.

Woo, T. L., & Pearson, K. Dextrality and sinistrality of hand and eye. Biometrika, 1927, **19**, 165-199.

Woods, B. T., & Teuber, H. L. Early onset of complementary specialization of cerebral hemispheres in man. Transactions of the American Neurological Association, 1973, **98**, 113-117.

Woolley, H. T. The development of right-handedness in a normal infant. Psychological Review, 1910, **17**, 37-41.

Yakovlev, P. I. Teleokinesis and handedness: an empirical generalization. Proceedings of the Eighteenth Annual Convention of the Society of Biological Psychiatry, June, 1973.

Yakovlev, P., & Lecours, A. R. The myelogenetic cycle of regional maturation of the brain. In A. Minkowski (Ed.), Regional Development of the Brain in Early Life. Philadelphia: David and Company, 1967.

Yeni-Komshian, G. H., & Benson, D. A. Anatomical study of cerebral asymmetry in the temporal lobes of humans, chimpanzees and rhesus monkeys. Science, 1976, **192**, 287-389.

Yin, R. K. Face recognition by brain injured patients—a dissociable ability. Neuropsychologia, 1970, **8**, 395.

Zaidel, E. Linguistic confidence and related functions in the right cerebral hemisphere of man following commissurotomy and hemispherectomy. Unpublished doctoral dissertation, California Institute of Technology, 1973.

Zangwill, O. L. Cerebral Dominance and Its Relation to Psychological Function. London: Oliver & Boyd, 1960.

Zangwill, O. L. The current status of cerebral dominance. Research Publications of the Association for Research in Nervous and Mental Disorders, 1962, **13**, 103-118.

Zangwill, O. L. Speech and the minor hemisphere. Acta Neurologica et Psychiatrica Belgica, 1967, 67, 1013-1021.

Zoccolotti, P. Inheritance of ocular dominance. Behavior Genetics, 1978, 8, 377-379.

Zurif, E. F., & Carson, G. Dyslexia in relation to cerebral dominance and temporal analysis. Neuropsychologia, 1970, 8, 351-361.

Author Index

Subject Index

This index is organized by the specific topic headings that have been dealt with in relation to the four types of lateral preference (handedness, footedness, eyedness, and earedness). The reader should consult the specific headings of interest, rather than look under the more global lateral preference topics.